W9-BWY-161

Ethics in Nursing

Joyce Beebe Thompson, R.N., Dr.P.H.

Director, Graduate Nurse Midwifery Program
School of Nursing
University of Pennsylvania
Philadelphia, Pennsylvania

Henry O. Thompson, PH.D.

Director of Education
Institute of Personal and Family Relations
Boonton, New Jersey

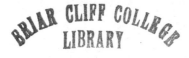
BRIAR CLIFF COLLEGE
LIBRARY
SIOUX CITY, IOWA

Macmillan Publishing Co., Inc.
New York

Collier Macmillan Publishers
London

DEDICATED TO:

My brother and sisters:
Gerald R. Thompson
Verna M. Dobbertin
Helen L. Christopherson
Nancy J. Young
Sharon K. DeMaris
Mavis L. Fitzgerald
                    H. O. T.

My brothers and sisters:
James G. Beebe
Carol M. Miller
Jeanne K. Bergin
and my parents:
Glen E. and Ida M. Beebe
                    J. B. T.

RT
85
.T48
1981

Copyright © 1981, Macmillan Publishing Co., Inc.
Printed in the United States of America

All rights reserved. No part of this book may be reproduced or transmitted in any form or by any means, electronic or mechanical, including photocopying, recording, or any information storage and retrieval system, without permission in writing from the Publisher.

Macmillan Publishing Co., Inc.
866 Third Avenue, New York, New York 10022

Collier Macmillan Canada, Ltd.

Library of Congress Cataloging in Publication Data

Thompson, Joyce Beebe.
  Ethics in nursing.

  Includes bibliographies and index.
  1. Nursing ethics. I. Thompson, Henry O. (date)
joint author. II. Title. [DNLM: 1. Ethics, Nursing.
WY85 T473e]
RT85.T48 1981   174'.2   80-17341
ISBN 0-02-420690-3

Printing: 1 2 3 4 5 6 7 8   Year: 1 2 3 4 5 6 7 8

Ethics
in
Nursing

C422014

Preface

"The nurse acts to safeguard the client and the public when health care and safety are affected by the incompetent, unethical, or illegal practice of any person." ANA Code for Nurses, Statement Three, 1976.

Discussion of the ethics of professional nursing practice is becoming more evident in educational and practice settings. There are many reasons for this, among them the individual nurse's desire to practice and care for other human beings in an ethically sound, competent manner. In addition, such things as the development of ever more sophisticated diagnostic procedures and life support systems for use in the provision of health and illness care now means that we can do more than ever in predicting the quality of life as well as prolonging life for some people. Should we? Who decides? Where does the nurse stand among these issues and what should her/his role be in such decisions?

The answers to these and other equally difficult questions are unclear and complicated by differing views among society, religious groups, institutions, individuals, and professions. A further source of frustration for the student and practitioner of nursing is that most writings and texts on the subject of bioethics and its dilemmas such as the foregoing questions, do not include comments or participation from nurses or discussion of the roles that nurses may play in such critical ethical situations. If one were to judge by today's current literature on the subject of ethical decision making, it oftentimes seems that nurses do not have a part in such decisions.

Nurses have a *large* part to play in ethical decision-making and other aspects of ethical dilemmas. Nurses are the largest group of care givers in the health care delivery systems, and they provide the majority of health and illness care on a day-to-day and minute-to-minute basis for clients. In sheer time spent in interaction with clients, the nurse is more likely to face the wide variety of ethical issues and dilemmas in health and illness care than any other single group of professionals in this field. Consider the following examples of nursing involvement. The nurse is often the person left with the responsibility of caring for the newborn while it is starved to death or for the comatose person whose relatives or doctor have likewise decided to "pull the plug." The nurse is rarely asked to participate actively in decisions on the quality of life though she/he certainly does have impact on the decisions being made. It is often the nurse to whom patients turn when faced with difficult ethical decisions, if given that choice by the physician, and how the nurse responds represents an ethical action. And just what are the rights of the nurse in these difficult situations? These and other important questions will be discussed throughout this text.

Modern nursing requires that the nurse be concerned with both adults and children, colleagues in the medical field, the institution or employer, and society as a whole as well as the self. All of these relationships and responsibilities have ethical as well as legal components. The competent professional is concerned with them all, recognizing that at a given moment one or another of these people might have priority. We suggest that today's nurse can maintain an ethical perspective by being aware that *all* decisions in practice have an ethical dimension. A concern prior to the time of decision-making or involvement can help by using that concern to examine one's self and the issues abroad in today's world that will influence one's view of the ethical nature of practice.

The purpose of this text, then, is to provide the knowledge of ethical issues from a perspective or nursing practice and responsibilities, including a focus on the many roles of nurses and case situations involving nurses that are illustrative of the various roles they may assume in the provision of health and illness care. A set of guidelines for self-study of the cases is included in Chapter One, and their use is encouraged throughout the text as one learns of the issues, their historical foundations, and how nurses may be concerned or involved in them.

It is important to understand from the outset that we are *not* writing this book to give answers to the perplexing ethical dilemmas and questions that are raised constantly today in nursing. There are few absolute right or wrong answers when one is dealing with a variety of human beings. In fact, we firmly believe that the purposes of the study of ethics are to facilitate the efforts of individuals to ask better questions when ethical issues are operant as well as to gain a better understanding of one's own moral code as a basis for professional practice actions and decisions. This book is written with these purposes in mind.

The ethical issues discussed in detail in this book follow the biological sequence of events across the life cycle, from genetics (preconception) to aging and death. Chapters Two through Eight each include the historical, religious, and philosophical background of the ethical issues, modern technology and its effects, the roles/rules conflicts specific to nursing practice including discussion of "who decides" when appropriate, how the ethical issues relate to nursing practice, and case studies involving nurses that illustrate application of the issues to professional practice.

Because of the frequent interface of ethical and legal aspects of nursing practice, a separate chapter on Rights of Individuals (Chapter Nine), contributed by Dr. Lucie Kelly, is offered to further clarify some of the legal aspects of professional practice. It will become obvious to the reader that it is often difficult to separate the ethical and legal aspects of practice, just as many ethical issues reappear in several of the chapters. Thus it is that our decision to place the discussion of research issues in the time span of childhood and the discussion of issues of dying in the time span of aging is somewhat arbitrary, though intended to aid the reader in understanding the specific ethical issues through application to a tangible period of the life cycle.

We also hasten to add that not all ethical issues involved in caring for other human beings have been included in this text. We have been selective so that the text would appeal to the nursing audience it is intended for, and yet not seem an overwhelming task for the student new to the study of ethics.

A glossary of terms is included to facilitate understanding of the various concepts and terms of an ethical nature. Consistent with our belief that students and graduates alike can be stimulated to do further research on the various issues presented, extensive footnotes and some additional bibliography are included at the end of each chapter, and a selective annotated bibliography of books is included at the end of the text. Hopefully, these will help to facilitate the nurse's self-study efforts in a field which is often looked upon as difficult to understand. Because we are dealing with an area of study that has many conflicting points of view, the bibliographic references selected attempt to represent the various sides of the issues at hand.

We have discussed what this text is supposed to do for the reader. We would like to briefly state what this book does *not* do. This book does not offer the reader specific, absolute rules to be applied in every clinical situation so that the nurse will know how to act ethically. It would seem that it is unethical to do so. This is also not a text on the specifics of how to provide nursing care, though occasionally suggestions may be offered as they relate to the issue at hand. It is expected that the reader will gain the knowledges necessary for competent nursing practice in other texts and clinical experience. Likewise, the glossary does not include medical and nursing terms common to the practice of these professions.

Suggestions on How To Use This Text:

This text is written to be used in a variety of ways depending on the needs of the individual learner. We offer the following guidelines for its use, however, recognizing that some readers may benefit from some initial guidance. The textual portion of each chapter can stand alone; that is, it can be read without footnotes and without referring to any other chapter. The exception is that Chapter One provides the background information and the Guidelines for analyzing case situations, so it is suggested that one read that first. As noted above, the extensive footnotes are provided for additional study and research for those who desire to continue their study of ethics. One may begin with any of the chapters according to interest, and proceed from these to complete the book. The case studies are consecutively numbered and titled for ease of reference and indexing, so that one could also decide which chapters might be of primary interest based on the case studies included.

For added understanding, Chapters Two through Eight each has a summary of ethical issues prior to the discussion of the roles of the nurse. This means that the reader may also choose to read the summary of issues to gain an idea of what the chapter includes. The individual chapter texts, however, are written to be read from front to back, because the understanding of history and issues is presumed in the nursing roles sections and case studies.

The cases are suitable for group or individual study and, in our teaching experience have proven most valuable when several people are available for study, reflection, and sharing. This usually enhances one's understanding not only of one's own perspective on the issues, but the variety of beliefs, moral stands, and perspectives held by others.

We trust these suggestions will facilitate your use of this text and your venture into the study of ethics applied to nursing practice.

JOYCE BEEBE THOMPSON, R.N., Dr.P.H.
HENRY O. THOMPSON, Ph.D.

Acknowledgments

The writing of any book requires the efforts and cooperation of many people. This book is no exception. We would like to especially note the participation and invaluable assistance from the following persons.

For their sensitivity and insight into caring for clients and families during each phase of the life cycle, we thank Stephanie L. Rochester, CNM, Warren E. Knowsley, RN, Ann F. Surratt, RN (Genetics); Rochelle Goldstein, CNM, Kathryn Rosasco, RN (Neonatology); Dorothy Allbritten, RN, PNP, Dolores Jackson, RN, PNP (Childhood and Adolescence); Dr. Geri Lynch, RN, Rita Ryan, RN, Elizabeth Mahoney, RN (Adults); and the many clients, families, and professional colleagues who provide the bases for the case situations.

We have received encouragement and editorial assistance from many friends and colleagues. We wish to extend our gratitude especially to Warren E. Knowsley, RN, Dr. Diane McGivern, RN, Dr. Eunice Messler, RN, and Dr. Warren G. Thompson, M.D., for their willingness to read and critique our efforts.

The completion of this book depended a great deal on the untiring efforts of several people. We thank Edna Rainone Knowsley, Alice W. Chiariello, and Nancy Kulb for their technical assistance. We also acknowledge the support and encouragement of our family and friends.

Our final expression of gratitude is extended to our guest author, Dr. Lucie Y. Kelly, RN, who most graciously gave of her time and efforts during a most busy period of her professional career. We appreciate these efforts and are pleased she has contributed her expertise in legal aspects of nursing to this text.

The Authors
JOYCE BEEBE THOMPSON, R.N., Dr.P.H.
HENRY O. THOMPSON, Ph.D.

Index of Case Studies

Case 1: Amniocentesis   35
Case 2: Consanguinity   37
Case 3: Artificial Insemination   37
Case 4: Case of Genetically Defective Adults   38
Case 5: Oral Contraception   59
Case 6: Informed Consent—Sterilization of
       Mentally Retarded   61
Case 7: Vasectomy   61
Case 8: Hospital Policy—No Contraception   62
Case 9: Postabortion Counseling   87
Case 10: Request for Abortion   88
Case 11: Referral for Abortion Counseling   89
Case 12: Very Premature Infant   117
Case 13: Congenital Disease   119
Case 14: Viable Product of Abortion   120
Case 15: Infants and Research   146
Case 16: A Child's Consent   146
Case 17: Child Neglect   147
Case 18: Child Abuse   147
Case 19: Adolescent Pregnancy   148
Case 20: Adolescent Sexuality   149
Case 21: Dialysis   172
Case 22: Transplant   172
Case 23: Women As Patients   173
Case 24: Sexual Identity and Care Giving   174
Case 25: Distributive Justice   174
Case 26: Patient's Right to Die   194
Case 27: Truth Telling   194
Case 28: Death with Dignity   195
Case 29: Allocation of Lifesaving Resources   195

Table of Contents

Dedication   iv

Preface   v

Acknowledgments   viii

Index of Case Studies   ix

Chapter

1

Why Bother with Ethics?   1

DEFINITIONS   1

WHY STUDY ETHICS?   2

WHY HISTORY?   6

APPROACHES TO ETHICS   8

WHY A PROFESSIONAL CODE?   10

GUIDELINES FOR STUDY   12

NOTES AND REFERENCES   13

Chapter

2

Ethics and Genetics   23

HISTORY   23

THE PRESENT   24

THE ISSUES   31

THE NURSE AND GENETICS   31

CASE STUDIES   35

NOTES AND REFERENCES   38

Chapter

3

Ethics and Birth Control   49

INFANTICIDE   49

ABORTION   50

INTRAUTERINE DEVICE (IUD)   50

MISCELLANI   51

THE PAST   51

THE PRESENT SCENE   54
STERILIZATION   56
THE ISSUES   58
ROLE OF THE NURSE IN CONTRACEPTION   58
CASE STUDIES   59
NOTES AND REFERENCES   62

Chapter

4

Abortion As an Ethical Issue   *73*
INTRODUCTION   73
HISTORY   74
WHEN IS LIFE, LIFE?   76
THE LAW   77
ATTITUDES   78
NURSES AND ABORTION   82
CASE STUDIES   87
NOTES AND REFERENCES   90

Chapter

5

Neonatology and Ethics   *105*
INTRODUCTION   105
VIABLE PRODUCTS OF ABORTION   106
ORDINARY VERSUS EXTRAORDINARY
TREATMENT   107
SPECIAL CASE OF NEONATES   108
RESEARCH   112
THE ISSUES   113
NURSES, NEONATOLOGY, AND ETHICS   113
CASE STUDIES   117
NOTES AND REFERENCES   120

Chapter

6

Childhood and Ethics   *131*
INTRODUCTION   131
CHILDREN AND RESEARCH   132
CHILD ABUSE   134
ADOLESCENT SEXUALITY   136
THE ISSUES   138
NURSES AND THE CARE OF CHILDREN AND
ADOLESCENTS   139
NURSES AND THE ABUSED CHILD   141
NURSES AND ADOLESCENT SEXUALITY   144
CASE STUDIES   146
NOTES AND REFERENCES   149

Chapter

7

Bioethics and Adults *161*
INTRODUCTION 161
DISTRIBUTIVE JUSTICE 161
SCARCE RESOURCES 162
ETHICS AND WOMEN 164
THE ISSUES 166
NURSES CARING FOR ADULTS 167
SEXUAL DISCRIMINATION 170
CASE STUDIES 172
NOTES AND REFERENCES 175

Chapter

8

Ethics and the Later Years *183*
INTRODUCTION 183
ALLOCATION OF RESOURCES 184
ORDINARY/EXTRAORDINARY MEANS 185
EUTHANASIA 187
THE ISSUES 188
NURSES AND CARING FOR PEOPLE IN THEIR
LATER YEARS 188
CASE STUDIES 193
NOTES AND REFERENCES 196

Chapter

9

Legal Aspects of Patients' Rights and Unethical Practice *211*
PATIENTS' RIGHTS 212
TRENDS IN INFORMED CONSENT 214
THE RIGHT TO DIE 217
THE RIGHTS OF THE HELPLESS 219
RIGHTS OF PATIENTS IN RESEARCH 221
PATIENT RECORDS: CONFIDENTIALITY AND
AVAILABILITY 222
PRIVACY 224
ASSAULT AND BATTERY 224
FALSE IMPRISONMENT 225
ABORTION, STERILIZATION, AND
CONTRACEPTION 226
DEALING WITH INCOMPETENT
PRACTITIONERS 227
THE RIGHTS OF NURSES AND EMPLOYERS 228
NOTES AND REFERENCES 229

Annotated Bibliography (Selected) 233
Glossary of Terms 245
Index 253

Chapter 1

Why Bother with Ethics?

DEFINITIONS

Ethics has been "easily" defined as the attempt to state and evaluate principles by which ethical problems may be solved.[1] That looks like circular reasoning. It's like saying a circle is a geometric form that is circular. At moments, health personnel concerned with the ethics of their practice may indeed feel as if they are going around in circles. But then, most of us have such moments, whether we are housewives, ditchdiggers, lawyers, business people, professionals, or laity.

Ethics and Morals

The word *ethic* comes from the Greek *ethos*, whereas the word *moral* comes from the Latin *moralis*. The words are synonymous and some ethicists and moralists use them in this way.[2] We follow another strand of usage in which we see morals as the *oughts* and *shoulds* of society, whereas ethics are the principles behind the *shoulds*, the *whys* of moral code or statement.[3] In this sense, one might say that the American Nurses' Association's *Code for Nurses* is a moral code and the *Interpretive Statements* are the ethical principles, the explanation, the *why* behind the code.[4] In practice, morals and ethics often run together. Our concern is not a consistent, exact, rigorously correct usage, which does not exist anyway, but rather an awareness of the ethical dimension of life and professional practice.[5]

Bioethics

Bioethics might be seen as a subdivision of ethics. Ethics includes business ethics, political ethics, and so on. Bioethics in current usage follows more the idea of *bios*, or *life*, so that bioethics tends to refer to the life sciences. In practice, it has extended to the physical sciences and the technology that affects the life sciences. One view of bioethics in this light concerns the use of the life sciences for improving the quality of life.[6] As such, it includes environmental ethics and a broader scope than health and medical care. We use it here in the narrower sense of health care. Traditionally, medical ethics has been concerned with fee setting, how big to make the doctor's sign, and such other items as might today be listed under etiquette. Now the term has taken on the concerns of bioethics and is sometimes replaced by the words *biomedical ethics*. Generally, we use bioethics, medical ethics, and biomedical ethics, interchangeably.[7]

Metaethics

Metaethics is of some interest to us also. This is the attempt to analyze the reasons behind the reasons. If morals are the shoulds and oughts, and ethics the principles behind the shoulds, metaethics asks whence the ethical principles? Greek *meta* means behind, beyond, higher. One can derive intermediate inclusive principles and then ask what is behind those.[8] At some point, one may get to final or supreme principles such as nature or God. For some, the "good" is an ultimate without further definition.[9] For some people, life, the individual, or society is the final value upon which all other values depend. Kieffer has suggested that our conceptualization of human nature is where our ultimate values rest. For some, science is such an ultimate norm, whereas others find it in tradition. For yet others, the only ultimate is, "All things are relative."[10] We touch on ultimates from time to time in this text, but our concern is more at the level of interaction between ethics and morals and the situations in which people interact.[11]

WHY STUDY ETHICS?

Nurses have struggled long and hard to attain professional status, and the formal acceptance of a Code of Ethics in 1950 was one step in achieving this professional growth. The goal of nursing is to care for people with the respect and dignity accorded every human being. Nurses work with people, and people are the central focus of nursing care.[12] As a professional, the nurse accepts responsibility for making decisions and taking actions regarding the health and illness care of other individuals. Nurses also work in a variety of settings and assume a variety of roles that require interaction not only with clients and families, but with other team members as well. It is not uncommon for individuals to vary in their approach to solving patient care conflicts, and the nurse's exposure to such a wide variety of clients and professionals often involves her/him in such conflicts. In addition, the professional commitment to competence in practice requires the nurse to continually update her knowledge base for practice, and a significant portion of this knowledge is related to the development of new technologies that enhance or prolong life, with the inherent ethical dilemmas these create.

Each of these statements about nursing practice today forms the basis of our reasoning that nurses should study ethics. A study of ethics and the issues/conflicts that may arise in nursing practice can provide the nurse with the groundwork for a systematic approach to ethical behavior as a nurse. It can also provide for an increased awareness of the variety of moral positions and ethical issues involved in health and illness care. Today's nurse can maintain an ethical perspective by being aware that all decisions in practice have an ethical dimension,[13] principally because nurses are working with other human beings and making judgments about what *should* be done for them. Let us examine each of these reasons for the study of ethics a bit closer.

Nurses Work with People

Nurses enter into relationships with clients in order to carry out their professional responsibility to provide nursing care when requested and/or needed. Clients bring a variety of beliefs, values, and moral stands with them to the nurse-patient relationship.[14] Likewise, nurses bring a variety of personal beliefs, values, and moral stands to such a relationship in addition to their professional responsibilities for practice.

Kelly[15] notes that individuals who choose nursing as a career make a commitment to their clients that goes beyond their own personal feelings and moral stand. This professional commitment is delineated in the *Code for Nurses*, and states, among other things, that the "nurse provides services with respect for human dignity and the uniqueness of the client. . . ."[16] This implies that nurses know what beliefs, values, and moral stands are held by the client and family (in order to respect them) and how these might influence the client's ability to request, receive, or refuse medical and/or nursing care.[17] One way to understand another's morals and values is to study the historical development of these, as is provided in this text.

Values Clarification: In addition to nurses' understanding and respecting what morals/beliefs the clients bring to the care situation, it follows that nurses would also benefit from knowing their own values—both personal and professional—and how these can potentially influence the nurse-patient relationship and the manner in which professional services are provided.[18]

Several authors agree that understanding the nature of values and one's personal values is central to the study of ethics.[19] Therefore, one reason for nurses to study ethics is to begin to identify their own moral positions and biases so as to explore ways to prevent these biases from unconsciously interfering with one's ability to provide care for a given individual. A specific example of such prevention is operant when the nurse who cannot support elective abortion and the right of others to choose it deliberately avoids employment in settings where she/he will have contact with people requesting or receiving an abortion.

Another important aspect of values clarification for nurses is allowing the nurse to test out the limits of her/his ability to care for people with opposing values/moral stands because she/he now knows what those positions are. Caring for drug addicts, suicidal people, prostitutes, or people electing plastic surgery to alter body appearance may be difficult for a given nurse who cannot accept these individuals' choice of activities. Both nurse and client stand to benefit when the nurse determines ahead of time what behaviors and decisions she/he can tolerate and be truly supportive of in care situations, and when she/he needs to withdraw from or avoid a given situation, making sure another colleague will assume care responsibilities. It seems ludicrous to assume that all nurses can work well with all patients, even though the *Code for Nurses* may imply such action. How seriously the nurse takes her/his professional responsibilities outlined in the ANA *Code for Nurses* is of value in knowing, however. A nurse who needs to work and takes whatever job is available will probably not be the one caught in the dilemma of choosing between responsibility to the patient or her job; she has already chosen the job as priority. We must be quick to add, however, that most nurses at one time or another will probably compromise their professional responsibilities for personal gains or values, just as clients may also compromise their health with unhealthy behaviors, though they claim to value health.

We note that although values clarification is important for nurses who strive toward making ethical decisions, it is *not* synonymous with ethical decision making. That is, a nurse who is aware of her own values and moral positions will not necessarily always make ethical decisions in her clinical practice. Circumstances (care of the patient) might require action inconsistent with the nurse's values or the nurse's values might be inconsistent with those of others—colleagues, patients, or other health team members.

Nurses Make Decisions

There are a lot of decisions required in nursing practice and, as nurses expand their scope of practice to include primary care, more decisions and clinical judgments are required.[20] There are also several ways nurses may make decisions. The more traditional nursing stance was to accept one's role as care giver, but not decision maker, and then proceed to covertly make decisions anyway. Most nurses quickly learned to "work the system" to get what they wanted for patients if the first person asked refused their request. When nurses got caught in the heat of a critical care debate and were asked by other team members or client "What would you do in this situation?" they often deferred to the physician or client with, "It's your decision, not mine."

Accountability: Today's nurses have more readily accepted the concept of accountability for their nursing actions and clinical judgments and, as responsible professionals, are learning about the legal and ethical implications of their practice. We recognize, however, that there are institutions and colleagues who interfere with some nurses' willingness to make decisions, but we submit that nurses are learning to work through these difficulties in order to carry out their professional responsibilities to the client.[21] To admit that one did something to another person because someone else (physician, nursing supervisor) told one to do it is not reflective of the responsible, accountable nursing practice of today. To openly decide and to admit that one took a specific action because "in my best judgment it was what the patient needed" is being accountable for one's decision-making behavior. Please note, however, that "in my best judgment" is a value-laden statement and involves a value decision. Whether the judgment and resultant action were ethical depends on many other factors—clear and accurate identification of the client's needs and desires, extent to which the professional's values were imposed on the patient with informed consent, the ethical perspective one is applying to the situation in order to decide on the "ethicalness" of action (deontological, utilitarian, situational).

Decision-Making Situations: Some of the common questions that arise in nursing practice and require some sort of ethical decision making, either by nurses, or team members, or clients, or all together, are as follows. What ought to be done in this situation? Who should do it? Who decides who decides? What is the right thing to do? What harm or benefit will come from the decision and the resultant actions? If we can, should we?

During the course of nursing individuals and families, ethical dilemmas may arise as clients' and professionals' moral positions come into conflict.[22] These dilemmas require a responsible choice between two or more actions, often of equal rightness. Responsible choices require a clear understanding of the values that motivate behavior, their sources, and implications.[23] Some of the questions that arise out of value conflicts are as follows. If the nurse is not comfortable about a decision made by another colleague or client, what steps, if any, should she/he take? Does she/he have the right to take any further actions? Does the scientifically proven treatment always take precedence over the maybe not-so-scientific holistic and natural approach? If a patient has not been told of her condition and the doctor refuses to do so, does the nurse tell her when asked? How the nurse deals with any one of these questions necessitates an understanding of ethics and morals and setting priorities in decision making, which is also an ethical decision. The study of ethics can help the nurse understand what is going on in such situations and allow her to participate in the process knowledgeably.

Ways to Make Decisions: Given a practice situation, there are many ways a nurse can influence clients in their decision making. One way is to simply impose the nurse's own values on the patient. Another way is to share the nurse's values with the patient in such a manner that the final decision is still based on the nurse's values. A third way to influence client decisions is to share one's own values and listen and respond to the patient's values with a resultant decision that may reflect either or both sets of values. A fourth way is to base decisions totally on what the patient values. How an individual nurse decides among these choices or others for decision making is also a value decision, recognizing that each choice may have both positive and negative effects for the client and the nurse.

Decision-Making Context: Even when no apparent dilemma or conflict exists between nurse and patient, it does not follow that the path of action is always clear or ethical. Compare the results of nurse and patient agreeing on abortion, and a Catholic view of this action held by another nurse. In the nurse-patient agreement, abortion is seen as ethical; in the latter situation, abortion is unethical (by Catholic doctrine). This illustration serves to point out that the ethical nature of a decision may vary from situation to situation, depending on the individuals involved and their values/moral positions. And what is ethical action today may not be so ten years from now because of changing value orientation and technology, or other factors. This variable nature of ethical decision making is another reason that nurses can benefit from the study of ethics—to gain an understanding of ethical principles that tend to have a longer life-span than one's values/beliefs of the moment.

Roles and Relationships

Modern nursing requires that the nurse assume a variety of roles and enter into a variety of collegial relationships with other professionals. Nurses may be advocate, counselor, confidant, care giver, decision maker, or colleague, either separately or in combination, at any given time. The nature of nursing requires that the nurse be concerned with clients and families, colleagues in the health and medical field, institution and/or employer, and society as a whole, as well as the self. All of these roles and relationships have ethical as well as legal components within which actions might be taken.[24] They all also can give rise to conflicts for the nurse. The competent professional is concerned with them all, recognizing that at a given moment one or another of these roles and people may have priority. How these priorities are established represents value judgments and involves ethical decision making. This is one more reason that nurses may choose to study ethics.

Respect for Colleagues: Many of these role conflicts will be discussed throughout

this book. The point we wish to emphasize here is the importance of knowing and respecting one's colleagues' value/moral positions. We speak often of the priority of nursing responsibility to the client, but without mutual respect for other health team members, the client will likely receive less than optimum care. It is important for health team members to realize that often when they are fighting among themselves for power or control of decisions because *"they* know best," it is the client who suffers from the battle.

Nursing has reached the level of professional stature that requires and promotes supportive, collegial working relationships. Is it too much to ask for the nurse who spends time and energy learning about, understanding, and respecting the client's dignity and uniqueness to also do the same for his/her nursing or medical colleagues? We think not. Just as there are varying value systems among clients, there are varying value systems among nurses and other team members. What works or is "right" between one patient and one nurse may not be "right" for another set of individuals in a nurse-patient relationship or the doctor-patient relationship.

Team Decision Making: Some authors suggest that one of the best ways to ensure that health and medical care decisions are ethical and in the "best" interests of the client is to submit these decisions for team discussion and action.[25] This team might include the client, family, and professional staff, and, in order for such a team to function, mutual respect for all is required. No longer are we in an era of health and medical care in which the physician is always the "captain of the ship." We are moving toward the client as captain, with health professionals as the competent navigators.[26] Team discussion and decision making for crucial ethical dilemmas may more readily support this newer approach to care, and all participants can learn from one another what it means and "costs" to make ethical decisions. Because there are rarely absolutes in ethics, that is, a variety of "right" answers may be possible, teamwork also illustrates the difficulties in making such decisions.

Professional Competence

The field of biomedical ethics is rapidly expanding and is of vital concern to nurses. The need to continually update one's nursing knowledge to maintain competency is taken for granted. The fact that ethics is still relatively new to nursing curricula may indicate a need for expanding the nurse's knowledge in this area as well. The very development of new ways to keep people alive or to enhance the quality of their life or potential life has created some new ethical issues to be dealt with in professional nursing practice. Other ethical issues or dilemmas are as old as the dawn of time, tempered only by the societal values of the present day.

Nurses who work in critical care units or research may be more familiar with the kind of dilemmas raised by technology. When to put a person on a respirator can be just as difficult a decision as when to pull the plug. Whether amniocentesis should be required of all pregnant women over thirty-five is just as complex as whether a genetically defective child should be allowed (or helped) to die. These questions would never be raised if we did not have the technology to offer such options for care. And nurses, because of their constant and ofttimes continuous contact with clients, are frequently in a position to participate in such decisions. They have data on the client and family and their reactions to the current condition of the patient that often provide the basis for making a decision on treatment. Responsible decision making, however, requires knowledge, and this book is an attempt to provide some of that knowledge—ethics—needed for making ethical decisions.

Summary

Nurses who study ethics can increase their effectiveness as care givers and decision makers as they increase their understanding of the variety of value systems/moral positions operant in care situations, from client, self, and other professionals. They may also be able to recognize potential conflict situations and work through them before actual conflict arises. Ethics can no longer be considered as an adjunct to nursing practice. It is an integral part of each nurse's day-to-day interaction with people.[27] Nurses are involved in ethics daily whether they admit it or not, and they have an important role in determining solutions to ethical dilemmas.[28] In their interactions with clients, nurses can make a substantial contribution to the growth and development of the society of the future if they are willing to clarify and put their own ethical behavior on the line. The greatest good may be to find the means to reduce the conflict between the use of science (technology) and the growing awareness of the need for humanness and dignity (the art) in health care. By helping other people to find richer lives and greater dignity, nurses can considerably enrich their own feelings of self-worth.[29] The study of ethics and nursing practice is one avenue toward reaching such a lofty goal for clients and self.

WHY HISTORY?

In a way, asking why bother with history is an extention of the question of why bother with ethics. The professional person's knowledge base is much broader than that which is immediately involved in putting on a band-aid or practicing any other skill. A nurse-practitioner may spend a lot of time putting on band-aids but she/he knows when to use a band-aid and when to check for a brain tumor. There is a knowledge of legalities involved such as when putting on the band-aid is assault and battery (unconsented touching). There is a knowledge of psychology and human relations involved in what it means to put on band-aids. There is an ethical perspective in knowing why we should or should not put on band-aids in caring for people, whether out of respect for the Golden Rule, professional conduct, God's commandment to love our neighbor, the utilitarian belief in the greatest good for the greatest number, and so forth.

The actual history of the band-aid might not be as important as the history of nursing and medical care for people. The history of sanitary technique and sterilizing procedures might be even more important. But all such perspectives can also be a part of the ever present "Why are you doing what you are doing?" A practical approach or an existentialist (for the moment) approach might be to forget the why. Just do what comes to hand and don't think about it. Hierarchical systems, including male domination of women, have been particularly prone to this latter view. The system or the superior expects us to do or die, but not to question why. We are often to simply do what we are told to do. One way to relate to such a system is to live with it, to accept it. It's easier in a way. When we want to change or do something about it, we need to think. There are those who don't like to think. It's too much work. There are others who are willing to accept responsibility for themselves and their work. They think. One of the things they think about is the historical perspective.[30]

There's a famous line attributed to the philosopher George Santayana: those who do not know history are doomed to repeat it. A variation is that those who do not know the mistakes of the past are doomed to repeat them. There is then a negative value in knowing history. Knowing history can help us to avoid mistakes. Norman E. Himes believes that panicky observers may steal our emotional gyroscope and induce us to lose our historical perspective. If we do, "we shall most certainly adopt unwise policies."[31] More positively, knowing history can help us understand how we came to be where we are. If we want to change, knowing our history can help us to change. If we do not want to change, knowing our history can help us to stay where we are, to the degree that that is possible in a world of change.

Increased Understanding: The historical knowledge may not lend itself to change, pro or con. It may simply help us understand. Victor Frankl found that the people who survived in the concentration camps of Hitler were often the people who had meaning in their lives. One way of distinguishing humans from other animals is this concept of meaning. One aspect of meaning is understanding. Understanding can be a goal in itself. It can be a factor in our survival. The aged and suicides and various other categories of people may not be interested in survival. There are often complex factors, but certainly one of them is meaning. Faced with the uncertainties, life may be devoid of meaning. But if we can only understand, even uncertainties can

be taken in stride. One of the great classical examples of this is a man called Job. He suffered more from his lack of understanding than from his boils. When God answered him out of the whirlwind, there was no answer for the physical suffering and loss, but there was a new perspective that helped Job to meaning, to acceptance, to life. History can help with such perspective, whether we are theist or nontheist.[32]

Health personnel, like other human beings, need meaning and perspective for their own lives. Health personnel, by definition, are not in isolation, hermits, in a vacuum. They are in relationship with people. Sometimes it is a rather mechanical relationship. The line forms at the clinic. You slap on a band-aid here and pour on some iodine there, and the assembly line moves on. Even the most mechanistic of lines, however, contains human beings. A scientific approach to medical care requires a consideration of the human factor, the practitioner's own, that of other practitioners, and that of the patients. The art of health or medical care brings this concern even more strongly to the fore. One cannot practice scientific health care, let alone the art of health care, without having some understanding of others.

One cannot understand others without having some knowledge of the morals, ethics, values, beliefs, and customs of those around one. And where did these come from? The strictures against abortion, for example, go back very nearly to the dawn of history, the beginning of writing. The efforts to obtain an abortion are equally ancient, if not even older. There would have been no need for laws against abortion if it were not being practiced. As noted, one aspect of ethics is to study the reasons, the principles behind a moral code or law. Are these principles still valid? Many say yes, but others say there are other (higher?) principles to be applied, if not in every situation, then at least in some. Whether we approve or do not approve, the thrust to meaning suggests it is helpful to know why we hold our position and why others hold theirs. We may agree or disagree, even as society, religion, our professional integrity, the welfare of our patients, the soundness of our health care, and numbers of other perspectives expect us to know what we are doing. Jean-Paul Sartre examined bad faith and told us to take it or leave it, but first understand clearly what it is that we are taking or leaving.[33]

APPROACHES TO ETHICS

Jones and colleagues list eleven main types of ethical theory, with several subdivisions. Not all would agree with their listing. As you move through these pages, it will seem at times that ethicists do not agree on much of anything. In such a complicated subject, this is hardly surprising. They note that like any intellectual discipline, ethics is difficult to characterize for those unfamiliar with it. Yet it is the job of any discipline to help the understanding of the complexities. They do this through the presentation of selections of writings from the history of ethics.[34]

Our Approach

Their concern is with the whole field of theoretical ethics. Our concern is more practical ethics, or applied ethics, and even a rather narrow segment of that. Bioethics is but a fraction of the whole, and medical or biomedical ethics is but a part of that, though we tend to use them interchangeably.[35] That helps with the simplification. We do not present here an entire course in the whole field of ethics, but an introduction to one portion of it. We combine it with an approach to education. One technique that is at least as old as Socrates, and maybe as old as the human race, is to move from the known to the unknown. We have taken the life cycle and brought to bear some (not all) of the ethical questions related to health care. No doubt there are those who would choose other ethical questions or who would add or subtract data from those we have considered. That is good. One of our educational concerns is dialogue and discussion and even debate as a way of getting to know the perspectives and issues. This will be most clear in the questions related to the case studies. It's more subtle in the very selection of the cases to be studied. On occasion, we have tried to objectively present different views on an issue. At other times, our own perspective stands out clearly.[36]

We have focused primarily on two ethical approaches: the utilitarian and the deontological.[37] This is not to say that other main types are without value or substance for bioethics, but only to say that we, too, need to simplify the complexities, to get some "handles" to approach it all. The discussion is intended to allow other main types and perspectives to be brought to the issues.

Deontology

The deontological approach (formalism) derives its name from the Greek *deon*, meaning duty, and *logos*, or discourse. It's of some considerable appeal to the health care field for, historically, ethical positions related to medicine have been articulated in sets of rules.[38] Kurt Baier[39] notes four major examples of the rules approach to ethics. One is the Hebrew-Christian tradition, which sees the ideal life for people in obedience to God or a law that expresses His will.[40] The point here and in all deontological approaches is that of rule that establishes the right or wrong without regard to anyone, or their personal situation, or time, and without regard to the circumstances.[41] Immanuel Kant (1724–1804) is a second major example. It is duty that determines the moral worth of an action. Kant believed in a *categorical imperative* independent of human desires that is universally applicable to all. We are to submit to this absolute, unconditional imperative, as the Jewish or Christian person submits to God. Our submission is not to the will of another but to our own will insofar as we are rational and respect the law. Kant stressed several liberal values such as autonomy, freedom, dignity, self-respect, and respect for individual rights. Although these are compatible with the Judeo-Christian ethic, it is only in modern times that they have become widely accepted.[42] Baier cites the Oxford intuitionists such as Harold Arthur Prichard (1871–1947) as a third category. Right and wrong are a matter of intuition. We know intrinsically what to do.[43] His fourth category involves a revival of classical contract theory. Originally, the social contract was a political concept on how society is bound together under some kind of rule or ruler. Under such ethicists as John Rawls, the social contract is more a matter of the just distribution of resources. We will take note of this in Chapter Seven on adults and the allocation of scarce resources. The covenant concept of medical care, that once medical care has begun the care giver is obligated to continue, is another aspect of this rule for morality.[44]

Utilitarianism

Utilitarianism is concerned with the end product of our actions. What are the consequences? This concern with the end or the goal is sometimes described as teleological (Greek *telos*, or end, and *logos*) ethics. Some see utilitarianism as a form of teleological ethics.[45] The concern with the end or consequences or results has led some to accuse utilitarians of practicing an ethic of "the end justifies the means."[46] The accusation is that we can do anything we want to do so long as our intent is a good end. This may mean ignoring or going against the rights and needs of many people. The positive statement of the utilitarian ethic is that of achieving the maximum good. The usual phrase is, "the greatest good for the greatest number." This means that the many who would be overridden would presumably be a minority, but that depends on who decides what is the greatest good, and whether the greatest number is simply a mathematical percentage or, if by greatest, the deciders mean greatest in quality, that is, themselves. This might be a matter of ethical elitism, ethical egoism, or ethical parochialism, in which the standard is a special group, oneself, or one's own group. In another sense, utilitarianism refers to an ethical universalism with concern for the good of humanity or the nation.[47]

Another way to express this is as a utilitarian calculus. That is, one can calculate, perhaps even in a pseudoscientific manner, or figure out to the traditional "T," what is good in a "by the numbers" method. But this cold calculation is balanced by what some call a rule utilitarianism. This tends to merge into deontology. One could say that traditionally that which has been thought best is best, tested by time, and shown to be indeed the greatest good for the greatest number. The conventional wisdom of the past just might be the best after all. So Kant's idea of the universal quality comes in here as a test for the rightness or wrongness of an action or a position. We can ask what would happen if the act or attitude were to be adopted by humanity or a major segment thereof? But while deontology tends to be concerned with authority (the Bible, a famous philosopher, Pope, rabbi, an ethicist), utilitarianism tends to be a matter of consensus.[48]

A consensus of a different kind is that which comes from the dialectic or Socratic method. Socrates used to ask questions and then demand reasons even as he asked more questions.[49] The consensus, if ever achieved, comes from some agreement on which questions are important and which reasons are acceptable. A society may be closer to a consensus than the initial appearance would indicate. In our discussion of contraception and abortion, for example, we note that American women practice both, at least statistically, without regard to their religious preference. That is a statistical datum, even though some religious groups are against both. In fact, socioeconomic level is a better indicator of the two practices than is religion. The consensus or practice may not be acceptable to some ethicists, but it is there. Are these practices right?[50] By the consensus, or utilitarian, approach of the greatest good for the greatest number, apparently they are right. By the deontological approach of rules that apply regardless of the people involved, they may or may not be right. It depends on whose rules are being applied. Fletcher agrees that it may or may not be right, depending on the rule of love.

The Situation

Joseph Fletcher, an Episcopal clergyman with a background at Yale and more recently professor of medical ethics in the School of Medicine at the University of Virginia, has gained some fame for espousing situation ethics. He describes this as act utilitarianism. The situation determines how we will act, what is right or wrong, what is ethically acceptable or no. Yet, at the heart of his ethics is a rule, the rule of love, congenial to Judaism and Christianity.[51] We offer Fletcher here for consideration not simply because Rabbi Joshua of Nazareth (Jesus, called the Christ in Christianity) considered love the summary of all Jewish law (635 laws in the Hebrew Scripture), as Rabbi Hillel considered the Golden Rule. It is rather that all ethics are influenced by the situation in which the principles and the rules or moral codes are formulated. Some Roman Catholic ethicists, for example, are quite aware that the historical situation influenced, if it did not determine, the formulation of deontological rules that now form an official part of their tradition. This historical awareness or depth is not so apparent among other ethicists.[52]

This combination of situation and rule is perhaps the most common to the human condition. In the clinical situation of many, if not all, practitioners, in the case studies to follow, in the real world (as contrasted to the abstraction of theory), many people try to apply rules taking the situation into account. Sometimes rules are followed regardless of consequences, as may happen in a neonatal intensive care unit where heaven and earth are moved to save a defective child without regard for what happens to the child during the rest of its life. Sometimes research is carried out without regard for the welfare of research subjects because "the end justifies the means." However, some see the carrying out of a rule without mercy as a denial of the very thing the rule supposedly represents. Some suggest the "tyranny of the majority" may indeed achieve the greatest good for the greatest number, but a good that ignores the individual and perhaps many individuals, at that, may in the end be seen as a questionable kind of good.[53]

Summary

In summary, we again emphasize that we do not pretend here to have touched on all the major approaches, or even on the favorite approaches of selected individuals or groups. We do take this opportunity to pay tribute to one group. Roman Catholic ethicists have done so much for so long in the field of ethics, and bioethics in particular, that the subject can not be considered without taking Catholic thought into perspective, even if it is only to disagree. Religious and nonreligious ethics stand in their debt.[54] In earlier centuries, they blended Greek and Roman philosophical ethics with the Semitic traditions of Judaism to the point where the two at times cannot be distinguished. The Catholic scholastics of the Middle Ages formulated the doctrines on which much of today's thinking (Protestant, Jewish, and secular) is still based. On the current scene, some Catholic ethicists are swinging with the situation, even as some non-Catholics dig in and try to hold onto an essentially Catholic formulation. Without stopping to count footnotes, one could get the impression of considerable attention to Catholic thought in the following pages, and probably be correct.[55]

WHY A PROFESSIONAL CODE?

Turning from ethics in general to nursing ethics in particular, it is helpful to start with the existing codes.

Health care ethics are concerned with the rights, duties, and obligations of professional personnel, institutions of care, and clients. Statements of codes of behavior for doctors and nurses have developed to help define the standards of the professions in keeping with the duties, obligations, and rights of the professionals.[56] The code of ethics is often considered an essential characteristic of a profession and provides means for the exercise of professional self-regulation.[57] A code indicates the professional's acceptance of the responsibility and trust invested in him/her by society. The true ethics of all health care codes are based on the rights and dignity of individuals—treating the patient as a person.[58]

When one enters the profession of nursing, he or she not only accepts the responsibilities and trust that have accrued to nursing over the years, but also the obligation to adhere to the profession's code of conduct.[59] The *Code for Nurses* and especially the Interpretive Statements of the American Nurses' Association (ANA) provide valuable guidelines for the professional nurse regarding the duties and obligations to clients, the profession, and society.

The ANA Code

The 1976 Code is as follows:

ANA Code for Nurses

1. The nurse provides services with respect for human dignity and the uniqueness of the client unrestricted by considerations of social or economic status, personal attributes, or the nature of the health problems.

2. The nurse safeguards the client's right to privacy by judiciously protecting information of a confidential nature.

3. The nurse acts to safeguard the client and the public when health care and safety are affected by the incompetent, unethical, or illegal practice of any person.

4. The nurse assumes responsibility and accountability for individual nursing judgments and actions.

5. The nurse maintains competence in nursing.

6. The nurse exercises informed judgment and uses individual competence and qualifications as criteria in seeking consultation, accepting responsibilities, and delegating nursing activities to others.

7. The nurse participates in activities that contribute to the ongoing development of the profession's body of knowledge.

8. The nurse participates in the profession's efforts to implement and improve standards of nursing.

9. The nurse participates in the profession's efforts to establish and maintain conditions of employment conducive to high quality nursing care.

10. The nurse participates in the profession's effort to protect the public from misinformation and misrepresentation and to maintain the integrity of nursing.

11. The nurse collaborates with members of the health professions and other citizens in promoting community and national efforts to meet the health needs of the public.

Historical Background

In 1897, when the ANA's first constitution was adopted, it included a reference to the need to establish and maintain a code of ethics.[60] Between then and 1950, several attempts were made to formulate and adopt

such a code. The purpose of developing a code of ethics was to create a sensitivity among nurses to the ethical nature of practice and to offer principles to guide the nurse in exercising clinical judgment.[61] Well over half a century after the need for a code of ethics was stated, a Code for Nurses was formally adopted by the ANA in 1950.

The 1950 code was revised on three separate occasions and updated to reflect the change and growth in the profession of nursing as a whole.[62] A shift from emphasis on personal ethics to an emphasis on professional ethics is evident. The *Code for Nurses* speaks to the very philosophy of nursing practice—respect for human dignity, rights and value systems of others, and protection of the patient from the "incompetent, unethical, or illegal practice of any person." It is important to note that the code may often exceed but can be no less than the requirements of the law for the practice of nursing. Violations of the code may not be punishable by law, but the ANA may reprimand, censure, suspend, or expel members on the basis of these violations.

The ICN Code

The International Council of Nursing (ICN) *Code for Nurses* (1973) is similar to the foundations of the ANA Code.[63] It speaks to the responsibilities of the nurse to other people, to practice, to society, to co-workers, and to the profession as a whole. It, too, is offered in its entirety for study and reflection.

ICN Code for Nurses (1973)
Ethical Concepts Applied to Nursing

The fundamental responsibility of the nurse is fourfold: to promote health, to prevent illness, to restore health, and to alleviate suffering.

The need for nursing is universal. Inherent in nursing is respect for life, dignity and rights of man. It is unrestricted by considerations of nationality, race, creed, color, age, sex, politics or social status.

Nurses render health services to the individual, the family and community and coordinate their services with those of related groups.

Nurses and People

The nurse's primary responsibility is to those people who require nursing care.

The nurse, in providing care, promotes an environment in which the values, customs and spiritual beliefs of the individual are respected.

The nurse holds in confidence personal information and uses judgment in sharing this information.

Nurses and Practice

The nurse carries personal responsibility for nursing practice and for maintaining competence by continual learning.

The nurse maintains the highest standards of nursing care possible within the reality of a specific situation.

The nurse uses judgment in relation to individual competence when accepting and delegating responsibilities.

The nurse when acting in a professional capacity should at all times maintain standards of personal conduct which reflect credit upon the profession.

Nurses and Society

The nurse shares with other citizens the responsibility for initiating and supporting action to meet the health and social needs of the public.

Nurses and Co-Workers

The nurse sustains a cooperative relationship with co-workers in nursing and other fields.

The nurse takes appropriate action to safeguard the individual when his care is endangered by a co-worker or any other person.

Nurses and the Profession

The nurse plays the major role in determining and implementing desirable standards of nursing practice and nursing education.

The nurse is active in developing a core of professional knowledge.

The nurse, acting through the professional organization, participates in establishing and maintaining equitable social and economic working conditions in nursing.

The professional codes of ethics in nursing serve as standards for the behavior of nurses and provide general guidelines for nursing

actions in ethical dilemmas. They do not, however, provide specific guidelines for how the nurse should act in a given situation. In theory, ethical codes are clear and unambiguous; in practice, the nurse must draw upon his/her own resources and judgment to select the proper course of action.[64] In addition, the codes do not offer guidance for the nurse in dealing with conflicts between professional and personal values, though the statements on patient's priority may subsume this idea. For these reasons we offer the following suggested guidelines for studying ethics, and we encourage application of the Code for Nurses to each case study.

GUIDELINES FOR STUDY

One of the major difficulties in ethical study is that often no definite, clear-cut, single answer exists for a given dilemma, or at least not one on which everyone can agree. For this very reason, we have found it helpful for nurses to submit themselves to critical reflection of values and moral positions and the study of principled actions in the calm of a classroom or workshop.[65] Here nurses can study actual or hypothetical cases involving clients and professionals. They can examine what decisions were or ought to be made, who made or should make them, the basis for the decisions, and the benefits and risks of alternative actions taken or that might be taken. Assuming the role of the nurse in each case study may help the student to clarify how he/she may or would react in a similar situation.

There are many ways to approach the study of ethics and nursing practice.[66] Some approaches were discussed earlier in this chapter. The following guidelines were developed to facilitate this needed critical reflection and study of ethical components of decision making. We have tested their use and noted success in application during four years of joint teaching of ethics for nurses. We found that use of the guidelines can help raise the consciousness of the individual nurse to his/her own beliefs and moral positions, to the variety of beliefs and moral positions of other people involved in the case study, as well as to the existence of ethical dimensions in all of nursing practice. The guidelines were also developed to encourage nurses to apply a certain thought process to the analysis of case studies in ethics. The guidelines are as follows:

Guidelines for Identifying and Analyzing Ethical Dilemmas in Nursing Practice [67]

1. Review the situation as presented and
   a. determine what health problems exist;
   b. identify what decision(s) need to be made;
   c. separate the ethical components of the decisions from those decisions that can be made solely on a scientific knowledge base;
   d. identify all the individuals/groups who will be affected by the decision(s).
2. Decide what further information is needed before a decision on a course of action can be made, and gather this information.
3. Identify the ethical issues involved in the situation as presented. Discuss the historical, philosophical, and religious bases for each of these issues.
4. Identify your own values/beliefs (moral stand) regarding each of these ethical issues and your professional responsibilities dictated by the Code for Nurses.
5. Identify the values/beliefs operant in the other people involved in the situation. Use knowledge of historical, philosophical, and religious bases of ethical issues to enhance understanding of other people's moral stands on the issues.
6. Identify the value conflicts, if any, in the situation.
7. Discuss who is best able to make the needed decision(s) and identify the nurse's role in the decision-making process. (Who owns the problem?)
8. Identify the range of decisions/actions that are possible and the anticipated implications of same for all people involved in the situation. Identify how closely the suggested actions conform to the Code for Nurses.
9. If appropriate, decide on a course of action as the nurse in the situation and follow through.
10. In retrospect, evaluate/review the results of the actions or decisions and keep in mind for future situations of this type.

We encourage the reader to use these guidelines with the case studies presented at the end of each chapter. We have provided some examples of how the guidelines can be used in the first three chapters and trust they will facilitate your introduction and further study of the ethical dimensions of nursing practice. At some point in study, you may wish to deal only with the additional questions following each case, though it is hoped that consistent application of the guidelines will broaden your perspective and understanding of what the study of ethics can mean for the practicing nurse.

NOTES AND REFERENCES

1. W. T. Jones, Frederick Sontag, Morton O. Beckner, Robert J. Fogelin, eds., *Approaches to Ethics* (New York: McGraw-Hill Book Company, 1962), p. 1. George H. Kieffer says ethics deals with the good, and the ethical decisions are to promote the good. Kieffer, *Bioethics* (Reading, Mass.: Addison-Wesley Publishing Co., Inc., 1979), p. 45. The next question might be, "What is good?" See metaethics following. For a fuller discussion, see Alasdair MacIntyre, "Why Is the Search for the Foundations of Ethics So Frustrating?" *The Hastings Center Report*, no. 4 (Aug. 1979), 9:16–22. The report is cited hereafter as *HCR*. At one point, MacIntyre says that all modern moral philosophers are against all others except himself. This is reminiscent of the biblical statement in Judges 17:6 that everyone did what was right in his own eyes. Actually, the confusion is not that bad for there are broad areas of agreement and disagreement, but the article emphasizes the ongoing struggle to understand, to seek, and to follow the "right." Douglas Sloan, "The

Teaching of Ethics in the American Undergraduate Curriculum, 1876–1976," *HCR* no. 6 (Dec. 1979), **9**:21–41.

2. John Ladd, "Ethics I: The Task of Ethics," *Encyclopedia of Bioethics* (1978), **1**:400–407. The encyclopedia is cited hereafter as *EB*. Jacques Barzun claims the professions need to recover mental and moral force. By moral he means not merely honest. He sees moral as the nature of encounter between two human beings. Barzun, "The Professions Under Siege," *Harper's Magazine*, no. 1541 (Oct. 1978), **257**:61–68, and reprinted, *Reader's Digest*, no. 681 (Jan. 1979), **114**:15–20. His remark has overtones of Natural Law. See following. Jacques P. Thiroux distinguishes *ethos* as character and *morals* as custom or manners. Thiroux, *Ethics* (Beverly Hills, Calif.: Glencoe Press, 1977), p. 2. He agrees, however, that in ordinary language the two are used as synonymous. Shirley Maurice and Louise Warrick, "Ethics in Professional Nursing Practice," *Journal of Obstetrical, Gynecological, and Neonatal Nursing* no. 6 (Nov./Dec. 1979), **8**:327–329, distinguish between morals and ethics. Moral precepts are derived from religion and culture and are externally imposed. Ethical principles are emotionless derivations from natural law, facts, and evaluations that reflect conscience, reason, responsibility, and choice. They see ethics as the highest level of duty. This reflects Kant and deontology (see later), although they reject the rules approach to ethics in favor of personal responsibility in relation to the situation (see Fletcher and situation ethics following, as well as Donald Jones and professional ethics).

3. Kieffer, op. cit., pp. 61–62, lists as examples of principles such things as honesty, truth telling, self-restraint, love, responsible action, benevolence, individual rights, distributive justice, equality, reduction of pain, double effect (an evil side effect is tolerated if the intended good comes from a good means and outweighs the bad), and fraternal charity (Golden Rule). Utility is a principle in utilitarianism. Paul Taylor, "Utilitarianism," pp. 12–22, in *Contemporary Issues in Bioethics*, ed. by Tom L. Beauchamp and Leroy Walters (Encino, Calif.: Dickenson Publishing Co., Inc., 1978). The Hippocratic oath's *primum non nocere*, "first, do no harm" is an important medical principle. Kieffer, p. 46, puts *must* on the level of morals, whereas ethics answers the question of what *ought* to be done. Paula Sigman unites *should* and *ought* under the theory of obligation. "Ethical Choices in Nursing," *Advances in Nursing Science*, no. 3 (Apr. 1979), **1**:37–52. William K. Frankena uses the theory of obligations term. The two main foci of this theory are good deeds and equality. Frankena, *Ethics*, 2nd. ed. (Englewood Cliffs, N.J: Prentice-Hall, Inc., 1973), p. 47. Our distinction between action (morals) and principles (ethics) parallels his foci. See also Ladd, op. cit., p. 401, Anne J. Davis and Mila A. Aroskar, *Ethical Dilemmas and Nursing Practice* (New York: Appleton-Century-Crofts, 1978), pp. 1–2, 24–25, and Kathleen M. Fenner, *Ethics and Law in Nursing Professional Perspectives* (New York: D. Van Nostrand Company, 1980), pp. 8–16.

4. *Code for Nurses with Interpretive Statements* (Kansas City, Mo.: American Nurses' Association, 1976). It is reprinted in *EB*, **4**:1789–1799. The source of the rules and explanations is a question of metaethics.

5. K. Danner Clouser, "Bioethics," *EB*, **1**:115–127. See also Fenner, op. cit., pp. 8–9, 21–26.

6. Van Rensselaer Potter is credited with the origin of the term "bioethics". *Bioethics: Bridge to the Future* (Englewood Cliffs, N.J.: Prentice Hall, Inc., 1971). Clouser, op. cit., p. 118. Lewis P. Bird, "Dilemmas in Biomedical Ethics," pp. 131–155, in *Horizons of Science*, ed. by Carl F. H. Henry (New York: Harper & Row Publishers, 1978). Carl Wellman, "Ethics IX: Naturalism," *EB*, **1**: 442–447. Anthony Shaw, "Defining the Quality of Life," *HCR*, no. 5 (Oct. 1977), **7**:11. Richard A. McCormick, "The Quality of Life, The Sanctity of Life," *HCR*, no. 1 (1978), **8**:30–36. Peter Steinfels, "Against Bioethics," *HCR*, no. 2 (1976), **6**:18–20, spoofs the use of the term while defining it as interdisciplinary, mostly philosophy, but also religion, law, and medicine. One might add biology. Beauchamp and Walters, op. cit., Preface and p. 1. Eric Fromm has said that there is no such thing as medical ethics, only human ethics applied to specific situations. Quoted by Elisabeth Kubler-Ross, *Questions and Answers on Death and Dying* (New York: Macmillan Publishing Co., Inc., 1974), p. 75.

7. Clouser, op. cit., pp. 119–120. We will not consider the ethics of animal care though we appreciate the concern for animal life.

One approach to a discipline is to look at what its practitioners do, at the issues bioethicists consider. Many see behavior modification as a major issue. We appreciate its importance but have generally excluded it from our concerns. See Robert Neville, "Behavior Control: Ethical Analysis," *EB*, 1:85–93. Kieffer, op. cit., pp. 262–312. Beauchamp and Walters, op. cit., pp. 503–566. Davis and Aroskar, op. cit., pp. 137–156. Robert Hunt and John Arras, *Ethical Issues in Modern Medicine* (Palo Alto, Calif.: Mayfield Publishing Co., 1977), pp. 341–402. Thomas A Shannon, *Bioethics* (New York: Paulist Press, 1976).

Beauchamp and Walters, pp. 49–51, see medical ethics as the oldest branch of bioethics, going back to Hippocrates (460–377 B.C.). For them, research ethics was next to develop (seventeenth century) with public policy (for example, allocation of scarce resources) as the third development (1960s). They see three major themes in bioethics—beneficence (do no harm; do good), justice, and self-determination. Gary Marotta says the term *medical ethics* was introduced by Thomas Percival in 1803 in his *Code of Ethics*. This book was the basis of the American Medical Association's *Ethical Principles*. "The Enlightenment and Bioethics," pp. 62–65, in *Bioethics and Human Rights*, ed. by Elsie L. and Bertram Bandman (Boston: Little, Brown and Company, 1978). Robert M. Veatch thinks the old medical ethics still important for they help define the role of the physician. However, the new set of problems represented by bioethics has come upon us. *Case Studies in Medical Ethics* (Cambridge, Mass.: Harvard University Press, 1977), p. v. Apparently, he thinks the doctor's role is well established for his cases are on bioethics rather than the size of signs and fees. The role of the nurse receives minimal attention: one passes the buck, one doesn't know what to say, and one is on a transplant team. However, he feels (p. vi) that the case studies will be helpful to nursing schools. It is not clear how. In a listing (p. 3) of a wide range of decision makers, there are no nurses.

8. Both rules and reasons change. Reuben Appet, a lawyer friend, notes the reason de-

parteth, but the rule persists. The reason may even be lost in the mists of the past. Here we might make a distinction among sources. The ANA Code was formulated by a committee, as were the Interpretive Statements. One could say the committees are the immediate source. They had a context so the situation is a source. One can trace the history of the code and one can trace the history of the ideas in it and thus have historical sources. One can also look at psychological, sociological, religious or theological sources. Here, we mean a process of questioning, such as that used by Socrates (469–399 B.C.). Someone says we *should* do something. Why? Because it's good. Why should we do the good? What is good? Where does *good* come from? Who or what decides what is good? Jones and colleagues, op. cit., p. 19. Raziel Abelson, *Ethics and Metaethics* (New York: St. Martin's Press, Inc., 1963).

9. Others, such as the utilitarians Jeremy Bentham (1748–1832) and John S. Mills (1806–1873), see pleasure as the only good and pain as the only evil. The philosopher Thomas Hobbes (1588–1697) saw man as a pleasure-pain machine. Jones and others, op. cit., pp. 178–192. Gerald J. Hughes, "Natural Law," pp. 30–32, in Beauchamp and Walters, op. cit. The modern world is perhaps most familiar with this from the pleasure/pain principle of Sigmund Freud (1856–1939). See his *Civilization and Its Discontents* (New York: W. W. Norton & Company, Inc., 1962). The Epicureans are the most famous among the ancients for this position. Epicurus (342–270 B.C.) was a Greek philosopher who founded his school in Athens. Plato (428–348 B.C.) and his student Aristotle (384–323 B.C.), among others, objected to this view. It may be a matter of what one sees as pleasure, which may include helping others or writing a book. The issue of what is good involves a huge volume of philsophical and religious literature. It remains a basic issue, if not *the* basic issue.

10. This is sometimes expanded to mean relative to society. What is right in one culture may be wrong in another. Related to this is the concept of consensus ethics. The right is simply what most people think is right. Carl Wellman, "Ethics XII: Relativism," *EB*, 1:454–457. Thiroux, op. cit., pp. 56–77. Sigman, op. cit., pp. 38–39. Donald G. Jones, ed.,

Private and Public Ethics (New York: The Edwin Mellen Press, 1978). This consensus is probably not to be confused with the excuse that "everybody's doing it." A case in point is sexual ethics (see adolescent sexuality, Chapter Six). Half of American adolescents are sexually active. The cry of "everybody's doing it" focuses on this half, but not the other half that is not active. In deontology (see later) something can be right or wrong whether society approves or not. Veatch, op. cit., pp. 3–4.

Kieffer, op. cit., pp. 10–11, 47, 60, sees metaethics as a branch of ethics. The branch is concerned with logic, semantics, and knowledge. Another branch is normative ethics, which we call morals. Beauchamp and Walters, op. cit., pp. 2–3, note another non-normative branch of ethics. Historians, anthropologists, and others study different ethical systems or beliefs to objectively describe them. By non-normative, they mean objective description of what people do, rather than telling people what they *ought* to do, which we call morals. The *ought* for them is applied normative or prescriptive ethics. Our concern with ethical principles is their general normative ethics. Thiroux, op. cit., pp. 3–4. Kieffer's "Human Nature" view is related to Natural Law (see later). The Catholic ethicist Bernard Häring also sees understanding human nature as crucial for understanding medical ethics. Häring, *Medical Ethics* (Slough, England: St. Paul Publications, 1972), pp. 42–64. So does Protestant Bird, op. cit., p. 134, and Eastern Orthodox Nicholas A. Berdyaev, *The Destiny of Man* (London: Goeffrey Bles, 1948). However, many, if not most, theists see God as the ultimate.

Science as an ultimate is perhaps better called Scientism. Christopher Lasch refers to those who come to medical science in a spirit of religious ecstasy. "Aging in a Culture Without a Future," *HCR*, no. 4 (Aug. 1977), 7:42–44. Modern advertising uses scientists and medical people as ultimate authorities in this religious sense. Owen Barfield, *Saving the Appearances: A Study in Idolatry* (New York: Harcourt Brace Jovanovich, Inc., 1965) suggests that such scientism is idolatry from a traditional Judeo-Christian perspective. Our point here is simply that science viewed as an ultimate value is a religion. See also

Walter R. Thorson, "The Spiritual Dimension of Science," pp. 217–257, in Henry, op. cit.

11. Henry D. Aiken has suggested levels of concern. The expressive level is the gut reaction, based upon belief that something is true. The moral and ethical level is as our usage. The fourth level is the postethical, somewhat equivalent to our metaethical, but also on a level with Kant's universal law, and with Natural Law. *Reason and Conduct* (New York: Alfred A. Knopf, Inc., 1962), pp. 65–88.

The term *values* may also be noted. It is sometimes used to cover a wide range and even all ethical thought. It may be loosely used for anything of value—books, trees, antiques. And it may also be used for the ultimate on which all else rests, a final principle worthy of esteem for its own sake. Kieffer, op. cit., p. 46. In values clarification theory, the concept is more elaborate. Values are personal guidelines that change with new data but provide a frame of reference for ideas, events, and relationships. Diane Uustal, *Values and Ethics: Considerations in Nursing Practice* (South Deerfield, Mass.: Uustal, 1978), p. 46. Values are personal beliefs about the truth or worth of thoughts, objects, or behavior. Some prefer to think of a process of valuing. Louis Raths, Merrill Harmin, Sidney B. Simon, *Values and Teaching* (Columbus, Ohio: Charles E. Merrell Publishing Company, 1966), pp. 3–37. While acknowledging the confusion and the debate over values, Krathwohl et al., distinguish three levels of value: acceptance, preference, and commitment. See David R. Krathwohl, Benjamin S. Bloom, Bertram B. Masia, *Taxonomy of Educational Objectives: Handbook II: Affective Domain* (New York: David McKay Company, 1964), pp. 139–153.

In practice, the line between ethics and metaethics is not hard and firm. As with morals and ethics, the terms may either blend into each other or be used interchangeably. Beauchamp and Walters, op. cit., p. 5.

12. Kay Partridge, "Nursing Values in a Changing Society," *Nursing Outlook*, no. 6 (June 1978), 26:356–360. Barbara A. Carper, "The Ethics of Caring," *Advances in Nursing Science*, no. 3 (Apr. 1979), 1:11. Leah Curtin, "The Nurse as Advocate: A Philosophical Foundation for Nursing," *Advances in Nurs-*

ing Science, no. 3 (Apr. 1979), **1**:1–10. Judith P. Swazey, "Professional Protectionism Rides Again," *HCR*, no. 2 (Apr. 1980), **10**:18–19.

13. Davis and Aroskar, op cit., pp. viii. Sigman, op. cit., p. 37, 38, 40, 41, 42. See Barzun. The encounter of two human beings is of a moral nature. Veatch, op. cit., pp. 2, 17, 35. To be sure, he notes some are trivial value choices, but many are choices between life and death.

14. Myra E. Levine, "Nursing Ethics and the Ethical Nurse," *American Journal of Nursing*, no. 5 (May 1977), **77**:845–849. Carper, op. cit., pp. 11, 18. Jones and others, op. cit., pp. 8–9.

15. Lucie Kelly, *Dimensions of Professional Nursing*, 3rd ed. (New York: Macmillan Publishing Co., Inc., 1975). See Chapter 13, "Professional Ethics and Accountability," pp. 208–220. See S. S. Coletta, "Values Clarification in Nursing: Why?" *American Journal of Nursing*, no. 12 (Dec. 1978), **78**:2057.

16. *ANA Code for Nurses*, op. cit., p. 4.

17. R. C. Dilday, "The Code for Nurses: An Educational Perspective," in ANA *Perspectives on the Code for Nurses*, Publication #G–132, 3m (March 1978), pp. 10–17.

18. Diane B. Uustal, "Values Clarification in Nursing: An Application to Practice," *AJN* no. 12 (Dec. 1978), p. 2059. Carper, op. cit., p. 18. Sigman op. cit., pp. 41–42. Diane Uustal, *Values and Ethics: Considerations in Nursing Practice*, op. cit. Fenner, op. cit., pp. 63–74.

19. Shirley M. Steele and Vera M. Harmon, *Values Clarification in Nursing* (New York: Appleton-Century-Crofts, 1979), Preface, p. vii. Davis and Aroskar, op. cit., p. 20. Carper, op. cit., p. 18.

20. Steele and Harmon, op. cit., p. 21. K. M. Sward, "The Code for Nurses: A Historical Perspective," in ANA *Perspectives on the Code for Nurses*, op. cit., p. 8. Sigman, op. cit., p. 38. Lucie Kelly, "Endpaper: Can't Can't," *Nursing Outlook*, no. 7 (July 1979), **27**:496.

21. B. Durand, "The Code for Nurses: A Nursing Practice Perspective," in ANA *Perspectives*, op. cit., p. 18. See Edna L. Neumann, "ANS Open Forum," *Advances in Nursing Science*, no. 3 (Apr. 1979), **1**:95, for discussion of problems with nurses' acceptance of responsibility for ethical judgments. Larry Churchill, "Ethical Issues of a Profession in Transition," *AJN*, no. 5 (May 1977), pp.

873–875. See also Lucie Kelly, "Endpaper: In Our Imperfect State," *Nursing Outlook*, no. 5 (May 1979), **27**:368. Sister A. Teresa Stanley, "Is It Ethical to Give Hope to a Dying Person?" *Nursing Clinics of North America*, no. 1 (May 1979), **14**:69–80, for discussion of case involving Ms. Tuma, RN.

22. Rita Payton, "Nurse-Practitioners and Ethics in Practice," tape recording of a speech made to the National Conference for Nurse-Practitioners, Keystone, Colorado, June 1979. H. L. A. Hart speaks of "role responsibility" along with causal, liability, and capacity responsibility. "Responsibility," pp. 32–38 in Beauchamp and Walters, op. cit.

23. Claire L. Jacobi, "Dilemmas for Educators: Values or Valuing," *Kappa Delta Pi Record*, no. 2 (Dec. 1975), **12**:50–51. Sigman, op cit., p. 42.

24. Andrew Jameton, "The Nurse: When Roles and Rules Conflict," *HCR*, no. 4 (Aug. 1977), **7**:22–23. "Nursing Ethics: The Admirable Professional Standards of Nurses—A Survey Report," *Nursing*, no. 9 (Sept. 1974), p. 35. Sally Gadow, "ANS Open Forum," *Advances in Nursing Science*, no. 3 (Apr. 1979), **1**:92–95. Curtin, op. cit., pp. 1–9.

25. Sylvia C. Gendrop, "The Order: No Code," *Linacre Quarterly*, no. 4 (Nov. 1977), **44**:313. See Albert Jonsen and Michael Garland, eds., *Ethics of Newborn Intensive Care* (San Francisco: Health Policy Program and Institutes of Governmental Studies, University of California, 1976. (See chapter on Grand Rounds, in particular.) Dagmar Cechanek, "Nursing Reactions," in *Ethical Dilemmas in Current Obstetric and Newborn Care*, Report of the Sixty-fifth Ross Conference in Pediatric Research, Columbus, Ohio, 1973, pp. 59–60. N. Fost and J. Robertson, "Letter to the Editor," *New England Journal of Medicine*, no. 20, **295**:1141. The literature on team decision making is notable for its lack of reference to nursing staff as members of such a team.

26. Rita Payton, "Information Control and Autonomy," *Nursing Clinics of North America*, no. 1 (Mar. 1979), **14**:23–33.

27. Levine, op. cit., p. 846. Sigman, op. cit., p. 38. Carper, op. cit., p. 11.

28. Payton, "Information Control. . . .," op. cit. Neumann, op. cit., p. 95.

29. Luther Christman, "Moral Dilemmas

for Practitioners in a Changing Society," *Nursing Digest*, Summer 1978, pp. 47–49. Anne J. Davis, "Ethical Dilemmas and Nursing Practice," *Linacre Quarterly*, no. 4 (Nov. 1977), **44**:302–303.

30. Lasch, op. cit., pp. 43–44, notes a dramatic shift in our current sense of historical time. He ascribes this to the prevalence of the narcissistic personality in our time. Narcissism cuts us off from past and future.

31. *Medical History of Contraception* (New York: Gamut Press, 1963), p. 422. Swazey, op. cit., p. 18.

32. Himes suggests that apart from learning nature's laws, there is no other way of determining the future except by studying the past through the historical method, op. cit., p. 423. Kübler-Ross sees a sense of history as necessary for peace. We need to know that we are part of what has come before and part of what is yet to be. The urgencies of the present are thus put into perspective, in *Death, The Final Stage of Growth* (Englewood N.J.: Prentice-Hall, Inc., 1975), p. 167. Ernest Lefever claims man is a creature of history. We are products of the past. To reject the past is to reject the fabric of human continuity that gives moral meaning to our present. "Morality versus Moralism in Foreign Policy," pp. 21–40, in Jones, op. cit.

33. Jones and others, p. 9. This is one way of describing informed consent, a main issue in health care today. The consent is not informed without understanding, or at least a reasonable attempt to understand. People may morally and legally give or withhold consent, but without clear understanding, neither taking it or leaving it, is informed. A similar urge to learn ethics is in the suggestion of Alfred N. Whitehead that the simple-minded use of "right and wrong" is one of the main obstacles to progress in understanding. Davis and Aroskar, op. cit., p. viii.

The Catholic Theological Society of America's report, *Human Sexuality: New Directions in American Catholic Thought*, prepared by Anthony Kosnik and others (New York: Paulist Press, 1977), is a study in ethics. It is concerned with the reasons behind moral codes, including origins. To the extent that it also prescribes or tells what people should do, it is a study in morals.

34. W. T. Jones, op. cit., pp. xviii–xx. Wellman, "Naturalism," op. cit., p. 443.

George E. Moore, *Principia Ethica* (Cambridge, England: Cambridge University Press, 1903), p. 7. Philippa Foot, "Ethics IX: Moral Reasoning," *EB*, 1:450–454, notes that it is all so confusing to the philosophers themselves that some do not think moral action is possible. Structural ethics tries to answer this metaethical question by an hypothesis of deep structures with which we are born. The concept of good and the innate sense of obligation to obey moral laws are examples of deep structures. The moral codes are surface structures. Kieffer, op. cit., p. 29. George E. Pugh, "Human Values, Free Will, and the Conscious Mind," *Zygon*, no. 1 (1976), **11**:2–24. Gunther S. Stent, "The Poverty of Scientism and the Promise of Structuralist Ethics," *HCR* (Dec. 1976), **6**:32–40. See Intuitionism. For a clear, brief (113 pages) overview of ethical theory, see Peter Baelz, *Ethics and Belief* (New York: The Seabury Press, 1977).

35. Clouser, op. cit., p. 116. Davis and Aroskar, op. cit., p. 4.

36. Clouser, op. cit., p. 117. Kieffer, op. cit., p. 40.

37. Kieffer, op. cit., pp. 52–53, calls these two main types of normative ethics. Ruth Macklin, "Moral Concerns and Appeals to Rights and Duties," *HCR*, no. 5 (Oct. 1976), **6**:31–38.

38. William D. Solomon, "Ethics II: Rules and Principles," *EB*, 1:407–413. Hunt and Arras, op. cit., pp. 4–5. It is common to other professions, too, of course, and is sometimes seen as equivalent, so professional equals ethical and unprofessional equals unethical. Personal communication, June 1979, Donald G. Jones. See also, David Little, "Duties of Station vs. Duties of Conscience: Are There Two Moralities?" pp. 125–157, in Jones, op. cit. This concern is reflected by Paul F. Camenisch when he claims that the role of a public servant is not a moral elective but a moral duty. Society has given rights to the professions in support of education and a licensed monopoly. The professions now have a responsibility, a duty to society. "On the Professions," *HCR*, no. 5 (Oct. 1976), **6**:8–9. See also, Eliot Freidson, "The Perils of Professionalism," *HCR*, no. 3 (June 1978), **8**:47–49.

39. "Ethics III: Deontological Theories," *EB*, 1:413–417. There are other ways to consider deontology. The theory is sometimes

divided between an act deontology and a rules deontology. In the first, the duty is determined in each act. This is somewhat like the inductive approach common in clinical education—here's the situation; now what do we do with it? The rules approach is more a deductive method. For example, you treat diabetes with insulin. So when you find a case of hyperglycemia, that's what you do. You apply the rule.

40. Some aspects of the Judeo-Christian ethic are interpreted as utilitarian. In the wider sense here, we might include all religions, including such faith and commitment systems as Science, Marxism, and Secular Humanism. See Frederick S. Carney, "Ethics VII: Theological Ethics," *EB*, 1:429–437. Jones and others, p. 8. Stent, op. cit., p. 32. Hunt and Arras, op. cit., pp. 38–43, see religious ethics as having a variety of these philosophical perspectives. Protestant Paul Ramsey is deontologist but Protestant Joseph Fletcher is utilitarian. Catholics Thomas Aquinas (A.D. 1225–1274) and Daniel Maguire are in the latter group. Traditionally, Roman Catholic ethicists have been interested in Natural Law, which Hunt and Arras see as yet another theory alongside of deontology and utilitarianism. For some theists, Natural Law equals the Will of God. Fletcher and others reject Natural Law, or at least the Catholic interpretation of it. Nontheistic proponents of Natural Law can see it as the law of nature without a deity as the author or creator of nature. It was part of ancient Roman Law and is also traced to Aristotle. Macklin, op. cit., pp. 33–34. The principles of double effect and ordinary/extraordinary treatment (more on this later) may be seen as part of Natural Law. Natural Law considers rules essential (the good is objectively determined through an understanding of nature), so it is deontological. It also considers consequences, so it is utilitarian. The concern is for human good, whereas duty is to God or nature. See also Beauchamp and Walters, op. cit., pp. 3–4. Veatch, op. cit., pp. 4–7. Hughes, op. cit., p. 31, suggests that the natural state of people is health with the whole person functioning in harmony (Aristotle, St. Thomas Aquinas). Natural Law then suggests health personnel are either trying to keep people natural or restore them to their natural state. This, of course, tends to break down in working with the permanently handicapped or the dying. Shannon, op. cit., p. 6, notes the claim of the Roman Catholic Magisterium to be the sole interpreter of Natural Law. The claim is based on the New Testament in the Bible. He suggests an unsubstantiated claim weakens the concern. Non-Catholics, of course, do not recognize the claim of the Magisterium, but their thinking is influenced by its influence in Western culture. Health personnel concerned with colleagues and patients will also want to be aware of the claim.

One of the riddles of theological ethics was asked long ago by Socrates. Is something good because deity does it, or does deity do it because it is good? The latter implies an ultimate greater than deity. Health personnel face this constantly. Is something good because it was ordered? Or was it ordered because it was good?

41. Daniel Maguire suggests that saying something is right or wrong in all possible circumstances implies divine knowledge. It is "non-sense" to say something is good or bad regardless of reality. "The Freedom to Die," pp. 171–180, in Shannon, op. cit. Traditionally, religions and religious organizations have often claimed divine knowledge or authority, either through direct revelation or in an intermediate form such as Scripture. For circumstances, see situation ethics.

42. One might see these values as relative rather than absolute. Kieffer, op. cit., pp. 12–13, suggests that Darwinian evolution has put a permanent doubt into any absolute deontology. Absolute or not, we do live by rules. A theist might see God as absolute, even as our view of the will of God changes with the situation. See Wellman, "Relativism," op. cit. Kantian thought appears in biomedical ethics in the idea of truth-telling and the prohibition on using people as a means to an end, even a worthy end or a good cause. Among bioethicists today, Paul Ramsey represents Kant's concern for the dignity of individuals. See his *The Patient as Person* (New Haven: Yale University Press, 1978). The whole deontological approach is sometimes called the Kantian theory. Hunt and Arras, op. cit., pp. 12, 24–38. They see the Golden Rule as an example of Kant's Categorical Imperative.

43. Macklin, op. cit., p. 35, calls intuitionism the most common deontological posi-

tion today. One could argue, of course, that what we "know" is culturally or environmentally conditioned. This relates to an old argument on nature and nurture. Kant stands for nature and might be classed as an intrinsicist or a nativist. Kieffer, op. cit., pp. 21–37, argues for an evolutionary ethic that is not dependent on the nonhuman, either natural or supernatural. Following the sociobiologists such as Edward O. Wilson, the evolutionary biologists George G. Simpson and C. H. Waddington, he suggests we are born with a capacity for ethics as for language. The particular language we speak and the particular ethic we accept are another matter. Arthur Caplan notes wide disagreements as well as enthusiastic acceptance of sociobiology. "Ethics, Evolution, and the Milk of Human Kindness," *HCR*, no. 2 (Apr. 1976), **6:**20–25. Caplan, Robert S. Morison, Bernard D. Davis, and Larry Miller, "Sociobiology: The Debate Continues," *HCR*, no. 5 (Oct. 1976), **6:**18–19, 48–50. In some ways, intuitionism resembles the so-called law of nature and Natural Law. We are supposed to know naturally what is right and wrong. See Eric D'Arey, "Natural Law," *EB*, **2:**1131–1137. It also relates to egoistic hedonism. If it feels good, do it. See utilitarianism judged by the individual. Hunt and Arras, op. cit., pp. 10–12. Lawrence Kohlberg in his theories of moral development is building on the work of Jean Piaget who sees the child developing through an interaction of natural endowment (the nativist theory) and the environment (nurture). Kohlberg has six stages of moral development. The last and presumably highest is universalism (compare Kant and Natural Law). Kohlberg's Stage 5 is the social contract level (see Rawls following). Stage 4 is the law and order level, sometimes compared to moral rules such as the Ten Commandments, and to the deontological level in general. Stage 1 is the punishment and obedience level, which is not a respect for authority but simple fear of power and retaliation. Kohlberg, "The Development of Moral Character and Ideology," pp. 396–399, in *Review of Child Development Research*, ed. by M. L. Hoffman and L. N. W. Hoffman (New York: Russell Sage Foundation, 1964). Piaget, *The Moral Judgment of the Child* (New York: The Free Press, 1965). Intuitionism is also related to the concept of conscience and to the Freudian concept of superego. Willard

Gaylin, "From Twain to Freud: An Examination of Conscience," *HCR*, no. 4 (Aug. 1976), **6:**5–8. Donald E. Miller, *The Wing-Footed Wanderer: Conscience and Transcendence* (Nashville, Tenn.: Abingdon Press, 1977).

44. John Rawls, *A Theory of Justice* (Cambridge, Mass.: Harvard University Press, 1971). He suggests, pp. 130–136, five concepts of right. Principles should be general, universal (compare Kant), public, orderable (can decide between conflicting claims), and final (higher than law or custom). Kieffer, op. cit., pp. 58–59, sees Rawls as a mix of deontology and utilitarianism with his concern for equality and good for the many. Some see Rawls as a Kantian. Where he emphasizes justice, Ramsey emphasizes dignity for the individual. Davis and Aroskar, op. cit., pp. 26–27. Roger D. Masters, "Is Contract an Adequate Basis for Medical Care?" *HCR*, no. 6 (Dec. 1975), **5:**24–29. William F. May, "Code, Covenant, Contract or Philanthropy," *HCR*, no. 6, **5:**29–38. Foot, op. cit., p. 450. Veatch, op. cit., p. 8, notes informed consent, self-determination of patients, and "do no harm" as deontological principles in medical ethics. Thomas Jefferson's "man is endowed with certain inalienable rights" (Declaration of Independence) is a principle now influencing medical practice.

45. Kurt Baier, "Ethics IV: Teleological Ethics," *EB*, **1:**417–421. R. M. Hare, "Ethics VI: Utilitarianism," *EB*, **1:**424–429. Note that in an absolute sense we do not know the consequences until after the fact. This itself has ethical implications. In our discussion of the IUD (Chapter 3), we note the uncertainty principle. When in doubt, some say follow the rules (see rules utilitarianism). Others say we are free to follow our conscience (Intuitionism? Kant's Categorical Imperative?). Because medical care can rarely guarantee consequences, the contract is not the same as a purchase in which the merchandise can be returned or the politician be voted out of office. Masters, op. cit., p. 25. Kieffer, op. cit., pp. 52–53. Jones and others, pp. xviii, xxiii–xxiv. Hunt and Arras, op. cit., pp. 12–24. See note 9. John S. Mill, *Utilitarianism* (New York: The Liberal Arts Press, 1957). Thiroux, op. cit., p. 20.

46. The principle of double effect is an example here. A cancerous uterus is removed to save a woman's life. She happens to be preg-

nant. In effect, this is an abortion, but it is a secondary effect. The primary purpose was treating the cancer. Traditional Roman Catholic ethicists tend to allow this under the principle of double effect, even though they are against abortion. Hare, op. cit., p. 425. Richard A. McCormick and Paul Ramsey, *Doing Evil to Achieve Good* (Chicago: Loyola University Press, 1978). In the history of politics, the view that the end justifies the means is associated with Machiavelli (1469–1527) and is sometimes labelled Machiavellian. See Michael Walzer, "Political Action: The Problem of Dirty Hands," pp. 96–124, in Jones, op. cit.

47. Hare, op. cit., p. 428, calls this a universalized prudence. He sees the Golden Rule as an example. Just what is good is a matter of considerable and continuing debate. See metaethics. Taylor, op. cit., p. 15, notes a further distinction between altruism, that is, good for others without the self, and good for everyone including the self. He thinks one of the great values of utilitarianism is that it provides a standard of value that is impartial and universal. This, of course, sounds like deontology. The principle or rule is that of utility. John S. Mill, *On Liberty* (New York: W. W. Norton & Company, Inc. 1975, original 1859), p. 12. Robert M. Veatch makes a distinction between individual utilitarianism as in the nurse-patient relationship, and social utilitarianism with its concern for the larger society. *Ethical Dilemmas in Current Obstetric and Newborn Care*, report of the Sixty-fifth Ross Conference on Pediatric Research, ed. by Tom D. Moore (Columbus, Ohio: Ross Laboratories, 1973), pp. 71–72. Frankena, op. cit., p. 19, calls egoism a third theory compared to deontology and utilitarianism. Davis and Aroskar, op. cit., pp. 20–23. Thiroux, op. cit., p. 21, sees egoism and utilitarianism as two theories within the consequentialist (teleological) viewpoint.

48. Baier, op. cit., both articles. Hare, op. cit. Joseph Fletcher, "Ethics V: Situation Ethics," *EB*, 1:421–424. Ladd, op. cit., p. 402. Foot, op. cit., p. 456.

49. Ladd, op. cit.

50. We are touching here on an old philosophical problem. David Hume (1711–1776) formulated it as the gap between what is and what ought to be. Because something exists, it does not follow that it is right. War exists.

Some have tried to say there is such a thing as a just war. Others say war is evil. We may not be able to stop having wars, but that does not mean they are moral or ethical or right. The *is* is not the same as the *ought*. Another term for this is the *naturalistic fallacy*. It is false to assume that because it exists in nature, it is morally required. Hume, *A Treatise of Human Nature* (1739) (Oxford, England: Oxford University Press, 1941). W. D. Hudson, *The Is-Ought Question* (New York: Macmillan Publishing Co., Inc., 1969). Arthur J. Dyck, "Moral Requiredness: Bridging the Gap Between 'Ought' and 'Is,'" *The Journal of Religious Ethics*, no. 2 (Fall 1978), **6**:293–318. Foot, op. cit., p. 452. Wellman, "Naturalism," op. cit., pp. 443–444. In bioethics, the question arises in the form, "Because we *can* do it, must/ought we do it?" We can sometimes keep a body functioning on machinery long after it would have naturally died. Because we can do it, must we? Some say yes and others say *is* does not mean *ought*. Clouser, op. cit., p. 115. Kieffer, op. cit., pp. 11–12.

51. Fletcher, op. cit. Kieffer, op. cit., p. 35, derives the love ethic through the scientific development he calls evolutionary ethics.

52. Shannon, op. cit., p. 5. James M. Gustafson, "A Protestant Ethical Approach," pp. 101–122, in *The Morality of Abortion*, ed. by John T. Noonan (Cambridge, Mass.: Harvard University Press, 1970), p. 101. Kosnik and others, p. 112, note the history of Catholicism's insistence on procreation as originating in Stoicism, supported by other factors. These included economics, war, high infant mortality, short life span, plague, and famine.

53. Fletcher, op. cit., p. 424. Lisa H. Newton, "No Right at All: An Interpretation of the Abortion Issue," pp. 113–118, in Bandman and Bandman, op. cit.

54. We might argue that all positions are religious. The atheist and agnostic hold a faith position as much as the theist. Religion in this broad sense of the term covers far more than the Judeo-Christian ethic. See Carney, op. cit., p. 429. Paul Ramsey notes that the Supreme Court has accepted secular humanism as a religion. He wonders if nonreligious positions still exist. "Reference Points in Deciding about Abortion," in Noonan, op. cit., pp. 60–61. Ultimate concern has been equated with deity and religion through the writings of Paul Tillich. *The Courage to Be*

(New Haven: Yale University Press, 1952), pp. 46–51. On this basis, science, Marxism, one's job, or car, or family, or anything that becomes a major or ultimate concern becomes a religion.

55. Carney, op. cit., pp. 429–430, sees ethics as a critical reflection. Theological ethics is reflection on theory/theology. Moralists are concerned with morals, normative, applied, or practical ethics in some systems of thought. We remain concerned with the principles or reasons behind the moral concerns as well as the practical application of the principles.

For indebtedness to Catholic thought, see Gustafson, op. cit.

56. Kelly, op. cit., p. 208. Davis and Aroskar, op. cit., p. 8. Barzun, op. cit., p. 68. See also Fenner, op. cit., pp. 29–43.

57. *ANA Code for Nurses*, op. cit.

58. Kelly, op. cit., p. 209.

59. ANA Code . . . op. cit., p. 1. The Code is reprinted with permission of the American Nurses' Association, Kansas City, 1976. Our appreciation is extended to the ANA for this permission, dated August 8, 1979.

60. Sward, op. cit., p. 2.

61. "A Suggested Code: A Code of Ethics Presented for Consideration of the American Nurses' Association," *AJN*, no. 8 (Aug. 1926), **26**:599–601.

62. A. J. Davis, op. cit., p. 306. M. E. Doona, "The Ethical Dimension in 'Ordinary Nursing Care,' " *Linacre Quarterly*, no. 4 (Nov. 1977), **44**:322–323.

63. B. L. Tate, *The Nurse's Dilemma: Ethical Considerations in Nursing Practice* (Geneva: International Council of Nurses, 1977).

The Code is reprinted with permission of the International Council of Nurses, Geneva, Switzerland, 1973. Our appreciation is extended to the Council for this permission, dated 28 August 1979.

64. Sward, op. cit., p. 8. S. Maurice and L. Warrick, "Ethics and Morals in Nursing," *The American Journal of Maternal Child Nursing* no. 6 (Nov./Dec. 1977), **2**:343–345. Mary C. Silva, "Science, Ethics, and Nursing," *AJN*, no. 11 (Nov. 1974), **74**:2004–2007.

65. Henry O. Thompson and Joyce E. Beebe, "Nurse-Midwifery and Ethics—A Beginning," *Journal of Nurse-Midwifery*, no. 4 (Winter 1976), **21**:7–11. Rosemary Krawczyk and Elizabeth Kudzma, "Ethics: A Matter of Moral Development," *Nursing Outlook*, no. 4 (Apr. 1978), **26**:254–257. Joyce Beebe and Henry O. Thompson, "Teaching Ethics to Nurse-Midwives," *Journal of Nurse-Midwifery*, (Spring/Summer 1978), **23**:31–35.

66. Tate, op. cit., pp. ix—xi. R. Bergman, "Ethics—Concepts and Practice," *International Nursing Review*, no. 5 (1973), **20**:140–141, 152. M. A. Murphy and J. Murphy, "Making Ethical Decisions—Systematically," *Nursing*, no. 6 (May 1976), **6**:CG13–14. M. B. Ryden, "An Approach to Ethical Decision Making," *Nursing Outlook*, no. 11 (Nov. 1978), **26**:705–706. Davis and Aroskar, op. cit., Chapter Two, "Ethical Approaches," pp. 19–30. Silva, op. cit., p. 2007. Mila A. Aroskar, "Anatomy of an Ethical Dilemma: The Practice," *American Journal of Nursing*, no. 4 (April 1980) **80**:661–663.

67. Adapted by Beebe from Rebecca Bergman, op. cit., and Murphy and Murphy, op. cit. See David Belgum, op. cit., pp. 44f.

Chapter 2

Ethics and Genetics

The ethics of genetics[1] is in one sense newer than this morning's newspaper, which has not caught up with the laboratories which, in turn, have not caught up with the creative minds of the geneticists. In another sense, genetic ethics is so old that the origins are lost in the mists of time. It may help to get a handle on the modern scene if we take a look at our ancestors.

HISTORY

Bentley Glass has pointed out that virtually all societies have controlled both marriage and procreation.[2] There have been both laws and taboos on incest, for example. Abortion was so common in the Roman Empire that Seneca publicly thanked his mother for not aborting him. Infanticide is common in primitive societies, both ancient and present-day. Social ostracism and confinement in prisons and mental hospitals have controlled and sometimes prevented reproduction by criminals, the mentally ill, the retarded, and the diseased (leprosy, tuberculosis). Compulsory sterilization has been practiced on slaves (eunuchs for the harem) and *castrati* singers (so boys would keep their falsetto soprano).[3] There are still laws on the books in some of the United States for the sterilization of mental defectives. These have not been widely enforced since the 1930s but, over a period of several decades, thousands of people were sterilized. "Voluntary" sterilization of sex offenders is a current issue.[4]

Strictly speaking, these examples from history are not all a matter of genetics. The Bible, for example, is somewhat inconsistent in its taboos on incest. The sons of Adam married their sisters (Apocalyptic Book of Jubilees 4), Lot sired children with his daughters (Genesis 19), Abraham was married to his half-sister (Genesis 20), Amnon raped his half-sister but before that she seemed to think their father would give her to him in marriage (II Samuel 13), and a son might inherit his father's wives along with the kingdom (II Samuel 3). Yet, elsewhere, marriage and sexual intercourse with "any one near of kin" was forbidden on pain of death, childlessness, or being cut off from one's people (Leviticus 18 and 20; Deuteronomy 27). Among those listed as near of kin are the categories just mentioned.[5]

Apart from divine revelation, we do not know the exact origins of incest or marriage taboos. Still, it would be reasonable to suppose that ancient peoples were well aware of some of the problems of inbreeding. We know that ancient peoples were keen observers of nature. That includes astronomy (Babylonia, especially), the flood levels of the Nile (Egypt), the results of selective breeding of livestock (Genesis 30), and human personality (Proverbs). Thus marriage taboos may have had a genetic component even though ancient peoples lacked knowledge of modern genetics. In any event, such practices had a genetic effect.[6]

The same can be said for the practice of infanticide that usually included children with defects (genetic and otherwise) when they survived pregnancy and birth, as well as children who were unwanted for whatever reason.[7] Similarly, the confinement or ostracizing of the mentally and physically ill had a genetic effect in reducing or preventing their reproduction. We should note here, too, that life expectancy was much shorter prior to the twentieth century. There were fewer pregnancies among older people and a lower incidence of genetic-related problems such as Down's syndrome.

Incest taboos continue into the present and are written into law in some cultures. As with the Bible, there is some variation in the law as to what constitutes consanguine (blood-related) marriage. Infanticide has continued into the present in some societies.[8] In Western culture, it has been condemned since the early centuries of the Common Era. Histo-

rians argue over the reason for the condemnation. Some ascribe it to the Judeo-Christian respect for life as a gift from and sacred to God.[9] Others point out that empires needed troops for their armies and workers for their fields, so the reasons were military and economic.[10] Our point here is that the banning of infanticide and the encouragement to have children (still part of the income tax structure) also have a genetic effect.

It is of some importance to note here that the "right" to marry or the "right" to have children has, at best, a checkered history. Denmark's laws allowing marriage after sterilization for carriers of genetic defects has a long history, even though both the reason and the means of dealing with the problem are quite new. "The reason departeth but the rule persists." Alternately, one might say the reason changes but the form persists. Marriage and procreation have usually had controls, which, in turn, have had genetic effects.[11]

THE PRESENT

In the twentieth century we are faced with the astounding success of two movements: democracy and technology. The triumph of democracy has focused on human rights, including the right to marry and have children.[12] It has also focused on human responsibility, which has included self-government and education. Several years ago, Sir Alan S. Parkes suggested a Declaration of Human Obligations. These included the obligation not to produce unwanted children and not to take substantial risks of producing children with mental or physical defects.[13]

Into the midst of rights and obligations come enormous changes in technology. These changes are remarkable in most fields of human endeavor. In medicine they border on the miraculous. Pacemakers and metal or plastic joints have already given us a version of the cyborg, the part man and part machine of science fiction. Many of the medicines prescribed by doctors and nurses today did not exist ten years ago. The pace appears to be accelerating rather than slowing down.

In genetics, by 1970, more than sixteen hundred genetically related disorders could be detected. By the mid–1970s, there were twenty-three hundred detectable problems, and by McKusick's 1978 edition, there were more than twenty-eight hundred.[14] Like the national debt, the sheer volume overwhelms the mind. We have already come a long way from the work of Gregor Johann Mendel (1822–1884), the Austrian monk who worked out the laws of heredity.

But Mendel is still very much with us. In fact, he provides a kind of anchor in the inundation of this new flood of genetic information. Mendel's laws help us to move from the traditional medical diagnosis to prediction. Certain characteristics are dominant in heredity, such as blue eyes and brown hair in northern Europeans. Other characteristics are recessive. A person with a genetic disorder can be so diagnosed. In addition, a person might be a carrier; that is, the disorder does not appear outwardly, but it is recessive in the genetic makeup of the individual. If two carriers of the same recessive trait reproduce, there is a one-in-four chance that offspring will be afflicted. Statistically, if there are four children, one will have the disorder, one will be free of it, and two will be carriers. Walters notes that about fifty of these recessive conditions can be detected in the carrier state.[15]

It is with these predictions that "the plot thickens" in genetic ethics. As long as we were ignorant of the process, human beings took their chances, hoped for the best, and took what came, with the exceptions noted earlier. We had little choice but to play what Joseph Fletcher calls "reproductive roulette."[16] Our choices are now vastly increased. Note that one choice is to continue Fletcher's roulette, to continue letting nature take its course according to the natural law concepts of the past. Others say this is irresponsible and ethically indefensible.

Rights and Choice

Ethical dilemmas abound in this whole process. For example, where do we start with our genetic concerns? One obvious place is wherever people happen to be when we find them or they come to us with genetic concerns. Alternatively, we might reach out and

begin by choice. As noted, Denmark has laws requiring sterilization prior to marriage for carriers of some genetic defects. If we start before the marriage choice is made, such compulsion may not be necessary. This would point to high school and college level health education and testing as the entry point for our concern with genetic disorders.

The coercion issue is a basic ethical principle. As with marriage in general, freedom of choice has never been absolute in human history. However, it is a cherished tradition, especially in the West. There are those who argue it is essential to be really human. Still, we require such things as vaccinations for contagious disease and testing for venereal disease in premarital examinations. Can we require testing or screening, including mass screening for detectable genetic disorders? These are certainly not contagious. But society does have a concern in the matter.[17]

We will consider rights more thoroughly in a later chapter. Here we can note an old cliché, my rights end where your nose begins. I may claim a right to freedom of choice, even to taking the risk of producing a defective child. But society will have to pay for this child in increased educational and hospitalization costs. So some would argue that my right to produce a child is not an absolute one.[18] Does society have a right to stop me or anyone else from reproducing without regard to genetic disorders?

Some would say not, while others say yes, and still others say maybe. How do we weigh the rights of society and the individual? How do we compare the rights of potential parents with the rights of potential children? For those who follow absolutely the "natural order," the individual may be free to proceed. But very few see this as an absolute right. It may be a matter of the severity of the problem, for instance, diabetes (readily treatable) versus Tay-Sachs disease (always fatal within a few years, at most) versus sickle cell anemia (considerable potential for a normal life though abnormal pain and suffering). It may be a matter of the statistics, as in Mendel's laws. Is this the first child or the fourth? Whether formally or informally engaged in genetic counseling, health professionals will find it helpful to have some understanding of these aspects.

Judeo—Christian Tradition

In the Western world, a major portion of the Judeo-Christian tradition (generally speaking, the conservative side of the tradition) does not want us to "play God." Whatever happens naturally is what is to be. Carried out consistently, this would, of course, eliminate most health care. We do not know of any religious tradition that requires a couple to knowingly produce a defective child. Some may sound that way in their insistence upon saving a fetus or child, even when it is known to be defective.[19] Life itself is sacred. The quality of life is of secondary importance for some.

Another major portion of the Judeo-Christian tradition (generally speaking, the liberal side of the tradition) sees humanity as co-creators with God. We are permitted and even obligated to control the genetic makeup of people. Without the creator concept, this position is similar to that of secular humanists. Here, too, we have Bentley Glass' oft-quoted dictum that every child has the right to be free of genetic defect and abnormality insofar as this can be achieved. The right of the individual to procreate must give way to a greater right: the right of every child to enter life with an adequate physical and mental endowment.[20]

Either wing may approve of objective, nondirective counseling in which the counselor shares the data with the counselees. The latter can then make their own decision, perhaps with further advice from their spiritual advisor for approved or accepted procedures. There are those counselors, however, who understand their role to be that of advocate, a paternalistic role. This may be that of advocate for either of the positions described, but ethicists seem particularly concerned for those advocates of the no-defective-children school of thought. In either case, the counselor runs the risk of violating the freedom of choice, the autonomy, of the parties concerned. This is particularly so if the counselees are emotionally upset and hence more susceptible to persuasion as in a parent-child or doctor-patient relationship.[21]

Compulsion

Note that many genetic difficulties have no known cure or even treatment. Some do have treatment. One of these is phenylketonuria (PKU), which requires a special diet controlling phenylalanine. Lack of treatment results in severe retardation with resultant problems for the individual, the parent(s), and society. One might expect treatment would be welcomed once the condition is diagnosed. Some, however, would invoke the natural law principle that nothing should be done. Some religious traditions do not believe in medical treatment. A false "positive" could result in damage from the special diet. For whatever reason treatment is refused, we need to ask here, too, if compulsion is ethical. Many state laws now require testing for PKU, but the laws do not all provide for or require treatment.

Contraception

We are skirting the edges here of the issue of contraception if the counselees have reached the stage in life where reproduction is potential or planned. The counselor who does not believe in any kind of contraception may influence the client in that direction. The counselor who believes in some kinds but not in others and the counselors who believe in all kinds may influence in those directions, respectively. Contraceptive issues are discussed fully in Chapter Three.

Another frequent question that arises in the area of genetics is, should those with a genetic problem or carriers of one be sterilized? Sterilization is usually a permanent form of birth control. Our interest here is in its relationship to genetics. It is ethically wrong from the religious and philosophical traditions that view the sterilization procedure itself as a violation of nature. For some, it is wrong because it prevents reproduction, may tempt one to sexual license, and involves mutilation of the body. Bernard Häring suggests it may sometimes be acceptable as a minor evil compared to an abortion as a way of preventing defective children.[22] For others, it is more acceptable for people past the young adult stage. Some see it as acceptable under any circumstances. The major concern, however, has been whether it is compulsory sterilization or a free choice. We noted earlier the laws for mental hospital patients or the retarded. Sometimes such persons may be incapable of giving their free and informed consent to the procedure. Informed consent will be considered later. We note here that it is both an ethical and a legal issue: *Who* is to be sterilized? *Who* decides on the sterilization? These are central problems for genetic and other cases as well.[23]

Amniocentesis

Here we want to note the development of *in utero* examination of the fetus. The most well known of these is *amniocentesis*, the surgical procedure of withdrawing amniotic fluid through the abdominal wall of the pregnant woman. The fluid is analyzed for disease, genetic defects, and fetal maturity. Although it carries some risks to both mother and fetus, amniocentesis is still less risky than the birth process. Amniocentesis is now so widely practiced that it is nearly routine. Some would argue that amniocentesis, like vaccinations, should be compulsory. Others suggest that because of the risks, it remains contraindicated unless family history, or genetic tests on the parents, or other factors such as age of the woman suggest the technique.[24]

The ethical concerns are abortion and the question of compulsion versus freedom of choice. This choice may be in having the procedure at all. Or it may be a matter of further decisions. Some clinics that perform amniocentesis will not do the procedure without prior commitment from parents to abort if the fetus is defective. Still others are more permissive, recognizing other factors such as relief of anxiety (not knowing may be worse than knowing even if the knowledge is of a defective child-to-be), or preparing parents or staff for the birth. The ethical issues of abortion are considered in Chapter Four.[25]

Confidentiality

One of the rights that is sometimes claimed is the right to privacy. In genetic counseling, testing, screening (including mass screening), and related matters, the right to privacy and the right to confidentiality are important. Confidentiality is a long-established legal right in pastor-parishioner, lawyer-client, doctor-patient, nurse-patient, and other relationships. When genetic information has not been kept confidential, there have been cancellations of insurance policies (even though carriers do not "get" the genetic disease) or employment difficulties. Social ostracism has been a common experience when genetic disorders were known among school children, between races, and in whole communities. The discovery of a genetic disorder may induce psychological trauma and severe emotional disturbances. On a more personal level, counselors may face an ethical dilemma if the individual tests positive but then does not want this known to other family members who may be carriers also, or to a prospective spouse or a present one, or to children. What obligation does the counselor have to these other persons or to society as a whole? This question has no clear answer.[26]

Genetic Engineering

As noted earlier, genetic counseling and screening involve ethical considerations in privacy and confidentiality, compulsion, freedom of choice, and informed consent, individual rights versus the rights of society, the rights of the unborn, if any, and the potential rights of those yet to be conceived. The last concerns responsibility to future generations. Some biologists have pointed out that our technological capabilities are increasing the defectiveness of the gene pool.[27]

Gene Pool: The *gene pool* is an abstraction for the collective genetic quality of society or the human race. Thanks to insulin, the number of diabetics has increased. Diabetics have not only survived but have reproduced diabetic children. Because this genetic problem can be treated, it does not seem to be a major concern. Other disorders, such as Huntington's chorea, have no treatment. Symptoms do not ordinarily appear until after middle age and the reproduction of children who in turn may have the problem. Thus, genetic disorders are increasing.[28]

Some ethicists fear a steady deterioration

of the human race. They claim it is irresponsible for this generation not to do everything possible to prevent further pollution of the gene pool through counseling, screening, contraception, and abortion. Others point out that every one of us has three to eight or more defective genes and we would have to eliminate ourselves to effect a complete cure. Others point out that whereas diabetes might soon increase to 50 percent of the human race, it will take fifty generations for the more rare cystic fibrosis to increase from its present 5 percent to 7.5 percent. So they suggest the situation is not one of imminent disaster for the human race.

Theory or No: Some make a sharp distinction between therapy for the afflicted (often accepted even though it interferes with the natural order) and such procedures as abortion or letting the newborn die. They see the last two as elimination and even murder. It is not therapy even though letting defective neonates die might be natural. The no treatment approach has also been suggested as a way of eliminating genetic problems through natural selection. Although generally not acceptable to health professionals, a lack of treatment is not unusual for defective newborns[29] and the terminally ill. Some genetic disorders could theoretically be eliminated in one generation if afflicted persons and carriers would not have children. In sex-linked problems, this could involve selective abortion. In hemophilia, aborting each female fetus (identified by amniocentesis) would stop the disease in that family line. Others consider the strategies of no treatment and abortion as inhuman and reprehensible.[30]

A related issue is that some conceptions end before the woman knows she is pregnant. The fertilized egg fails to attach itself to the uterine wall. From 25 percent to 50 percent of all conceptions do not reach term. As many as one third of these have identifiable defects.[31] Joshua Lederberg notes that we "could in principle" save these conceptions.[32] Should we? A long-standing ethical principle is that an *is* does not mean an *ought*. Because we can do it, it does not follow that we should or must. A further distinction is made between allowing something such as death to happen and intervening actively. We will return to this in considering the problems of the post-

natal defective child and in considering the problems of death and dying in adults, particularly among the aged. The problem is also related to scarce resources (triage).[33]

Artificial Insemination

The problems related to artificial insemination and test-tube babies are also of interest. Artificial insemination is practiced in two forms: AIH in which the husband is the source of sperm, and AID in which a donor is the source. More than 20,000 AID procedures are carried out every year in the United States alone, and there are more than one million AID children, but the status of the procedure and of the child is ambiguous.

The Anglican church considers the children illegitimate. The Roman Catholic church condemns both AID and AIH although some Catholic thinkers have suggested that AIH might be acceptable under certain circumstances. A similar position is held in Eastern Orthodoxy. The more conservative groups in Judaism, Protestantism, and other religions tend to condemn, or approve in very limited ways. The concern is with conception in any other than the natural way, with the legal spouse. Thus, the woman who conceives in this way may be condemned for adultery, as is the donor. The donor may also be strictured for having pleasure without responsibility. The procedure is seen as disruptive of the traditional marriage-family, considered the rock of civilization.[34]

Others point out that statistically the families practicing AID and AIH have an extremely low divorce rate, suggesting greater stability than in the average family. People who claim that a woman has a right to have a baby see AIH (as when a husband's sperm count is low and needs to be concentrated, or the fallopian tubes are blocked) and AID (the husband is infertile or has a genetic defect) as solutions within the marriage bond and hence supportive of family life.[35]

The law is frequently ambiguous as well. In many states, the AID child has no more rights than an illegitimate one. The law occasionally looks upon AID as adultery. Oklahoma recently passed a law requiring both spouses to sign consent papers at the time of AID and to formally adopt the child so that

AID children will have as much right to support and protection as the adopted child.[36]

Genetic Control: Among those who approve of AID there are suggestions for improving the gene pool and the human race. For some, this is suggestive of the nineteenth-century eugenics movement, usually traced to Sir Francis Galton (1822–1911), Charles Darwin's cousin. By encouraging natural selection with the help of Mendelian laws, a more desirable human being might emerge. The "nature of man" (what is it really?) and hence what is the "desirable" or the optimum in humanity is a subject debated in philosophical, religious, and scientific circles throughout the history of thought. Ethicists point out the horrible example of Hitler's Nazi Germany as an attempt at eugenics. Thus, some are fearful of any suggestion for eugenics. Still others insist it is only commonsense to select the donor in AID for desirable characteristics on the one hand and freedom from genetic disease on the other.[37]

The latter proponents would encourage the intelligent or otherwise well-endowed human to contribute sperm (which can be preserved through freezing) or eggs (as in test-tube babies).[38] Opponents may call it "playing God," to which those in favor respond that human nature is to control nature rather than be controlled by it. Genetic screening of donors and prospective donors might seem a reasonable requirement, not merely to protect the gene pool but the immediate planned conception as well. Generally, privacy and confidentiality have kept the donor anonymous. Legally and ethically, there are those who claim that the need for genetic control requires at least a registry, if not open disclosure of the identities of donors and the children conceived by their sperm. Both legally and ethically, there are those who claim that the AID child has a right to know its biological father, as in current adoption debates. Some are concerned about potential harm to the child if or when it finds out about its AID origins. Legally and ethically, there are those who want the husband to give his informed consent, preferably in writing, both to protect the wife against charges of adultery and the child in terms of support.

Test-Tube Babies

Until a few years ago, test-tube babies were the subject of science fiction writings.[39] It has now been done. That is, a human egg was fertilized *in vitro* ("in glass"). The fertilized egg developed to the blastocyst stage. The embryo was then transplanted to the womb of the mother whose blocked fallopian tubes precluded normal conception. Those who condemn any form of conception except through "natural" sexual intercourse automatically condemn the conception of children outside the womb. Those who follow the old "static natural law" concept that virtually sacralizes the biological processes can only look with horror on all these phenomena.[40] Ramsey claims it is not a proper goal of medicine to help women have children by any means necessary.[41] Others see the process as simply a form of AIH or AID,[42] and consider the sanctification of biological processes as idolatry at best and inhuman at worst.

There are a number of issues that have either evolved in a new way or are indeed new in relation to test-tube babies. One of these is the fear that conception has now been separated from sexual intercourse. Others point out that this separation has existed from the first knowledge of contraception and probably since people's first awareness that intercourse did not automatically lead to pregnancy. The idea that marriage must produce children is part of the larger issue of contraception, but it has come up for renewed discussion in the light of test-tube conception.[43]

The experimentation that led to the first test-tube baby, and that will probably continue as the procedure is perfected, involves many failures. If conception equals ensoulment, the implantation of the human soul, or simply the beginning of human life, these failures constitute abortion. It is thus equated with murder by some people. Some Catholic theologians, however, have suggested that ensoulment does not take place until the blastocyst is attached to the uterine wall. Thus, there is no need to baptize the fertilized eggs that never attach, as noted by Birch. Others suggest that the sperm and egg are themselves the source of life and must be treated as such.[44]

Prevent Harm: One concern is to prevent harm to the unborn.[45] Again, the issue turns on the time of ensoulment or the question of when life begins. The conservative view is that the conception must be protected. The insistence varies. For some, it is at quickening. Others put the time at organ formation, the blastocyst stage, initial fertilization, or even earlier. The whole issue of harm is complicated for no one knows whether there is any more harm here than in conception by sexual intercourse. So far no one has suggested banning sex because of potential harm to future generations. And yet, if the fertilized egg is human life, as in the belief systems of Roman Catholics and others, then experimentation here is with a human subject. Generally, we want consent for experimentation, and fertilized eggs cannot give consent.[46]

Research

The Nuremberg Laws grew out of the trials of Nazi war criminals after World War II.[47] The Nazis experimented with humans without regard for the safety or the life of the subjects, many of whom were killed by the experiments, or maimed for life. The Nuremberg laws put restrictions on experimentation with human subjects. Informed (knowledgeable) consent is required, for example, and there shall be no unnecessary harm. For those who see the fertilized egg as a human subject, the test-tube experiments are thus forbidden. Obviously, the fertilized egg cannot give informed consent to the experiment. Ramsey suggests that we not venture into medical research when we don't know exactly what we are doing, for we need to know that there are no risks.[48] This would, of course, eliminate most research. If carried out consistently, it would eliminate most new things, including new developments in health care and, perhaps, health care itself.[49]

DNA: Human experimentation extends to the science fiction type of things underway or on the drawing boards. DNA experimentation has been receiving a great deal of criticism as federal legislation has been debated. Among the fears is that a particularly virulent form of bacteria will be created, will escape from the laboratory, and destroy humanity. Others fear the creation of monsters who would destroy us or at least create problems. Proponents point to the potential good of DNA research as in the development of insulin. They note that the argument here is as old as the first bow and arrow or perhaps the first flint knife. *Any* development can be used for good or ill.[50]

Gene Therapy: In the past, hereditary diseases have not been cured.[51] However, there are now several potentials. One is therapy[52] for someone with a genetic disorder. The therapy potential includes such things as viral infection, transformation, and cell fusion.[53] Another potential is changing the genetic makeup of the egg or sperm, replacing a defective gene with a healthy one. The potential for good is obvious. So is the potential for the destructive, such as creating abnormal human beings. These might be genetic defects as bad or worse than what we have now. The argument then continues for abortion, letting defective neonates die. Still others fear talk of abnormals, such as using genetics to create cyborgs (part human, part machine) or crossing humans with higher primates to get slaves for menial work or war.[54]

Cloning: Cloning (Greek "klon" = twig, slip; that is, asexual reproduction) has already been accomplished with some lower animals. The nucleus of the cell is removed (enucleated) and replaced with the nucleus from a cell of the selected individual. A book on the market claims that a human clone has been produced.[55] Some see the book as a novel, typical of the science fiction genre. Others claim that it will be done, if not within the decade, at least within this century. The process is applauded by some and condemned by others.[56]

Nurses: Generally speaking, nurses are not heavily involved in the kind of research represented by test-tube babies, genetic therapy, and cloning. But they will be more so in the future, if for no other reason than the increasing professionalization of the health field.[57] We have seen the nursing programs expand from doctor's assistant (apprentice) to two- and three-year programs, and now greater emphasis on the baccalaureate program as minimum entry level into nursing.

Specialists such as nurse-midwives have moved into the postbaccalaureate certificate and more heavily into the master's degree programs. The pressure is rising for nurse educators and others, as well, to have doctorates. In most fields of human endeavor, this growing educational demand has brought with it a corresponding demand for research. Doctoral programs do not teach people to teach. They teach people to do research. Research is heavily encouraged by the government, by drug companies, and other interested parties, as well as by educational and service-oriented institutions. Educational requirements and attractive grants will stimulate enormous growth in the numbers of health personnel in research in future decades.

The time to consider the ethical problems in this research and its results is now, claim many ethicists. The rapid development of technologies in recent decades has created a need for many ethical decisions. The development has been so rapid there has been no time to think about what Plato and Aristotle or the Bible or simple commonsense can give us in the way of guidance. I. Michael Lerner has noted that we get our "traditional ethical guidelines from religion, but the new religion of science and technology that is arising, with its hierarchy of scientists instead of priests, with its sacred language of mathematics instead of Latin, with its sacrifice of traffic casualties instead of heretics, and with space exploration for its Crusades, is as yet not capable of providing any" new guidelines.[58]

The growth of technology is geometric rather than linear. Issues will not develop merely twice as fast as in the past, but in multiple speeds. The time to think about what is ethical and what is not in research is now, even as we struggle to come to terms with the burgeoning new knowledge already at hand.

THE ISSUES

Ethical issues can be grouped in several different ways, such as duties, obligations, and moral issues.[59] Problems in genetics might be grouped under counseling and care, mass screening, and experimental interventions.[60] Almost any categorization plan involves extensive overlapping. Yet, some scheme of organization is helpful in getting a grasp on the subject or in identifying the issues. Several areas of our concern are treated in later chapters, such as contraception (Chapter Three), abortion (Chapter Four), and allocation of scarce resources (Chapter Seven). This chapter deals especially with the following:

Rights and Choices: For example, who decides (in counseling, screening, therapy, and research) who shall be born, who shall have children, and so forth, and on what basis? Who is competent? Concerns are human rights in general, including the individual versus society, the rights to control one's body, patient rights, and the rights of health care personnel. Screening that focuses on special groups such as blacks (sickle cell anemia) or whites (cystic fibrosis), older women (Down's syndrome) may violate their rights. Informed consent is both a legal and ethical concern (see Chapter Nine).

Do Good/Do No Harm For example, the greatest good for the greatest number (utilitarian ethics) may do harm to some. Is harm justifiable if society as a whole benefits? How much harm or benefit is involved? Care for the present may harm the future (gene pool, the unborn). Confidentiality is also a right.

Quality Versus Quantity of Life: For example, must life be preserved at all costs, or is the decision based on some judgment about the quality of life or potential life?

THE NURSE AND GENETICS

Introduction

Health personnel, and nurses in particular, are concerned with the field of genetics in several ways. Let us turn now to some of the various roles nurses assume in the field of genetics, the settings in which they provide care, and the interrelationships of nursing role, functions, and responsibilities involved in these ethical issues and dilemmas. Discussion of aspects of the ANA Code for Nurses and Interpretive Statements is included, when appropriate, as guidelines for nursing behavior in a given situation.[61]

Nurses and Genetic Counseling

The roles that nurses commonly assume in the area of genetic counseling are those of identifying and referring people for counseling, being the support person for clients struggling to make a decision about genetic counseling or its results, providing information to clarify the results of testing, or being the actual counselor in genetics.[62] The settings in which nurses might assume these roles are anywhere that people are concerned about health, especially the health of babies or babies-to-be. These may include public health clinics or visiting nurse services, family planning clinics, schools, prenatal centers, and inpatient settings—especially the intrapartum and neonatal units.

Referral: In order that nurses may appropriately refer a person or persons for genetic counseling, they must be able to identify those people who might benefit from such a referral. Rubin suggests five categories of people who might be referred for genetic counseling. These include:

1. A couple who have produced a child with a genetic disorder or who know of genetic disorders in their families.
2. A couple who are consanguineous (blood relatives).
3. A woman with an obstetrical history of two or more spontaneous abortions or a stillbirth.
4. A woman who has had early pregnancy exposure to a known teratogen such as rubella or X ray.
5. A woman who has been advised to have prenatal genetic screening such as amniocentesis or fetoscopy.[63]

Nurses also need to know who the genetic counselors are and where they are located. Resource people, once identified, can be listed in a directory kept in the work setting.[64]

If prenatal diagnosis is anticipated, amniocentesis is best performed between the sixteenth and seventeenth week of gestation,[65] so referrals need to be made before that time. The nurse working in a prenatal setting is most often the first professional person in contact with potential genetic counselees, especially if the nurse is involved in obtaining the initial health history and/or in managing the course of pregnancy (for example, a nurse-midwife). Rubin[66] also provides the following guidelines for identifying those pregnant women who might be referred for amniocentesis. Institutional policies vary somewhat, but these general guidelines appear to be comprehensive.

1. Women who are thirty-five or older, especially if this is the first pregnancy.
2. A woman who is a known balanced translocation carrier or whose partner is.[67]
3. A woman who has previously given birth to a chromosomally abnormal child such as one with Down's syndrome (Trisomy 21).
4. A woman who is a potential carrier of X-linked disease such as Duchenne muscular dystrophy.
5. A woman who with her partner may transmit one of the inborn errors of metabolism such as Tay-Sachs disease.
6. A woman who fears a genetically abnormal child because of family history of same.
7. A woman who has previously delivered a child with a central neural tube defect.

Support: The nurse is often called upon to be supportive of women or couples during the decision-making process about the need for genetic counseling and what to do, given the results of the diagnostic tests. An important aspect of this role is further interpretation and reiteration of information received from the genetic counselor.[68] This may necessitate the nurse's involvement in the counseling session so that support and information are based on an awareness of what has already been shared with the couple. It is important that information be accurate and understandable.[69] Patients who have a trusting relationship with the nurse may ask advice regarding the actions to be taken. This could create a difficult situation for the nurse who may need to decide whether answering this request with a suggested action or decision is preferable to encouraging the patients to decide for themselves.[70]

Counselor: Counseling is a large part of nursing practice. There is a movement underway in the United States to professionalize therapy, including genetic counseling. But therapy and counseling have gone on for centuries among friends and acquaintances. Chances are it will continue. Yet, among acquaintances, we might more naturally turn to the clergy for spiritual matters and to health personnel for health matters, including genetics. It becomes important that nurses know either the genetics involved or be able to direct the inquirer to a knowledgeable expert.[71] Such an expert might be a physician, and some physicians are claiming exclusive rights to genetic counseling. Others are graduates of masters' and doctoral degree programs in genetic counseling and may or may not have a medical background as such.[72] Some of these counselors are nurses as well.

The aims of genetic counseling may be summarized in two categories. These include establishing an accurate diagnosis of genetic disease and sharing the findings of investigation clearly and completely with the couple. This information includes the problems identified, risks, and options available to them.

Counseling Approaches: There are a variety of approaches to genetic counseling. One common approach is the nondirective technique that facilitates decision making by the clients through the objective provision of information and interpretation of results of diagnostic and predictive studies. In keeping with the Code for Nurses, it is the right of clients to make their own decisions, based on information from genetic counseling or diagnoses. To make an informed decision, they need both information and an understanding of that information. Each patient is evaluated as an individual. It should be noted, however, that whether the counseling is directive or nondirective, counselors still have the opportunity to insinuate their own religious, racial, eugenic, or other values into the counseling relationship.[73]

Decision Milieu: The field of genetic counseling involves a great deal of emotion-laden decision making. The nurse who works as a genetic counselor can benefit from awareness of his/her own prejudices and values positions relevant to the ethical issues in genetics and needs to perform with the highest level of communication skills and scientific knowl-edge of genetic diagnosis, risks, and potential treatment, if any, of disorders. One of the most difficult dilemmas as a counselor (or patient advocate) is when clients make a decision with which the nurse counselor personally disagrees.[74] Remaining neutral in such a situation may be very difficult. Awareness of this potential conflict can help nurses understand their reactions to the decision being made and, it is hoped, provide for mechanisms, such as removing oneself from the situation or refusing to comment, which will diminish the chance of improperly influencing the client's decision.

Nurses and Genetic Screening

Nurses are frequently involved in genetic screening programs in public health agencies, prenatal clinics, as school nurses, or as nurses in newborn units. These nurses may be involved in the ethical issues of privacy, confidentiality, and parental rights versus societal rights. Statement Two[75] of the Code for Nurses offers guidelines for nursing actions relevant to these ethical issues. It reads, "The nurse safeguards the client's right to privacy by judiciously protecting information of a confidential nature." The interpretive statements that follow explain potential actions in more detail.

Consent: Nurses are often the professional people responsible for obtaining the patient's informed consent for screening tests. Here it is helpful to know about the screening procedure in detail, including what it claims to identify, how it is done, what risks are involved and for whom, and what type of follow-up is needed for reporting and interpretation of results. They may find themselves in an ethical dilemma if they are asked for information about a test result and they are aware of certain findings such as XXY chromosomal pattern in addition to the sought-after results.[76] How do values of confidentiality, truth telling, and patients' rights that conflict with the nurse's judgment of caring and compassion get resolved?[77] Suppose a husband comes to the prenatal clinic and demands to know the results of amniocentesis in regards to the sex of the fetus. The nurse knows he prefers the opposite sex and will pressure his wife to opt for an abortion. What does the nurse do? This situation may be interpreted as a conflict of rights (husband and wife) and also involves the issue of confidentiality—who is to be told what about a given test?

Risks: Steele and Harmon[78] suggest that screening programs should be conducted with the knowledge that the results may have serious social and psychological risks for the people screened. Because of these potential risks, they suggest that genetic screening programs be conducted in a similar manner to human experimentation or research. The guidelines for human experimentation include the need for stating the amount of information to be given about tests and their results, the way the information will be given and by whom, and assurance of the confidentiality and privacy of all information. It is often the nurse who has to carry out these guidelines or to see that they are adhered to.

Nurses and Care of Genetically Abnormal Persons

Nurses who work in neonatal units, community centers, public health agencies, rehabilitation units, and private or state institutions for the mentally retarded constantly face dilemmas in caring for children and adults with genetic disorders. These disorders may range from treatable PKU to severe mental retardation to agonizingly painful degenerative diseases such as Huntington's Chorea. Here nurses daily face such issues as the quality of life versus quantity and the need to protect the rights of their clients who often are unable to identify or defend those rights themselves.

An example of the potential dilemmas nurses face in caring for genetically abnormal people is the situation of adults institutionalized with Down's syndrome. People often see the Down's baby as cute and loveable, but the adult with Down's syndrome in institutions is a different story. Physically mature, the latter pose many care-giving problems for nurses, including the actual threat of physical abuse. One might question how a conscientious nurse can cope with caring for an adult who needs basic physical care, constant reinforcement of self-help measures, maintenance of a safe environment, and control of their aggressive and dangerous behaviors. What should be the nurse's reactions to the parents who visit once a month and complain to the nurse that their son is not "neat and clean," let alone fully clothed? The Code for Nurses, Sections 1.3 and 1.4 of the Interpretive Statements,[79] offers some guidelines to the nurse in this type of patient care situation. Nurses might want to examine their own attitudes toward caring for such patients prior to being employed in such a setting. Once employed, personal and professional value clarification also may help the individual nurse work out some acceptable modes of action in order to maintain respect for these individuals and diminish the chances of reacting to genetically abnormal patients inappropriately on a purely emotional basis.[80]

Nurses and Artificial Insemination

Nurses who practice in private physician's offices may become involved in the procedure of artificial insemination. Ethical issues of privacy and confidentiality are most evident here. A nurse has the responsibility to protect this privacy. Statement Two of the Code for Nurses[81] speaks to this responsibility. One of the case studies will deal with artificial insemination in more detail.

Nurses and Genetic Research

As stated earlier, nurses are becoming increasingly involved in research. As this interest and involvement increases, more nurses may go into genetic research. Therefore, it is important for nurses to know the ethical and legal constraints on such research as well as to keep abreast of current developments. The Code for Nurses and Interpretive Statements Section Seven[82] provides guidelines for the nurse involved in research, either as researcher or caretaker of people who are subjects of research efforts. More detail on nurses and research is offered in Chapter six on children.

CASE STUDIES

The following case studies have been changed sufficiently to protect identifications but are presented here substantially as they took place. There are several overlapping concerns in each situation. The answers of the individual, group, the institution, society, the various religious groups, the health professional, and others may agree or disagree. We seek answers for the sake of understanding ourselves and others and to enhance our decision-making process, both now and in times to come.

Guidelines

It is suggested that the reader use the Guidelines for Identifying and Analyzing Ethical Dilemmas in Nursing Practice at the end of Chapter One as one approach to each case study. Students and teachers, practicing clinicians, and all interested parties bring to the decision-making process their own belief systems, their own experiences, and an awareness of others, among other things. It is further understood that especially in clinical practice, one will not have the time or the need to go through every single step of analysis in every situation that arises. In some cases, decisions will be made by others—the patient, the institution, the powers that be—whether we like it or not. Nonetheless, the guidelines can be helpful not only in analyzing the cases presented here but in many ethical decision-making situations. And even when the decisions are taken out of one's hands, the guidelines can be helpful for understanding alternate options and the decisions made by others. The first case is presented with selective analysis, and the succeeding cases are presented for self-study, as will be the pattern throughout the book.

Case #1

Amniocentesis

Dr. J. came out of one of the obstetric clinic examining rooms and headed for the charge nurse. He asked her to go into Room 408 and "talk some sense into Ms. R.!" When the nurse asked the doctor for further explanation, the doctor stated that Ms. R. needed to have an amniocentesis performed to see if her fetus was free of Down's syndrome and she refused to come for the appointment. Ms. R. was thirty-nine years old and pregnant for the first time. She was receiving care in a regional medical center where all first-time pregnant women over thirty-six years of age were encouraged to have amniocentesis performed for genetic screening. She had been scheduled for an amniocentesis three days ago but did not come for the procedure. The nurse decided to talk with Ms. R. and found her quietly crying alone in the examining room. After a few moments, Ms. R. looked at the nurse. The nurse stated that Ms. R. seemed very upset and asked if there was anything she could do to help. Ms. R. immediately responded that Dr. J. wanted her to have some test that would tell him if her baby was mentally retarded and, if so, he said she could have an abortion. When the nurse asked Ms. R. how she felt about knowing if her child were healthy or affected with Down's syndrome, Ms. R. said that she would never consent to an abortion so she would wait until the delivery to know the condition of her infant. She went on to say that she had always wanted a baby and this was her only chance, so she wasn't about to give up the pregnancy. The nurse was convinced that Ms. R. had made a firm decision about amniocentesis and suggested that she get dressed and ready to go home. Her next appointment for antepartal care was given for three weeks and the charge nurse cancelled the appointment for amniocentesis. The doctor was told of the patient's decision, and his only comment was, "She's crazy! I wouldn't willingly bring a Down's baby into this world!"

Analysis

1. a. One might identify the health problems as whether Ms. R. is carrying a genetically defective fetus and/or the potential risk of the amniocentesis procedure to Ms. R. and the fetus. What you identify as a health problem here may be relative to your definition of *health* or even your own beliefs about quality versus quantity of life.

   b. The decision to be made at this point was whether Ms. R. should submit to amniocentesis because of her age, and Ms. R. made the decision *not* to do so. The physician seemed to want to make the decision for her, and the nurse seemed to support the woman's right to choose or refuse the procedure.

   c. The ethical component of the decision appears to be who has the right and/or responsibility to make the decision.

   d. The individuals currently involved in the situation are Ms. R., the fetus, the doctor, the nurse, and, possibly, society as a whole, depending on one's view of who should care for defective children/adults.

2. Further information might be gathered about the father of this fetus and other circumstances surrounding Ms. R's pregnancy, as well as Ms. R's understanding of Down's syndrome.

3. The ethical issues involved in this situation include the patient's right to decide on the issue of genetics screening, quality versus quantity of life for the fetus, rights of the health professionals, rights of society, and rights of the institution.

4. Your own thoughts belong here.

5. It would appear that Ms. R. values her pregnancy a great deal and is currently not concerned about the potential quality of the outcome or her chances of producing a defective child. She believes in control over her own body and has exercised her right to decide against amniocentesis. The physician apparently has some preference for quality rather than quantity of life, though it's difficult to know how much he is influenced by an "institutional policy." The nurse appears to give priority to the patient's right to make a decision and could be interpreting her role as providing a caring support of Ms. R. in her decision.

6. The most obvious value conflicts appear to be between the physician and Ms. R. on the issue of whether genetic screening should be performed.

7. The "best" person to make the decision will depend on one's beliefs about whose rights should predominate in this situation—Ms. R's? Dr. J's? Nurse's? Society's? (It's unclear from the data given if anyone is speaking for society as a whole.)

8. The range of decisions possible includes yes or no to amniocentesis today or in the near future, especially if abortion were an acceptable option to a finding of Down's syndrome. The physician could support Ms. R. in her decision, but he may have difficulty going against his own personal value system. The nurse appears to be in conformance with section 1.1 of the *Code for Nurses*, "Self-Determination of Clients." On the other hand, the nurse could have tried harder to convince Ms. R. of the "value" cf amniocentesis.

9. How would you have responded if you were the nurse? the doctor? the patient (Ms. R.)? the fetus? State rationale.

10. Is amniocentesis ever warranted if the pregnant woman (family) has made a decision to do nothing if the baby is affected with a genetic disorder?

Consanguinity

Mrs. L., a twenty-nine-year-old woman, carrying her second pregnancy, is being followed in the prenatal clinic. She is pregnant by her first-cousin husband and reports their relationship to be long-term and caring. A first pregnancy resulted in a baby with cyclops and proboscus facial formation along with multiple other anomalies. This infant died shortly after birth. The couple had genetic counseling and were well aware that there was a 50 percent chance of having another child similarly affected. At the twentieth week of gestation, Mr. and Mrs. L. refused amniocentesis, stating that they would not terminate the pregnancy. They did, however, agree to ultrasound, and a twin pregnancy was detected. The parents held out hope that at least one of the twins might be normal. The physicians kept hounding the nurse counselors to make sure the papers for tubal ligation were signed or vasectomy agreed to before birth. The nurse working with the couple found herself frustrated and confused as to how to proceed in supporting them through the rest of the pregnancy as the following thoughts kept going through her mind.

When do the rights of society (welfare recipients) take precedence over the rights of an individual (desire to procreate)?

Do the people caring for this couple have any right to encourage sterilization, or amniocentesis, for that matter?

What kind of anticipatory guidance can be given to this couple when you know that there is no guarantee that either child will be normal or abnormal?

Why does the physician push the counseling on sterilization off to the nurse, and what responsibility does she accept to carry out his wishes?

In addition to applying the Guidelines, consider the following questions during your study of the case:

1. How would you respond if you were the nurse in this situation, and why?
2. Does any couple have the right to produce defective children in their quest for a normal child?
3. What are the possible actions that might be taken in this situation?

Artificial Insemination

Two nurses met for lunch one day and were discussing the events of the morning. Both nurses worked for obstetricians in an office setting. One nurse seemed particularly upset as she was telling about the events of that morning. The story was as follows. The physician she worked for was noted for his support of and practice of artificial insemination, both husband and donor. Through an unexplained mechanical failure in the freezer holding the frozen donor sperm, these spermatozoa were unfit for use. It required the combined efforts of doctor and nurse to contact appropriate donors for the scheduled procedures that day. The nurse suggested they delay the appearance of recipients for a couple of hours while donor sperm was being collected. The doctor refused and noted they would stagger the appointments and use separate examining rooms. All went well until about 11:30 when one of the couples needed some extra time with the physician. Consequently, the nurse noted that this couple left the office at the same time as one of the donors. She mentioned this to the physician, but he brushed her aside and said he was certain that the couple had more important things to think about than wondering who that gentleman was they passed in the waiting room. The nurse felt ignored and angry at the physician and asked her friend what she should do about this incident. She added that she basically supported the use of AID but thought that the doctor was becoming a bit careless.

In addition to applying the Guidelines, please consider the following questions:

1. Do you think the nurse is justified in her concern?
2. What are the possible actions that could be taken in this situation?
3. What are the implications of these actions on the couples? the doctor? the nurse? the donors?
4. Which course of action would you choose if you were the nurse, and why?

Case #4

Care of Genetically Defective Adults

Mr. W., a nurse working in a state mental hospital, has been recently assigned to a ward housing adults with Down's syndrome. He finds himself increasingly disturbed by the apparent lack of concern on the part of staff for stimulating the patients to keep clean and dressed. He decided to initiate efforts to encourage showering and dressing by rewarding those who do so with walks outside and even an occasional trip to a local fast food restaurant. After several weeks of these activities, one of his colleagues stopped him in the hall one morning with, "Why do you spend so much effort on those dumb people? I stopped caring a long time ago. If you ask me, those kind of idiots should never have been born!"

In addition to applying the Guidelines, consider these questions during study:

1. How would you respond to this comment if you were the nurse, Mr. W.? the parent of one of these institutionalized adults? a sibling of one of these institutionalized adults?
2. When is society justified in deciding who shall be born?

NOTES AND REFERENCES

1. By "genetics" here, ethical discussion includes a broad range of phenomena such as chromosomal and enzyme activity, the manipulation of cells, eugenics and related matters, as well as genetics in the sense of "genes." David Hendin and Joan Marks, *The Genetic Connection* (New York: The New American Library, 1979).

2. Bentley Glass, "Ethical Problems Raised by Genetics," *Genetics and the Quality*

of Life, ed. by Charles Birch and Paul Abrecht (Elmsford, N.Y.: Pergamon Press, Inc., 1975), pp. 50–58. Arthur L. Caplan, "Genetic Aspects of Human Behavior V: Philosophical and Ethical Issues," *Encyclopedia of Bioethics* **2:**541–548. The Encyclopedia is cited hereafter as *EB*.

3. Glass, op. cit., p. 51. Joseph Fletcher, *Morals and Medicine* (Princeton: Princeton University Press, 1954), p. 174. The boys were used in the Sistine choirs in Rome. Bernard Häring notes that this had strong papal approval. "The Encyclical Crisis," in *The Debate on Birth Control*, ed. by Andrew Bauer (New York: Hawthorne Books, Inc., 1969).

4. Phillip Reilly, *Genetics, Law, Social Policy* (Cambridge, Mass.: Harvard University Press, 1977), pp. 122–132. Such sterilization was condemned by Pope Pius XI in 1930 in his encyclical "Casti Connubii." John T. Noonan, *Contraception* (Cambridge: The Harvard University Press, 1965), p. 430. Robert M. Veatch, "Can Convicts Consent to Castration?" *The Hastings Center Report*, no. 5 (Oct. 1975), **5:**17. The Report is cited hereafter as *HCR*. George H. Kieffer, *Bioethics: A Textbook of Issues* (Reading, Mass.: Addison-Wesley Publishing Co., Inc., 1979), p. 48.

5. Otto J. Baab, "Incest," *Interpreter's Dictionary of the Bible* (1962), **2:**700, and "Marriage," *IDB* (1962), **3:**278–287. Charles R. Taber, "Marriage," *IDB*, supplementary volume (1976), pp. 573–576. The Biblical "anyone near of kin" is a broader concept than consanguineous or blood relation. It extends to some relationships by marriage, as well. Stanley S. Harakas, "Eastern Orthodox Christianity," *EB* **1:**347–356, notes a similar genetic result for the teachings of Orthodoxy.

6. Joseph Fletcher, *The Ethics of Genetic Control, Ending Reproductive Roulette* (New York: Doubleday & Company, Inc., 1974), p. 183, claims the taboos were only based on nonsense. Amitai Etzioni, however, notes the dramatic evidence that the risk of abnormality is great in children of incestuous unions. *Genetic Fix* (New York: Macmillan Publishing Co., Inc., 1974), pp. 159–160. Statistically, first cousins have 12 percent of their genes in common, greatly increasing the chances of recessive diseases. Michael M. Kabach, "Perspectives in the Control of Human Genetic Disease," in *Genetics and the Perinatal Patient:*

A Scientific, Clinical and Ethical Consideration (Vail, Col.: Mead Johnson Symposium on Perinatal and Developmental Medicine, no. 1, 1972), pp. 51–57. James J. Nagle notes that risks in first cousin matings as compared to random matings increase sixfold in Tay-Sachs disease and sevenfold in PKU (phenylketonuria). Closer relationships increase the risk even more. *Heredity and Human Affairs* (St. Louis: The C. V. Mosby Company, 1974), pp. 281–286. Immanuel Jakobovits suggests Talmudic law has a eugenic ideal. Partners should be neither too short or tall. One should not marry into a family with leprosy, epilepsy, deformities, or mental illness. *Jewish Medical Ethics* (New York: The Philosophical Library, 1959), pp. 153–158.

7. The ancient Spartans, for example, exposed unhealthy infants in the wilderness of Mt. Taygetos. Jan Wojcik, *Muted Consent* (West Lafayette, Ind.: Purdue University Press, 1978), p. 42. Wolf W. Zuelzer, "Relationship to Pediatrics," *Ethical Dilemmas in Current Obstetric and Newborn Care*, ed. by Tom D. Moore (Columbus: Ross Laboratories, 1973), p. 17. The Romans drowned abnormal or weak children, according to Seneca (quoted by Noonan, op. cit., p. 85).

8. Fletcher, op. cit., p. 159.

9. Orphanages for abandoned children remain a major effort of the Christian missionary movement today. The respect for life, oddly enough, does not usually extend to war.

10. Fletcher, op. cit., p. 139. Henry D. Aiken thinks we might make a case for infanticide in grossly overpopulated countries. The rights of the living take precedence over potential life, and the merciful termination of life is acceptable, perhaps obligatory, if there is no possibility of a truly human life. "Life and the Right to Life," *Ethical Issues in Human Genetics*, ed. by Bruce Hilton and others (New York: Plenum Publishing Corporation, 1973), pp. 173–183. Numerous writers besides Fletcher and Aiken have noted the inhumanity of bringing children into the world without adequate food, shelter, and clothing. Some suggest the whole concern with genetics is a Western middle-class phenomenon. In Third World areas, infant mortality is as high as 70 percent, with genetic disease accounting for only 4 percent of the total. Thus, poverty, malnutrition, overpopulation, and social deprivation cause

far more suffering than does genetics. The United Nations has said that 100 million children are growing up without a chance of becoming normal, healthy people. Israel R. Margolis suggests that here is the greater sin, to condemn an infant to deformity, slums, orphanage, the cold of being unwelcome. "A Reform Rabbi's View," *Abortion in a Changing World*, vol. 1, ed. by Robert E. Hall (New York: Columbia University Press, 1970), pp. 30–33. See Charles Birch, "Genetics and Moral Responsibility," op. cit., pp. 6–19; Birch and Abrecht, op. cit., p. 7; Robert F. Murray, "Problems Behind the Promise: Ethical Issues in Mass Genetic Screening," *HCR*, no. 2 (April 1972), **2**:10–13.

11. Traditional Judaism requires marriage and procreation as a commandment. David M. Feldman, *Marital Relations, Birth Control and Abortion in Jewish Law* (New York: Schocken Books, Inc., 1968), 1978.

12. Kabach, op. cit., p. 51. See the United Nations Declaration of Human Rights and the UN World Population Plan of Action, quoted by Bayles in Gaylin, Thompson, Neville, and Bayles, "Sterilization: In Whose Interests?" *HCR*, no. 3 (June 1978), **8**:38. Among "the most basic social needs or 'rights' . . . of men and women are freedom to love, marry, and procreate." P. M. Wald, "Basic Personal and Civil Rights," in M. Kindred and others, eds., *The Mentally Retarded Citizen and the Law* (New York: The Free Press, 1976), p. 6, quoted by Thompson, op. cit., p. 30. Historically, the concept is questionable. The freedom to marry whom we please has had gross restrictions throughout the ages. In many cultures today, such a "right" does not exist and even in Western culture it is more honored in theory than in practice.

13. Other obligations include those "(c) Not to produce children, because of irresponsibility or religious observance, merely as a by-product of sexual intercourse. (d) To plan the number and spacing of births in the best interests of mother, child, and the rest of the family. (e) To give the best possible mental and physical environment to the child during its most formative years and to produce children, therefore, only in the course of an affectionate and stable relationship between man and woman. (f) However convinced the individual may be of his or her superior qualities, not for this reason to produce children of numbers, which, if equalled by everyone would be demographically catastrophic." Quoted by Charles Birch, op. cit., p. 17. Kieffer, op. cit., p. 392. Parkes' comments assume a value system that approves of contraception, considered in Chapter 3. To his last point, those who believe in Zero Population Growth (ZPG) would say two children maximum. Those who believe in using artificial insemination for eugenics might suggest the superior person contribute sperm to that program (see further following).

14. Victor A. McKusick, *Mendelian Inheritance in Man*, 5th ed. (Baltimore: The Johns Hopkins University Press, 1978), p. xiv. Some 1,489 inherited disorders are dominant, such as Huntington's chorea and achondroplasia (a form of dwarfism). There are, 1,117 known recessive inherited disorders such as cystic fibrosis, PKU, sickle cell anemia, Tay-Sachs disease. Among the 215 sex-linked (X-linked) disorders catalogued are hemophilia, some forms of muscular dystrophy, and color blindness. McKusick's fourth edition listed 1,218, 947, and 171, respectively, totaling 2,336. See also Amy Selwyn, "Genetic Counseling," pp. 13–117. This is a booklet (n.d.) of the National Foundation/March of Dimes (Box 2000, White Plains, N.Y. 10600). LeRoy Walters, "Genetic Intervention and Reproductive Technologies," *Contemporary Issues in Bioethics*, ed. by Tom L. Beauchamp and LeRoy Walters (Encino, Calif.: Dickenson Pub. Co., Inc., 1978), p. 567. Nagle, op. cit., p. 293. Marc Lappé and Robert S. Morison, eds., "Ethical and Scientific Issues Posed by Human Uses of Molecular Genetics," *Annals of the New York Academy of Sciences* (23 January 1976), **265**:1–208. S. P. Rubin, "Who Is At Risk?" *The Female Patient* no. 8 (Aug. 1976), **1**:44.

15. Walters, op. cit., p. 567. Note the use of statistics here. This is an average. In practice, all four, or three, or two, or one, or none might be afflicted, or be carriers. American Academy of Pediatrics, The Task Force on Genetic Screening, "The Pediatrician and Genetic Screening (Every Pediatrician a Geneticist)," *Pediatrics*, no. 5 (Nov. 1976), **58**:757–764.

16. Op. cit. Cf. Also Kenneth Vaux, "New Moral Demands in Baby-Making," *The Interpreter*, no. 8 (Sept. 1977), **21**:36–38.

17. Fletcher, op. cit., p. 183. Leroy Augen-

stein, *Come, Let Us Play God* (New York: Harper & Row, Publishers, 1964), p. 33. The Institute of Society, Ethics and the Life Sciences (Hastings Center) had a research group draw up guidelines for screening. Their particular concerns were for confidentiality and nondirective counseling, informed consent, protection of subjects, community participation, and education. Screening programs should have proper goals and be properly conducted. "Ethical and Social Issues in Screening for Genetic Disease," *New England Journal of Medicine* (25 May 1972), **286**:1129–1132. The *Journal* is cited hereafter as *NEJM*. See also the "Recommendations from the Committee for the Study of Inborn Errors of Metabolism: Genetic Screening: Programs, Principles and Research . . . National Academy of Sciences, 1975," *Pediatrics*, no. 5 (1976), **58**:762–764. Bruce Hilton, "Will the Baby Be Normal? . . . and What Is the Cost of Knowing?" *HCR* no. 2 (1972), **2**:8–9. Willard Gaylin, "Genetic Screening: The Ethics of Knowing," *NEJM* **286**:1361–1362. Robert M. Veatch, "Ethical Issues in Genetics," *Progress in Medical Genetics* (1974), **10**:247–253. Murray, op. cit. Legal concerns are noted in Reilly, op. cit., and by Tabitha M. Powledge, "New Trends in Genetic Legislation," *HCR*, no. 6 (Dec. 1973), **3**:6–7.

18. Even the conservative theologian Paul Ramsey notes that no one has an unqualified right to bear children. He goes on to say that the freedom of parentage is to good parentage and not a license to produce seriously defective children. *Fabricated Man* (New Haven: Yale University Press, 1970), p. 57. Elsie L. Bandman and Bertram Bandman note, "There is Nothing Automatic About Rights," *American Journal of Nursing*, no. 5 (May 1977), **77**:867–872. The *Journal* is hereafter cited as *AJN*. Social monetary costs are several billion dollars a year in the United States, where lifetime institutionalization is estimated at between $250,000 and $400,000 per person. See Rosalee C. Yeaworth, "The Agonizing Decisions in Mental Retardation," *AJN*, no. 5 (May 1977), **77**:864–867. A family reports their Down's syndrome child costs $5,000 a year. *The Interpreter*, no. 10 (Nov.–Dec. 1977), **21**:67. Down's children now have the standard lifetime of seventy plus years. Daniel Callahan responds rhetorically, "What is society spending this year on cos-

metics?" in "The Meaning and Significance of Genetic Disease: Philosophical Perspectives," pp. 580–585 in Beauchamp and Walters, op. cit., p. 582. There is no dollar value on the suffering of the afflicted and their families although the courts have been asked to determine this (see later on "wrongful life"). The rights we exercise until we run into someone else's rights are known as *prima facie rights*. Lisa H. Newton, "No Right at All: An Interpretation of the Abortion Issue," *Bioethics and Human Rights*, ed. by Elsie L. Bandman and Bertram Bandman (Boston: Little, Brown and Company, 1978), pp. 113–118.

19. Augenstein, op. cit., p. 16. Wojcik, op. cit., p. 42.

20. Glass, op. cit., p. 57, and "Human Heredity and Ethical Problems," *Perspectives in Biology and Medicine* (Winter 1972), **15**:237–253. The World Health Organization Technical Report, Series No. 497 (1972), p. 5, notes that "in a world . . . increasingly concerned with the quality of human life, it will be taken for granted that children should be free from genetic disease." Quoted by Angelo Serra, "Ethical Issues in Fetal Diagnosis and Abortion," pp. 109–119, in Birch and Abrecht, op. cit. J. R. Kramer writes about "The Right Not to Be Mentally Retarded." Quoted by Thompson, op. cit., p. 32.

We note here an interesting legal concern. Several lawsuits have been instituted for "wrongful life." Genetically, this means parents who had genetic information but ignored it and brought a defective child into the world. Later, the child may sue for damages. So far, the suits have been dismissed. But the dismissals have been on grounds called flimsy, such as the fear that others might also sue and clog up the court calendar. Thus, it seems only a matter of time until someone wins a case for being given a "wrongful life" of suffering and disability. In a related way, a parallel has been drawn with a law in the Georgian Republic. There a person can receive two years' imprisonment for spreading venereal disease. Infecting two or more persons results in up to five years. Legal knowledge is not a prerequisite for the judgment of criminal negligence. Theoretically, a government could decide that transmitting an undesirable gene is a criminal offense. See Margery W. Shaw, "Discussion," pp. 13–17 in Hilton and others, op. cit., p. 16. See also

Harakas, op. cit., p. 355. The whole area of genetics and the law is thoroughly discussed in Reilly, op. cit. "Wrongful Life" is considered on pp. 169–175. George J. Annas, "Medical Paternity and 'Wrongful Life,' " *HCR*, no. 3 (June 1979), **9**:15–17. The concept is established by amniocentesis followed by abortion; that is, no life *is* preferable to life under some circumstances.

21. Veatch, op. cit., pp. 236–242. Margery W. Shaw, "Genetic Counseling," *Science* (1974) **184**:751. Marc Lappé and others, "The Genetic Counselor: Responsible to Whom?" *HCR*, no. 2 (Sept. 1971), **1**:6–11. Wojcik, op. cit., p. 2688. Anne J. Davis and Mila A. Aroskar, *Ethical Dilemmas and Nursing Practice* (New York: Appleton-Century-Crofts, 1978), pp. 170–171. Robert F. Murray, Jr., "Genetic Diagnosis and Counseling II: Genetic Counseling," *EB* **2**:559–566. Tabitha M. Powledge, "Genetic Screening," *EB* **2**:567–573.

22. Op. cit., p. 172. Anthony Kosnik and others, *Human Sexuality: New Directions in American Catholic Thought* (New York: Paulist Press, 1977), pp. 128–136, notes a gradual change from absolutely forbidden to acceptance by some Catholics under limited circumstances. A 1975 document (pp. 296–298) forbids the procedure in Catholic hospitals. The law of secondary effect allows removal of organs when the primary purpose is treatment, for example, cancer. "Ethical and Religious Directives for Catholic Health Facilities, United States Catholic Conference, 1971," *EB* **4**:1755–1757.

23. Charity Cooper, "Sterilization of the Mentally Retarded Minor," *Journal of Nurse-Midwifery* (Spring/Summer 1978), **23**:14–15. Patricia Urbanus, "Sterilization and the Mentally Retarded: HEW's New Regulations," ibid., p. 16. Gaylin, op. cit., p. 28, notes that in the past competence has been clearly defined legally. This is changing to a less clearly defined but more flexible criteria he calls "variable competence." Individuals (including the retarded) vary widely in the degree of competence." At what point is an individual competent to choose sterilization or anything else? Who decides? Who decides that the retarded person should be sterilized? See also Margaret O'Brien Steinfels, "Involuntary Sterilization: The Latest Case," *Psychology Today*, no. 9 (Feb. 1978), **11**:124. Jack Slater, "Sterilization: Newest Threat to the Poor,"

Ebony, no. 12 (Oct. 1973), **28**:150–153. The latter describes an issue of informed consent involving a twelve-year-old retarded girl and her fourteen-year-old sister. They were sterilized in a federally funded clinic. Subsequently, a federal judge ruled that minors and incompetent adults could not be sterilized. See Robert M. Veatch, *Case Studies in Medical Ethics* (Cambridge: Harvard University Press, 1977), pp. 184–185. Note that the concern for informed consent is so strong, very few are asking who is going to care for the children of these incompetent adults. The right of informed consent overrides the rights of children or society.

24. The risk is estimated at 1 percent to 2 percent. It includes spontaneous abortion, bleeding, and possible impairment of the child's vision. See Bernard Häring, *Ethics of Manipulation, Issues in Medicine, Behavior Control and Genetics* (New York: Seabury Press, 1975, pp. 190–191. On 20 October 1975, the National Institute of Health released a study of 1,040 women with prenatal diagnosis who were compared with 992 controls. There were no significant adverse effects. There were no differences in miscarriages. The amniocentesis women had a 0.3 percent higher incidence of bleeding and fluid leakage. Research on a new blood test has been reported, although a useful test is "still years away." Virginia Adams and Tom Ferrall, "Ideas and Trends: Mother's Blood May Signal Fetal Defect," *The New York Times* (Sunday, 15 April 1979), p. E7. Rubin, op. cit., p. 46. "NICHD National Registry for Amniocentesis Study Group: Midtrimester Amniocentesis for Prenatal Diagnosis: Safety and Accuracy," *Journal of the American Medical Association* (1976), **236**:1471–1476. Lewis B. Holmes, "Genetic Counseling for the Older Pregnant Woman: New Data and Questions," *NEJM*, no. 25 (22 June 1978), **298**:1419–1421. Mitchell S. Golbus and others, "Prenatal Genetic Diagnosis in 3000 Amniocenteses," *NEJM*, no. 4 (25 January 1979), **300**:157–163. Tabitha M. Powledge and John Fletcher, "Guidelines for the Ethical, Social and Legal Issues in Prenatal Diagnosis," *NEJM*, no. 4 (25 January 1979), **300**:168–172. "Statement on Amniocentesis," ACOG Statement of Policy, Oct. 1978. Between 1968 and 1978, forty thousand women in the United States had amniocentesis; fifteen thousand of these were

in 1978. Tabitha M. Powledge, "Prenatal Diagnosis: New Techniques, New Questions," *HCR*, no. 3 (June 1979), **9**:16–17. Fritz Fuchs, "Genetic Amniocentesis," *Scientific American*, no. 6 (June 1980), **242**:47–53.

25. According to Catholic moral doctrine, it is never licit to terminate a pregnancy because of genetic defects in the fetus. See Häring, op. cit., p. 191. Numbers of non-Catholics agree. However, the views here, pro and con, are in flux and some changes are taking place. See also John Fletcher, "The Brink: The Parent-Child Bond in the Genetic Revolution," *Theological Studies* (Sept. 1972), **33**:457–485. Lesley Oelsner reports on a case in which the New York State Court of Appeals ruled that doctors could be sued for not recommending amniocentesis. The case involved the birth of two children with birth defects. "Doctors Held Liable in Abnormal Birth," *The New York Times* (28 December 1978). Annas, op. cit., pp. 16–17, reports the one case was settled for $67,358 in damages.

26. F. Clarke Fraser, "Survey of Counseling Practices," pp. 7–13 in Hilton and others, op. cit. Wojcik, op. cit., pp. 34–35; Kieffer, op. cit., pp. 142–143; Murray, op. cit., p. 564; Powledge, op. cit., pp. 570–571. The U. S. Supreme Court eliminated laws against contraception (1965) and abortion (1973), based in part on a right to privacy. Margery W. Shaw, "Genetics and the Law," *EB* **2**:573–578. William J. Winslade, "Confidentially," *EB* **1**:194–200.

27. Thompson, op. cit., p. 31, notes that the President's Committee on Retardation gave extremely little attention to retarded persons' children. These are more likely to be retarded and more likely to lack adequate care and intellectual development. See the concept of wrongful life noted previously. Aiken, op. cit., p. 177, reminds us that people used to see life as a continuous cycle, so the rights of ancestors and successors differed little from their own. Modern nomadism changed that. Martin P. Golding, "Obligations to Future Generations," *EB* **2**:507–512. Marc Lappé, "Genetics and Our Obligations to the Future," pp. 84–93 in Bandman, *Bioethics and Human Rights* (Boston: Little, Brown and Company, 1978).

28. Nagle, op. cit., p. 293. Shaw, op. cit., p. 13, notes that 25 percent of the patients admitted to a large metropolitan hospital suffered from a genetically caused or influenced disease. Theodore Friedmann says more than 25 percent of the children hospitalized are such sufferers. See his "Pre-natal Diagnosis of Genetic Disease," pp. 573–579 in Walters and Beauchamp, op. cit. Davis and Aroskar, op. cit., p. 159. The daily lives of fifteen million Americans are affected by birth defects each year. More than one million are hospitalized. These are not all genetic problems, however. *Birth Defects* (New York: The National Foundation March of Dimes, 1977), p. 1. Selwyn, op. cit., p. 5, reports 220,000 babies born each year with physical and mental defects. This is about 7 percent of all births. See also Stephen Breyer and Richard Zeckhauser, "The Regulations of Genetic Engineering," *Man and Medicine*, no. 1 (Autumn 1975), **1**:1–9.

29. See Chapter 5.

30. Joseph Fletcher, op. cit., p. 157; Häring, op. cit., p. 176; Lappé and Morison, op. cit., pp. 13ff. Sissela Bok and Marc Lappé, "The Threat of Hemophilia," *HCR*, no. 2 (1974), **4**:8–10. Elizabeth F. Neufeld and others, "Gene Therapy," *EB* **2**:513–527.

31. Birch, op. cit., p. 6. Fletcher, op. cit., p. 51, claims that almost all such natural aborts are defective, genetically or congenitally. See also Silva, op. cit., p. 2005. Charles E. Curran, "Abortion V: Contemporary Debate in Philosophical and Religious Ethics," *EB* **1**:17–26. Rubin states that 50 percent to 60 percent of all spontaneous abortions are caused by gross chromosomal defects. Op. cit., pp. 44–45. She goes on to explain the problem of balanced translocation carriers conceiving embryos with unbalanced chromosomal material that is incompatible with life. The "balanced" carrier is an individual who has the normal complement of forty-six chromosomes, but in an atypical arrangement.

32. Introduction to Fletcher, op. cit., p. ix. Those who believe the fertilized egg is a full human person must now (to be consistent) insist we do all in our power to "save" these millions of miscarriages.

33. This *is-ought* dichotomy goes back at least as far as the Scottish philosopher David Hume (1711–1776). See Fletcher, op. cit., p. xvi; Beauchamp and Walters, op. cit., Chapters 1, 7, and 8.

34. Häring, op. cit., p. 195; Harakas, op. cit., p. 354; Ramsey, op. cit., pp. 128ff. "Donor Insemination: New Survey of an Un-

documented Practice," *HCR*, no. 3 (June 1979), **9**:2–3. G. R. Dunstan, "Moral and Social Issues Arising from A.I.D.," pp. 47–55 in *Law and Ethics of A.I.D. and Embryo Transfer*, Ciba Foundation Symposium 17, new series (New York: American Elsevier Publishing Co., Inc., 1973). Dunstan says that Orthodox Judaism is against AID. Feldman suggests AIH is acceptable. Op. cit., pp. 128 and 135n. Harmon L. Smith, *Ethics and the New Medicine* (Nashville, Tenn.: Abingdon Press, 1970), pp. 55ff. Pope Pius XII spoke against AI in "Acta Apostolicae Sedis" **43**:850 (1951). See Paul Ramsey, "Manufacturing Our Offspring: Weighing the Risks," *HCR*, no. 5 (Oct. 1978), **8**:7–9. The usual way of getting sperm is through masturbation, which has been strongly condemned. See Chapter 3. Kosnik and others, pp. 137–140 notes a greater openness to AIH in Catholic circles today. AID is still highly problematic. Cf. also George J. Annas, "Artificial Insemination: Beyond the Best Interests of the Donor" *HCR*, no. 4 (Aug. 1979), **9**:14–15, 43. Annas urges careful record keeping on the donors to control for defective genetic make-up, allow the AID child to trace its genetic parent, etc.

35. Charles Fried says pregnancy is a fulfillment of female nature. A woman can claim pregnancy as a basic fulfillment similar to education, decent housing, health care, and so on. "Ethical Issues in Existing and Emerging Techniques for Improving Human Fertility," pp. 41–45, Ciba Symposium 17, op. cit. Others, including some women, have a different view of female nature. Some deny that pregnancy is a "right."

36. Reilly, op. cit., pp. 190ff. Dunstan, op. cit., pp. 47ff.

37. Fletcher, op. cit. Ramsey, op. cit. An example of the difficulty of determining the nature of man and what eugenic improvement to strive for is the view of Thomas Aquinas who thought of women as misbegotten and defective (quoted by Fletcher, p. 195). This view of "defective" is not widely acceptable today.

38. Mark S. Frankel, "Human-Semen Banking: Social and Public Policy Issues," *Man and Medicine* no. 4 (Summer 1976), **1**:289–309. He notes that abnormal births and spontaneous abortions are fewer with frozen sperm than in the general population.

39. The U.S. Department of Health, Education, and Welfare banned such experiments in this country. Cheryl M. Fields, "Research on 'Test-Tube Babies' Likely to Stir Emotional Debate," *The Chronicle of Higher Education*, no. 4 (25 September 1978), **17**:1, 16. In March 1979, the Ethics Advisory Board of DHEW recommended lifting the federal moratorium. The board found ethically acceptable the research and procedure for ova fertilized by the husband's sperm when the woman could not conceive normally. "Washington Notes: Ethics Panel Approves Study of 'Test-Tube' Embryos," *The Chronicle of Higher Education*, no. 5 (26 March 1979), **18**:16. Margaret O'Brien Steinfels, "In Vitro Fertilization: 'Ethically Acceptable' Research," *HCR*, no. 3 (June 1979), **9**:5–8. She notes that respect for life is clearer if *in vitro* fertilization is with the intent to implant the embryo in the infertile woman as contrasted to fertilization for research on the fertilized egg. As of June 1980, *in vitro* research was not being federally funded. In its May 1980, meeting, the new President's Commission for the Study of Ethical Problems in Medicine and Biomedical and Behavioral Research, refused to consider *in vitro* research though requested to do so by Senator Edward M. Kennedy. America's first clinic is in operation at the General Hospital of Norfolk, Virginia. J. Robert Nelson, "The Government's New Bioethics Commission," *The Christian Century*, no. 21 (4–11 June 1980), **97**:630–631. Tabitha M. Powledge reports on a law suit involving a proposed test-tube baby in "A Report from the Del Zio Trial—Drama But Not Ethics," *HCR*, no. 5 (Oct. 1978), **8**:15–17. Le Roy Walters reviews opinions in "Human In Vitro Fertilization: A Review of the Ethical Literature," HCR, 9, no. 4 (Aug. 1979), 23–43.

40. Häring, op. cit., pp. 194–199.

41. "Genetic Therapy," p. 160, in *The New Genetics and the Future of Man*, ed. by Michael P. Hamilton (Grand Rapids, Mich.: Erdman's, 1972).

42. Nagle, op. cit., p. 301.

43. Conception has *always* been separated from intercourse for those ancient and modern people ignorant of the connection. Kosnik and others, op. cit., pp. 112, 113, 143, trace the history of the insistence on procreation to Stoicism. Child-free marriages are more acceptable now for medical, social, economic, and eugenic reasons.

44. Häring, op. cit., p. 199; Kieffer, op. cit., pp. 204–209; Kosnik and others, pp. 198–199. Kosnik and others, op. cit., pp. 198–199, note the Western tradition of ignoring women while reverencing semen as almost human. The "precious fluid" was regarded with superstitious awe. See further following on contraception and "wasteful emission of seed."

An additional issue is that of triage (allocation of scarce resources). The infertility tests alone cost more than $1,000, not to mention the process itself. Again, we may be talking here only of an issue for the wealthy (see the discussion on poverty versus genetics). James Sellers, "Test-Tube Conception: Troubling Issues," *The Christian Century*, no. 26 (16 to 23 August 1978), **95**:757–758. Judith L. Woodward, "Infertility Issues," ibid., no. 31 (4 October 1978), p. 934.

45. We note in passing that no one has insisted upon "no risk" for woman or fetus before "natural" reproduction is undertaken. Marc Lappé, "Ethics of In-Vitro Fertilization: Risk-Taking for the Unborn," *HCR*, no. 1 (Feb. 1972), **2**:1–3. Stephen Toulmin, "In Vitro Fertilization: Answering the Ethical Obligations," *HCR*, no. 5 (Oct. 1978), **8**:9–11. Marc Lappé, "Ethics at the Center of Life: Protecting Vulnerable Subjects," *HCR*, no. 5 (Oct. 1978), **8**:11–13. John A. Robertson, "In Vitro Conception and Harm to the Unborn," *HCR*, no. 5 (Oct. 1978), **8**:13–14. Gerard Elfstrom suggests that Ramsey's concern for risks to the unborn (*HCR* **5**:7–9) applies equally well to natural conception. "Risk-Taking and Artificial Conception," *HCR*, no. 2 (Apr. 1979), **9**:4. Ramsey replies (pp. 4 and 21) that his concern is "the *add-on* risks" of in vitro fertilization.

46. This was a major consideration in the deliberations of the Ethics Advisory Board for the National Commission for the Protection of Human Subjects. As noted previously (Steinfels, op. cit., pp. 6–7), the board could support in vitro fertilization for transplant but not for experiments. No embryos should be kept in glass beyond the fourteen days usually associated with implantation.

47. Beauchamp and Walters, op. cit., pp. 49, 404–405.

48. Op. cit., p. 169, "Screening: An Ethicist's View," pp. 147–161, in Hilton and others, op. cit.

49. Häring, op. cit., p. 179.

50. James H. Burtness, "Creation in Our Own Image: Ethical Questions," *The Christian Century*, no. 28 (13 September 1978), **95**:818–822, and "Creation in Our Own Image: Christian Perspectives, ibid., no. 29 (20 September 1978), pp. 855–858. Lappé and Morison, op. cit., pp. 59ff. Tabitha M. Powledge, "Recombinant DNA: The Argument Shifts," *HCR*, no. 2 (Apr. 1977), **7**:18–19; Daniel Callahan, "Recombinant DNA: Science and the Public," ibid., pp. 20–23; Key Dismukes, "Recombinant DNA: A Proposal for Regulation," ibid., pp. 25–30. "Liberalized Rules Published for Genetic Research," *The Chronicle of Higher Education*, no. 20 (4 Feb. 1980), 16. "Weaving The New Threads of Life," *Life*, no. 5 (May 1980), **3**:49–58.

51. Nagle, op. cit., p. 293; Wojcik, op. cit., p. 34.

52. This could include dietary or medicinal therapy. Our reference here is to euphenics: genetic manipulation.

53. Nagle, op. cit., pp. 293ff, discusses all three. The ethical dilemmas come mostly in the third: human experimentation (it's new and risky), informed consent (fetus, infant, incompetent, the unconceived) and altering nature. Walter Eckhart, "Genetic Modification of Cells by Viruses," *BioScience* (1971), **21**:171–173. Kaback, op. cit., pp. 51–53. Neufeld, op. cit.

54. Silva, op. cit., p. 2006. Fletcher, op. cit., pp. 172–173.

55. David Rorvik, *In His Image: The Cloning of a Man* (Philadelphia, Pa.: J. B. Lippincott Company, 1978).

56. Häring, op. cit., pp. 202ff., says sensible people will never do it. Fletcher, op. cit., p. 154, claims it avoids genetic disease and it's a waste of time to argue if we should do it. The moral question is when and why. James D. Watson, "Moving Toward the Clonal Man," *The Atlantic* no. 25 (May 1971), **227**:50–53. John J. Swetman humorously faces the scare of cloning. A corporation, proposing to sell to the government a cloned army of one million John Waynes, faces cutthroat competition from natural parents who produce babies at no cost to the government. He adds that merely reproducing genetic material will not automatically give a desired product years later. "Cloneconomics," *Psychology Today*, no. 6 (Nov. 1978), **12**:127. Albert Studdard speaks to the same issue in his

"The Lone Clone," *Man and Medicine*, no. 2 (1978), **3**:109–114. One of the fears, as in an army of John Waynes, is that cloning reproduces the original. This is to ignore the influence of environment, which may or may not be the total influence in the developing of the human personality but is at least of equal, if not of greater, impact than genetics.

57. Silva, op. cit., p. 2006. "The Nurse in Research, American Nurses' Association Guidelines on Ethical Values," *AJN*, (1968), pp. 1504–1507.

58. Quoted by Birch, op. cit., p. 7, from Parkes' *Heredity, Evolution and Society* (San Francisco: W. H. Freeman and Company, Publishers, 1968), p. 179.

59. John Lemmon, "Moral Dilemmas," pp. 6–11 in Walters and Beauchamp, op. cit.

60. Robert M. Veatch, *Case Studies in Medical Ethics* (Cambridge: Harvard University Press, 1977), p. 197.

61. ANA *Code for Nurses with Interpretive Statements* (Kansas City, 1976).

62. Mary L. Horan, "Genetic Counseling: Helping the Family," *JOGN*, no. 5 (Sept./Oct. 1977), **6**:25–29.

63. Rubin, op. cit., p. 46.

64. Horan, op. cit., pp. 27–28. Free information on genetic services is available to health professionals from Professional Education Department, The National Foundation March of Dimes, Box 2000, White Plains, N.Y. 10602.

65. Rubin, op. cit., p. 46. Henry Nadler, "Genetic Decision-Making in Early Pregnancy," in *Ethical Dilemmas in Current Obstetric and Newborn Care*, sixty-fifth Ross Conference (Columbus: Ross Laboratories, 1973), pp. 47–49.

66. Op. cit., p. 47.

67. See n. 31.

68. Horan, op. cit., p. 27.

69. Ramona T. Mercer, "Crisis: A Baby is Born with a Defect," *Nursing*, no. 11 (Nov. 1977), **7**:47. The Patient's Bill of Rights of the American Hospital Association, 1973, reminds us that patients have a right to accurate information in understandable terms, *EB* **4**:1782.

70. Note issue of self-determination in ANA *Code for Nurses*, Section 1:1, p. 4, and how this may influence decision making. See also Sections 3 and 6, pp. 8–9, 12–13.

71. Henrietta Eppink, "Genetic Causes of Abnormal Fetal Development and Inherited Disease," *JOGN*, no. 5 (Sept./Oct. 1977), **6**:14–22.

72. About half of the seven hundred (1975 data) genetic counselors are physicians. Kieffer, op. cit., p. 139.

73. Rubin, op. cit., p. 47; Kieffer, op. cit., pp. 138–139; Wojcik, op. cit., pp. 35–44. Shirley M. Steele and Vera M. Harmon, *Values Clarification in Nursing* (New York: Appleton-Century-Crofts, 1979), Chapter Seven, "Reproduction and Genetics," pp. 105–118.

74. Wojcik, op. cit., p. 28.

75. Op. cit., pp. 6–7.

76. There may be a greater risk of criminal behavior with this chromosomal pattern. See Robert S. Krooth, "Genes, Behavior, and What Will Become of Us?" *Man and Medicine* (Summer 1976), **4**:255–264. Kieffer, op. cit., p. 139.

77. Yeaworth, op. cit., pp. 865–866; Wojcik, op. cit., pp. 28, 37–39.

78. Steele and Harmon, op. cit., p. 109. See also Carol E. Thompson, "Legal Aspects of Genetic Screening," *JOGN*, no. 5 (Sept./Oct. 1977), **6**:34–38.

79. *Code for Nurses*, op. cit., pp. 4–5.

80. Davis and Aroskar, op. cit., pp. 173–174.

81. Code for Nurses, op. cit., pp. 6–7.

82. Ibid., pp. 14–15.

ADDITIONAL BIBLIOGRAPHY

Theodore Friedmann and Richard O. Roblin, "Gene Therapy for Human Genetic Disease?" *Science* (3 March 1972), **175**:949–955.

Michael Hemphill, "Pretesting for Huntington's Disease," *HCR*, no. 3 (June 1973), **3**:12–13.

James M. Gustafson, "Genetic Engineering and the Normative View of the Human," pp. 46–58 in *Ethical Issues in Biology and*

Medicine, ed. by Preston N. Williams (Cambridge, Mass: Schenkman Publishing Co., 1973).

Marc Lappé and Richard O. Roblin, "Newborn Genetic Screening as a Concept in Health Care Delivery," *Ethical, Social and Legal Dimensions of Screening for Human Genetic Disease,* no. 6 (1974), **10**:1–24.

John A. Osmundsen, "We are All Mutants——Preventive Genetic Medicine: A Growing Clinical Field Troubled by a Confusion of Ethicists," *Medical Dimensions* (Feb. 1973), pp. 5–6, 27–28.

Marc Lappé, "The Danger of Compulsion," *Medical Dimensions* (Feb. 1973), pp. 8, 26.

Bernard D. Davis, "Prospects for Genetic Intervention in Man," *Science* (1970), **170**:1279–1283.

James F. Danielli, "Industry, Society and Genetic Engineering," *HCR,* no. 6 (1972), **2**:57.

Marc Lappé, "Moral Obligations and the Fallacies of 'Genetic Control,'" *Theological Studies,* no. 3 (Sept. 1972), **33**:411–427.

Joseph Fletcher, "Ethical Aspects of Genetic Controls," *NEJM* (1971), **285**:776–783.

Robert Hunt and John Arras, ed., *Ethical Issues in Modern Medicine* (Palo Alto, Calif.: Mayfield, 1977).

Robert M. Veatch, "The Unexpected Chromosome . . . a Counselor's Dilemma," *HCR,* no. 1 (Feb. 1972), **2**:8–9.

Thomas A. Shannon, ed., *Bioethics* (Ramsey, N.Y.: Paulist Press, 1976).

Audrey Redding and Kurt Hirschorn, "Guide to Human Chromosome Defects," *Birth Defects,* Original Article Series IV, no. 4 (Sept. 1978), pp. 1–16.

Mila A. Aroskar, "Ethical Dilemmas and Community Nursing," *Linacre Quarterly,* no. 4 (Nov. 1977), **44**:340–346.

Chapter 3

Ethics and Birth Control

INFANTICIDE

People have been trying to limit the number of their children for as long as there has been any record of human activities.[1] One of the common methods has been infanticide, often by exposure—leaving the infant along the trail or in the town dump. It was so common the biblical prophet Ezekiel could use infanticide as a metaphor (Ezekiel 16:1–4).

In Chapter Two we noted this procedure for genetically defective and unhealthy children. Children who were unwanted for any reason could be disposed of under Roman law. The *patria potestas*, the father's unlimited power to kill his children, was not outlawed until A.D. 135. Infanticide was legal in the Roman Empire until A.D. 374. The need for men in the army may have combined with Christian teaching to produce the concern for limiting infanticide.[2] The practice has continued to the present day, illegal mostly, but still condoned in a few societies.

Some cultures value males more highly than females, so the latter were more likely to be left exposed. An Egyptian papyrus consists of a letter from a man traveling abroad. He wrote to his expectant wife that if the child was male, keep it. If it turned out to be female, put it out to die.[3]

More recently, Fletcher writes of Robert Louis Stevenson (1850–1894) being shocked when he found the Polynesians practicing infanticide. Their ignorance of contraception and obstetrics meant they had to resort to "abortion at birth" when a newborn turned out to be defective, or when the small islands could not produce food and shelter for more people. Stevenson came to realize that they practiced infanticide out of love for the children they already had.[4]

One might say the Polynesians chose infanticide as favoring the quality of life (including sheer survival) for the previously born. Such quality of life might be seen as a factor in virtually all attempts to limit the number of children.[5]

Generally speaking, infanticide has been condemned in the Judeo-Christian West. The Jewish philosopher Philo Judaeus (c. 20 B.C. to A.D. 50) called infanticide murder. He also condemned sexual pleasure without a willingness to accept the responsibility of parenthood. Early Christian writers followed this thought.[6]

Infanticide takes a new turn today in the neonatal ward where new technologies now make it possible to save babies who might have died quite naturally a few short years ago. This subject will be discussed further in Chapter Five.

ABORTION

A second major way of controlling the number of children has been abortion. This has been called one of the oldest and most popular methods of birth control. It was the most widely used method until it recently slipped to third place, after sterilization and the pill. Plato and Aristotle supported it as a way to control excess population.[7]

Legalized abortion has helped such countries as post-World War II Japan and Hungary to stabilize their population growth.[8] Since its legalization in the United States, several million abortions have been performed; prior to that many were performed on an illegal or semilegal basis. It is estimated that there are twenty-five to fifty million abortions a year on a worldwide scale. Obviously, this lowers the number of children being born. It is a reminder that abortion as a form of birth control is far more widely used than is generally recognized.[9] Abortion will be treated more fully in Chapter Four.

INTRAUTERINE DEVICE (IUD)

In addition to population control, one must take note of the contraceptive method called the intrauterine device, or the IUD. For centuries, Near Eastern camel drivers have inserted small pebbles in the uteri of their female camels to prevent pregnancy on long journeys. An ancient Egyptian papyrus records the prevention of pregnancy in women with the insertion of various items in the uterus. Hippocrates described the procedure more than two thousand years ago. The method was rediscovered by experiments on animals in the late 1800s. In 1928, a Berlin doctor, Ernst Gräfenberg developed an intrauterine ring of silver wire. The Grafenberg ring was less than 100 percent effective and sometimes caused injury.

Although Japanese doctors continued to prescribe it, Western medicine generally rejected the IUD. In 1959, new developments, including the use of plastics and stainless steel, brought new acceptance of the IUD. There are now several million users of IUDs in the United States. It is a main choice in family planning programs in India, Pakistan, South Korea, and Taiwan. Although 7 percent to 10 percent of the women using an IUD will expel it spontaneously within the first year, its great advantage is that once inserted, the woman need only check for its strings to be sure it is there. Other advantages include the relative ease of its insertion and the immediate return of fertility when the IUD is removed. Complications such as pelvic inflammatory disease, cramps, and excessive bleeding are serious and require supervision, but the advantage of continuing protection and low cost are often seen as much greater than the disadvantages.[10]

Ethically, problems arise because we don't really know how it works. One interpretation is that the IUD in the uterus prevents the implantation of the fertilized egg. Thus, the IUD could be seen as an abortifacient. If this is the case, the strictures against abortion would apply to the IUD as a method of birth control. However, the ethical principle of uncertainty suggests that in uncertain situations one is free to follow alternate methods of judgment, including one's own conscience.[11] So one could reason that because we do not really know the IUD is an abortifacient, its use is licit even by those who do not approve of abortion as such. Alternately, of course, one could reason that it is better not to use an IUD just in case it is an abortifacient.

Another interpretation of the action of the IUD is that it merely speeds the passage of the ovum and that fertilization does not take place. Because it does not interfere with the coital act and does not stop the functioning of any part of the body, there are those who would say the IUD is an acceptable form of contraception. Others consider the IUD unethical no matter what its action might be, for all artificial birth control is seen as wrong.[12]

MISCELLANI

More than one hundred plants appear in ancient literature as affecting human fertility. Some are supposed to increase and others decrease that fertility. They were sometimes mixed as potions. The Jewish Talmud (completed A.D. c. 500) speaks of these with at least some approval (for women). The Talmud also refers to a *mokh*, used as a tampon during coitus or as a postcoital absorbent. In its former use, it resembles the diaphragm invented by a German doctor, Willhelm Mensinger, about 1880. In its latter use, the *mokh* resembles the postcoital douche.

Spermicides, sometimes used alone today or with the diaphragm, have a modern form but an equally ancient origin. Egyptian writers (c. 1850 B.C. and c. 1500 B.C.) recommended such mixes as honey and vegetable gum (acacia tips), or crocodile dung in fermented glue.

The condom has sometimes been said to have originated with a Dr. Condom, whom Charles II of England (1660–1685) called upon for help in preventing further increases in his illegitimate children. The use of a penal sheath of linen, fish skins, or animal intestines probably predates the story. The name may derive from the Latin *condus*, a receptacle (condere: to conceal, to preserve). Its modern form is the cheaper and more convenient rubber sheath, which remains important as a contraceptive method in the United States, Europe, and Japan.[13]

Coitus interruptus or withdrawal remains an important contraceptive method in Europe and the Near East. It is sometimes credited with the decline in birthrate in Europe from its popularity in the Middle Ages through the eighteenth and nineteenth centuries. It is known to primitive tribes throughout the world.[14]

The effectiveness of these techniques and their history are not our chief concern, but they have a bearing on the ethical issues, as we will see in a moment.[15] The last-named method is one of special importance to the development of an ethic of contraception.

THE PAST

Coitus Interruptus

The biblical book of Genesis, Chapter 38, tells the story of Onan. His brother Er was killed by God. Their father Judah told Onan to fulfill the law of leviratic marriage.[16] Onan was to impregnate Er's widow, Tamar. The child would be Er's child by proxy, and Er's name would be continued among the Israelites. Onan was willing, according to the story, to have intercourse with Tamar. He was unwilling to produce a child in his brother's memory. So he practiced coitus interruptus and spilled his semen on the ground. "And what he did was displeasing in the sight of the Lord" so God killed him too.

Through the centuries, biblical scholars have argued about whether God killed Onan because Onan did not fulfill the law of leviratic marriage and his father's orders, or, because Onan spilled his semen ("improper emission of seed"). In this connection, people do not argue whether God *did* kill Onan and his brother Er. For the theology of this, the readers may consult their own spiritual advisors. It is on the basis of this story, however, that onanism has come to mean coitus interruptus, and by extension, masturbation, and by further extension, any form of birth control. It has led to such interesting views as that of Thomas Aquinas (1225–1274) who thought rape and incest a lesser sin than masturbation. The biblical story has been used to support the suggestion that all contraception is wrong.[17]

Jewish Tradition

Jewish interpretation of the story has been mixed. The commandment to procreate has been seen as a positive commandment. Genesis 1:28 says that God told Adam and Eve, "Be fruitful and multiply, and fill the earth . . ." This is not unusually balanced against the view that the marriage relationship is also a positive commandment and a man may do what he wants to do with his wife. From this comes the thought that contraception may be ethical when it protects the health of the woman and for a variety of other reasons. Because the commandment to procreate is given the male, women have had greater freedom to practice contraception. In fact, slaves, captives, proselytes, and remarried women, among others, have been encouraged to avoid conception for a time, to make sure that any pregnancy is the result of their present husbands or to avoid giving offspring to non-Jewish captors. Minors and lactating women have also been so encouraged to protect their own health and that of their children.

There have, however, been a variety of interpretations over the centuries. One Talmudic text refers to "threshing inside and winnowing outside" during the first twenty-four months of lactation. This is usually interpreted as coitus interruptus. A third-century A.D. text, however, refers to the deadly sin of Onan. This sin was in his contraceptive act.

Masturbation is condemned in the Talmud. This "improper" emission of seed is sometimes extended to the condom as well as to coitus interruptus. Here, as in Thomas Aquinas (his later writings), a basic concern is to not interfere with the coital act. The motive behind particular acts of contraception is frequently the key to acceptability. The commandment to procreate, for example, is given to the race rather than to the individual who may, on occasion, not fulfill it. Some suggest that economic reasons are not sufficient justification for contraception but medical reasons are. Others consider social and economic circumstances, such as a decent and wholesome life, appropriate reasons for family planning. Intercourse with a sterile person or in times of sterility (pregnancy, for example) is generally acceptable though barrenness is a cause for divorce, especially for men. It is worth adding that there is no commandment against contraception in any of the law codes of the Hebrew Scriptures.[18]

Early Christian Tradition

Early Christianity was faced with several philosophies and religious movements such as Gnosticism and Manichaeism that denigrated procreation. In contrast, Christianity saw procreation as part of God's commandments, as did Judaism. However, where Judaism saw the sexual relationship in marriage as itself good, Christianity borrowed from pagan philosophies the idea that sex itself is evil. The early Christians were often accused of immorality, a common charge against "out-groups" throughout the centuries and still today. The Christian leaders responded with, "rational men control the sexual appetites," a philosophy derived in part from the general control of the emotions taught by the Stoics. An ardent lover, even in marriage, was accused of committing adultery. The apostle Paul said, "it is better to marry than to burn" with sexual lust (I Corinthians 7:9). The end result was Augustine's concept that sex was permissible (*not* required) only in marriage and only for procreation.[19] Although the Hebrew Scriptures do not promote celibacy, for Christians, abstinence was the only legitimate means of contraception, an attitude still with us.[20]

It is said that the only 100 percent effective contraceptive is saying, "No." This has generally been the teaching of Judaism and Christianity for sex outside of marriage. One of the great traditional fears of contraception has been that it would encourage promiscuity. Present evidence on this point is unclear. Many think that it does or it might. At least one church has said flatly that the availability of contraceptives does not promote promiscuity. Another has said that contraceptives should be available to all peoples.[21]

Natural Law

In addition to the pro-procreation, anti-contraceptive views,[22] Christianity borrowed from Greek philosophy the concept of Natural Law. Only "natural" intercourse is acceptable, only for procreation, only in marriage. Birth control in any form was seen as wrong. Animals, for example, as "natural" creatures, do not practice it.[23] Frequently, as with Pope Sixtus V in 1688, contraception was declared murder, an idea at least as old as Tertullian (A.D. 200).[24]

Augustine was the backbone of Western moral theology in general ethics and sexual ethics, in particular, until well into the twentieth century. In the present day, this is forgotten and it is now common to contrast the official teaching of the Roman Catholic Church against contraception with Protestant positions favoring birth control. This contrast is largely overdone.

Contrasting Views

The Protestant leader John Calvin (1509–1564) called coitus interruptus a double monstrosity. Anglican Jeremy Taylor (1613–1667) condemned Onan. State laws against the sale or distribution of contraceptive materials were struck down by the United States Supreme Court in 1965 in the case of *Griswold* v. *Connecticut*. Catholic lawyers, with the Catholic Council on Civil Liberties, gave the winning argument that the Connecticut law violated the right to privacy.[25] These laws were largely Protestant in origin, inspired in part, at least, by fear that Roman Catholics with their large families would overwhelm Protestantism, which had a declining birthrate. Perhaps the laws would force Protestants to have large families by denying them the "pornographic" means of limiting births. It was President Eisenhower, a Protestant, who refused contraceptives and contraceptive information to India and Pakistan in 1956. Later, under President Kennedy, a Roman Catholic, federal funds were used to promote birth control.[26]

Pope Pius XI spoke against contraception in his encyclical "Casti Connubii" in 1930. He spoke to a broad consensus of thought, Catholic and non-Catholic alike. He spoke to a world that had barely left behind the belief that masturbation causes insanity and that sodomy causes earthquakes.[27] Whereas Kinsey and other researchers have shown that masturbation is the most common of human sexual activities, a Protestant ethicist recently said it is unpleasant and aesthetically objectionable, though not always wrong.[28] The contrast in these matters might more accurately be seen as a contrast between liberal and conservative perspectives.[29] This spectrum appears in most religious groups and in secular society as well.

About A.D. 1500, Western moral thought began considering the idea that affection in marriage might also be appropriate. The affection concept was hardly a novel idea in human thought. The Hebrew Patriarch Jacob, about 1700 B.C., loved Rachel so much he worked fourteen years for her hand in marriage (Genesis 29). However, in the Middle Ages, this idea contrasted sharply with the ascetic view that marriage was only for procreation. It took 500 years, but eventually the view that affection and companionship are also legitimate functions of marriage was officially added to Christian teaching. Pope Pius XI accepted it as a secondary end of marriage in "Casti Connubii." Mutual love had become the second of two essential purposes in marriage by the time of the Second Vatican Council in 1965.[30] A committee of the Protestant Federal Council of Churches in 1931 endorsed birth control and the idea of sex as an expression of mutual affection. A storm of protest stopped the report, but over the next decade the Protestant Churches began accepting the two concepts as a means of holding the family together.[31]

Rhythm

In the meanwhile, the total ban on contraception was also changing. In 1951, Pope Pius XII, in an address to the Italian Association of Catholic Midwives, declared the ethical acceptability of the rhythm method of avoiding conception. The method was acceptable because it is "natural," that is, the fertile and less fertile periods of the menstrual cycle are a natural part of the cycle. Because it is natural, use of this knowledge does not violate the will of God who created nature. By 1961, the Catholic diocese of Buffalo was operating a Family Life Clinic to teach the rhythm method. All this did not happen overnight either.[32]

About 400 B.C., the Hippocratic school of

medicine was aware that women had a fertile time in the menstrual cycle. They thought this was right after menstruation. Hence, conception might be avoided through coitus in the infertile time of the period. This form of contraception was still being practiced by the Manichees about A.D. 400. The method was condemned by Augustine.

By 1845, Felix Archimedes Pouchet had observed that animals conceive only during menstruation and one to twelve days afterwards. Applying this to human fertility, the Church cautiously replied that use of the infertile period for intercourse could be an alternative to the great sin of onanism. Some objected to this, because the purpose of intercourse was procreation, at least according to orthodox Augustinian doctrine. However, in 1930, Pius XI in "Casti Connubii" held that intercourse during natural times of infertility was lawful, providing the intrinsic nature of the act was preserved. St. Thomas Aquinas had long since held that intercourse with an infertile spouse (naturally sterile, already pregnant, postmenopausal) was licit because the coital act itself was preserved.

In the meanwhile, the Japanese Kyusaku Ogino (1924) and an Austrian, Herman Knaus (1929), refined the fertile period. Because body temperature rises slightly in ovulation, a daily temperature chart adds to the method's accuracy, estimated as 60 percent to 80 percent without the chart and up to 99 percent with it.[33] However, one of every six women are irregular in their cycles, leading Garrett Hardin to say, "Blessed are the women that are irregular for their daughters shall inherit the earth . . ."[34]

When birth control pills were being developed, a prime concern was that they would help regularize the cycle to make the rhythm method more reliable. John Rock, one of the developers of the pill and a Roman Catholic, described its action as a pill-established safe period.[35] A second major facet was the number of theologians, especially in Holland, who suggested that the Church should accept the pill on analogy with the rhythm method. The pills do not destroy the natural cycle but only regulate it. The ova are not destroyed and the naturalness of the sexual act is preserved. The pill has caught on very quickly. More than ten million American women use it.[36]

Humanae Vitae

Pope John XXIII appointed a birth control commission to study the whole matter in 1964. A majority of the Commission said it was legitimate and even a duty to regulate birth. The means people use is their decision. However, in 1968, Pope Paul VI issued his encyclical "Humanae Vitae." He ruled in favor of the rhythm method and against all mechanical and chemical means of birth control. The encyclical is not an "infallible" declaration and hence is subject to change. Nonetheless, it represents the Church's official teaching.[37]

The move engendered considerable discussion. Bernard Häring pointed out that previous encyclicals had justified torture and burning witches and that popes had approved of castrating choir boys.[38] A survey of American priests suggests that about half agree and half disagree with the new ruling on contraception. Only 15 percent demand conformity from their penitants in the confessional. There is a higher degree of agreement among older priests and in the hierarchy of the Church. Among the laity, about two thirds disagree with the encyclical.[39]

The contrast to "Casti Connubii" is obvious. It is suggested that the change comes because, in contrast to 1930, we now have very efficient means of contraception. As with medical technology in general, before, we had no choice. Now we do.[40]

THE PRESENT SCENE

However, it should also be noted that there were numbers of other changes. Among these is the change in Protestant thinking. In growing numbers since 1929, non-Catholic groups have been accepting varying degrees of contraception as ethical. Today, some form of birth control, at least some of the time, has become widely accepted and is even morally demanded by some. Love and mutual fulfillment in marriage have become for many not only permissible but the norm. Coitus is seen as part of that, whether procreation is involved or not. Instead of sex being evil, it is often now seen as a positive good, for we are not to call evil what God has created. And further, joyless and exploitive marital sex is seen as a moral failing. These views are now widespread among various religious groups, including Catholics, and among people with little or no religion at all. The atmosphere of 1968 was considerably different from that of 1930.[41]

In an earlier day, Thomas Robert Malthus (1766–1834) sounded the alarm on the population explosion. His *Essay on the Principle of Population* (1798) was a landmark with continuing influence. Although he was an Anglican clergyman, the movement that grew out of his study was secular. The first Malthusian League to promote birth control was started in England in 1878. The League spread rapidly to other countries. In Holland, the first woman doctor set up clinics where she taught midwives contraceptive methods that they could, in turn, teach in the homes. International conferences on birth control began in 1900. Margaret Sanger (1883–1966) published her first article in 1912. She opened her first clinic in 1916. It was closed and she was put in jail. But in less than ten years, she was traveling throughout the world promoting family planning. In 1921, she founded the American Birth Control League, forerunner of the Planned Parenthood Federation of America (1942). By 1930, the courts started to rule that birth control information is not pornography, a decision already made in 1876 in England.[42]

Another important change was in the view of "natural law" itself. In Greek thought, the natural was the ideal. The natural did not, in fact, exist except in the mind. In Christian thought, natural law became identified with what happens in nature. Because God created nature, this natural law must be the law of God. The apostle Paul speaks of the natural law as binding on all humanity (Romans 2:9,15), not just on Christians. It relates to the Noahide laws of the Bible and of Jewish thought as also binding on all mankind (Genesis 9). Today, many people see nature as more subject to the human will. If it is wrong to avoid or change nature, most modern technology is wrong, a point with which some agree, though most do not.

Most medical practice stops or holds off natural processes such as disease and even death. Biological and physiological processes are open to human intervention. Several of the Dutch theologians just mentioned refused to consider the sexual process differently. To put it another way, it has been suggested that God gave man intelligence as well as genitals, and we ought to use our brains at least as often as the other.[43]

Religious Perspective

Today, Catholics and non-Catholics alike continue to hold an ethic based on natural law. In some cases this is philosophical rather than theological.[44] Some insist the natural law is eternal and unchanging, and some note that although the law is eternal, our interpretation changes with time. Others, Catholic and non-Catholic, note that natural law ethics were contextual and aprioristic. That is to say, the ethics were not drawn from "the natural" at all, but from the legal, philosophical, and scientific thought of that age, prior to any consideration of the natural, which only came later. Natural law is neither natural nor law according to these views.[45]

At the present writing, the official teaching of "Humanae vitae" stands. Some Catholic health personnel and hospitals follow the official teachings. Some disagree. Some Catholic ethicists suggest, in our present situation of plurality of belief, that Catholic doctrine should not be imposed on patients. Of course, non-Catholic beliefs should not be imposed either. This is a much broader issue, the issue of patients' rights. According to this doctrine, health personnel should not impose any kind of belief (pro or con) on patients.[46] Health personnel also have rights, of course.[47]

On the other hand, it must be noted again that Catholic moral theology has already seen as licit the systematic and lifelong practice of birth control if there is sufficient reason.[48] The argument often turns on the method of control. Is it natural, as in rhythm? Does it interfere with the naturalness of the coital act? What constitutes sufficient reason? For some, as noted earlier, the chance of producing a defective child is reason enough. Others extend the reason to health, economics, the population explosion, personal convenience, and so on. Statistical surveys suggest that between 80 percent and 90 percent of American Catholic women are using artificial birth control. Which reasons they use are not clear, but they are supported by some teachings and not by others. Similarly, some conservative Protestants approve of contraceptives, but others do not. Liberal Protestants generally approve. This spread of perspective is also found in Jewish thought. The secular world reflects this spectrum as well.

Secular Perspective

From a secular perspective, it is evident that contraceptive practice varies with socio-economic status. In the United States, it has long been an axiom that the higher the income, the lower the birthrate. Education has also been a factor. At least one writer has commented on the anomaly of the state of Kerala in India. The birthrate has gone down as the economic security and education have gone up.[49] Sweden has also been cited as an example of a rising standard of living resulting in increased birth control.[50] American statistics suggest that smaller families increase with higher levels of income, regardless of the religious preference of the people involved.

Ethicists tend to be hesitant about putting a price tag on life. Secular values, of course, include money. The rights of society might be explored here. Society spends money through taxes and charitable agencies. These welfare costs have increased. Society might accept the increase, or, by deciding that contraception is preferable, save considerable sums of money. The amounts are not always clear, however. One estimate is that $10 million in family planning could save $700 million in public spending for unwanted children. For some, such saving is an ethical consideration, but others feel there is no problem here.[51]

Summary

Ethics is not just a matter of popular opinion polls.[52] It is rather a matter of reasoned thought, as noted earlier. But we have seen here how reasoned thought is influenced by the context in which it is carried out. Early Christian thought was developed in opposition to pagan philosophies that declared procreation wrong. Now the ethical perspective is influenced by the availability of effective contraceptive methods, the development of technology, and, in the area of birth control, by the population explosion.

In the beginning, the Bible says God told the man and the woman to be fruitful and multiply and fill the earth (Genesis 1:28). There are those who are saying the earth is now filled and it is time to stop multiplying. St. Augustine said the same thing over 1500 years ago. So did Eastern Orthodox St. John Chrysostom. Today we are influenced in this thinking by the high cost of caring for and educating children, by the lack of meaningful work for large numbers of people, by the specter of massive starvation. Two thirds of the world goes to bed hungry. In building the Aswan High Dam (1952–1972), Egypt was able to increase food production 20 percent but, in the time it took to do that, the population grew almost 60 percent. World population doubled from five hundred million to one billion between A.D. 1 and 1750. By 1910, it had doubled again to two billion. By 1976, it was four billion. By 2020, it will be eight billion, though the growth rate may be slowing.[53]

STERILIZATION

About 70 percent of the current population increase will be in the southern hemisphere. The country of India alone adds 14 million children a year. In centuries past, most of these children died. Now, most live, thanks to modern sanitation and medicine.[54] India has made massive efforts at birth control. These have included paying people to be sterilized and threatening jail for those who refuse, if they already have three children. This interference with the birth process is contrary to the Hindu concept of reincarnation. The prevention of birth might prevent the return of a dead relative, according to that belief. However, the chief objection has been that the rewards and threats were coercive and, hence, a violation of freedom of choice.[55]

Varying Views

The freedom of choice issue was noted earlier in relation to sterilization of the retarded or mentally incompetent. Both voluntary and involuntary sterilization were condemned by

Pope Pius XI in "Casti Connubii." Early Christians occasionally practiced castration. In A.D. 325, the Council of Nicea condemned the practice because it was common among the heretic Gnostics. However, the castration of choir boys (to maintain their soprano voices) had papal approval. Sterilization mutilates; that is, it mars the image of the Creator. As an ethical wrong, the ban on mutilation goes back to impairment for military duty and opposition to extreme ascetics who mutilated themselves as a sign of devotion. A liberal Catholic position is that sterilization is acceptable if it is mutual and responsible. Eastern orthodoxy opposes sterilization on the ground that it violates the purpose of marriage—to have children.[56] A conservative Protestant view notes that sterilization at times may be permissible, but it impairs the creative activity God has given to man. In favor of permissibility, they cite the acceptance of eunuchs by Jesus and the early Church (Matthew 19:10–12 and Acts 8).[57] On the present scene we need to add Paul Ramsey's thought on natural law. He suggests that a vasectomy may be a far less serious invasion of nature than the massive assault made upon a woman's generative organism by the pill.[58] Orthodox Judaism vigorously opposes and also allows sterilization. Tubal ligation is preferred if sterilization is allowed at all (groups within Judaism vary as do groups within Christianity). The tubal ligation does not interfere with the coital act and the commandment to the male to avoid improper emission of seed.[59]

Choice

Sterilization now appears to be the first choice of contraceptive method for many Americans who have achieved their desired family size.[60] Those who promote Zero Population Growth (ZPG) have suggested no more than two children per family. The ethical issue here may be a subtle societal pressure, already being felt by those with large families. In an earlier day, society approved of "big happy families." Now the pressure is on to have no more children than a couple can care for, both economically and psychologically, or, in ZPG terms, no more than two.[61]

The issue here is freedom of choice. The Association for Voluntary Sterilization has said that "voluntary sterilization should be the right of every adult who wishes it and can give his or her informed consent."[62] The association's name implies the group's approval of the procedure, with emphasis on its being voluntary. The organization has been active in investigating cases of sterilization abuse, as among the retarded or mentally incompetent and people on welfare, who are sometimes pressured into the procedure.[63]

An interesting development has appeared in some subcultures in which birth control is seen as a sin. Some see a tubal ligation or vasectomy as preferable to a series of sins in each act of contraception. Veatch reports a value conflict between a WASP (White Anglo-Saxon Protestant) doctor and a woman of Puerto Rican background. In the islands, the Church spoke out very strongly against sterilization. Since then, the procedure has become very widely practiced. The woman was twenty-eight years old and had two children. Her economic resources were very limited. The doctor refused to do the tubal ligation because she might want more children some day and sterilization is usually seen as permanent. Because neither person saw this as an ethical issue, Veatch interprets the doctor's value system as future-oriented, whereas the woman's concerns are for the present situation.[64]

The Women's Movement

Women's concerns represent another big change in recent decades. In centuries past, ethical principles were developed by men, many of whom were celibate.[65] Men do not have to go through pregnancy, the often fatal dangers of childbirth, and the debilitating effects of frequent pregnancies. Celibate priests did not have to provide either economic or psychological support to the women bearing children or to the children who survived the rigors of birth and the first risky years of life. Today, women are making more of their own decisions. The number of American Catholic women using artificial birth control was noted earlier. Today, women are not only surviving childbirth in greater numbers, but they are beginning to write the rules about having children. As more women become involved in the developing of ethical thought, we can expect even more changes in the concepts covered in this chapter.

THE ISSUES

The control of the number of children involves a number of ethical concerns. Infanticide is not generally approved in our culture. Abortion, for whatever reasons, limits the number of children. This issue is examined further in Chapter Four. The use of the IUD may be an abortion problem or may be objectionable because it is a mechanical, not "natural," interference with the reproductive process. The latter has been the general objection to birth control throughout most of the history of the Christian West. That children should be welcomed in whatever number is part of the thought of the Judeo-Christian tradition, the Islamic faith, Hinduism, and other religions and cultures. However, in the face of the lower infant mortality rates, greater longevity, the population explosion, the high cost of rearing children (food, clothing, education), mass starvation, and increasing problems such as defective children, more and more the religions have adjusted their views to include the permissibility of contraception and responsible parenthood, or else people have made their own adjustment without official religious approval.

The use of sterilization as a contraceptive method has brought out the old issues of mutilation, as well as the problem of informed consent.

ROLE OF THE NURSE IN CONTRACEPTION

The roles that the nurse assumes in the practice area of contraception, including sterilization, range from counselor to decision maker. The most common role, by far, is that of counselor or providor of information to clients about the variety of methods of contraception available, the actual procedure, side effects, and benefits of sterilization. Nurse counselors in family planning clinics fill a major role in seeing that all people seek-

ing contraceptive services receive the complete, understandable information about contraception that forms the basis of informed consent. That includes teaching about methods available, potential risks and benefits to the patient of each method, and encouraging and supporting the patient's choice, based on sound, unbiased, factual data.[66] From the outset, it is presumed that nurses who do not believe in contraception will not willingly work in family planning clinics.[67] The issues arise, however, in other areas of nursing practice, as the case studies illustrate.

Counselor

It is imperative to recognize the difficulty in providing information or teaching others in an unbiased manner on any subject. This difficulty is increased in the area of contraception with its many cultural, religious, and personal taboos. This increases the importance of the nurse recognizing her own personal preferences and potential biases concerning family planning before providing contraceptive counseling so that she can be sensitive to overcoming her own biases and cognizant of patient preferences for methods that may not be based on scientific fact.[68]

Decision Maker

Nurses who expand their scope of education and practice and become family planning nurse-practitioners will also assume the role of decision maker in contraceptive care. That is, it becomes the task of the nurse-practitioner to decide which contraceptive method is best suited to a given individual, based on his or her physical condition, sexual patterns, medical contraindications, as well as personal preference.[69] Whether or not to prescribe oral contraceptives or insert an IUD at a given time for a given woman is a decision the nurse-practitioner needs to make based on sound, scientific knowledge and physical examination findings. There are, however, more considerations that often influence these decisions, as will be illustrated in the case studies that follow.

Value Bias

None of us is ever value-free so that our own belief systems/values may enter into our decision making on the method of contraception prescribed at any given time. For example, one might be convinced that contraception is an acceptable, if not valued, method to prevent unwanted children, but also believe that contraceptive methods freely available to teen-agers only serve to encourage extramarital sexual relationships.[70] This belief system might interfere with the nurse's decision on contraception for a fourteen-year-old girl when there are no medical or scientific contraindications for use of certain methods.

Other Roles

The other roles that nurses assume in caring for patients who seek/use contraceptive services or choose to be permanently sterilized include patient advocate, confidant, and reinforcer of physician's regimens. Often the nurse is respected for her knowledge and judgment and is thought of as more approachable than the physician. Consequently, patients seek out the nurse for advice on what to do (whether to follow the doctor's suggestions on contraception). The nurse may find herself in a difficult position if she disagrees with the physician's prescription of a contraceptive method or feels that the physician did not clearly hear or interpret the patient's desires. The nurse assumes the advocacy role advisedly and with due respect for the physician as well as concern for the patient.[71] This often means that the nurse discusses the patient's concerns with the physician, so that together with the patient they come to a mutually agreeable decision.

The nurse is often called upon to listen to the concerns of women seeking contraception or sterilization who feel that their men are not supportive of or are completely against use of any method. Often, women feel trapped into childbearing or into a bad choice of contraception because they must have a method that "doesn't show." An equally sad commentary is the situation when a woman seeks contraceptive advice and it is refused because her source of health care chooses not to provide such information or services.[72] For a variety of reasons, nurses find themselves working in such settings even when they believe in contraceptive choice for individuals, so that value conflicts may arise between the nurse and her responsibility to the institution that employs her.[73] These are difficult situations, and how each nurse responds will depend to some extent on how she views her responsibility to the patient and to the employer. The reverse situation is also quite possible, that is, a nurse who does not believe in contraception but works in an institution that promotes it.

CASE STUDIES

Whatever role the nurse assumes in the provision of contraceptive services, there are ethical dimensions to her practice. The issues discussed previously and their application to the nurse and to contraception are illustrated in the following case studies. It is impossible to include every possible nursing situation in this book, so four cases have been chosen to illustrate some of the more common ethical concerns and value conflicts. As is consistent with the other chapters in this book, the "Guidelines for Identifying and Analyzing Ethical Dilemmas in Nursing Practice" should be used with each case. The first case will be analyzed briefly to illustrate how the guidelines can be used.

Case #5

Oral Contraception

Ms. R., a sixteen-year-old, comes to the family planning clinic requesting oral contraception (the pill). She states she has occasional sex but can't predict this activity and wishes to be certain that she is protected against pregnancy. She also expresses the concern that she is forgetful at times and hopes she will remember to take a pill every night. After careful review of her medical and sexual history, the family planning nurse-practitioner believes that the Copper 7 IUD is best suited to Ms. R. and discusses this with her. Ms. R. listens, hesitates, then says that she would rather take the pill. The nurse-practitioner explains her concern about the use of oral contraceptives (OC) in view of Ms. R.'s age and admitted concern about forgetting to take the pills. Ms. R. states that she does not want anything "put up inside her," so the nurse agrees to a trial period of the pill.

Analysis

1. The health problems that exist in this case involve the safety of the use of hormonal contraception in young girls whose menstrual cycles may not be fully established. In view of this, the nurse-practitioner explained her concern to the patient and suggested that the Copper 7 be used. The nurse may have thought of many reasons for this choice, among them effectiveness in preventing conception, safety of insertion in a nulliparous woman, as well as some value judgments, such as limited need for motivation for use, and so on. It would appear that consent for treatment of minors is not a problem in this setting and chances are the nurse goes along with this policy as she is willing to provide a contraceptive method.

2. Further information that might be of help in making such a decision in the future includes a complete menstrual history, more detail on the sexual activity patterns of Ms. R., whether Ms. R. knows and understands all methods of contraception including side effects and responsibilities of the user, and more detail on Ms. R.'s apparent fear of things "inside her." It is recognized that each item of information selected to follow up on will be useful in making a decision, but also directs the decision in a sense (value components).

3. The ethical issues involved include provision of contraception for minors, extramarital sexual activity, patient rights, and freedom of choice. One might also add, "Is it ever appropriate to 'change' a patient's mind?"

4. The ANA Code for Nurses Statements 1, 2, 4, and 6 apply to various aspects of this case. Sections of the Interpretive Statements that may lend guidance to the nurse's actions in this case include 1.1, 1.3, 1.4, 2.3, 4.1, 4.2, 6.1, 6.3, and 6.4.

5. The nurse's value system appears to include support for freedom of choice, because even though the patient disagreed with the nurse's best judgment, the nurse did not force her to accept the IUD. Weighing the relative risks of the use of a given method and unwanted pregnancy, the nurse appeared to support the patient's choice of contraception. It would also appear that the nurse's values did not conflict with the prescription of OC to an unmarried, teen-age woman; or, if they did, the nurse's belief in individual choice was the predominant value acted upon at this time. She also appeared to believe that a sixteen-year-old can make a responsible decision on contraceptive use.

6. The potential value conflict as to what method of contraception is "best" for Ms. R. was resolved when the nurse-practitioner agreed to prescribe what Ms. R. desired. Other physicians and nurses may have decided otherwise if they believed that Ms. R.'s age was an absolute contraindication to the use of oral contraceptives.

7. Ms. R. made the decision on the choice of contraception. The nurse appeared to assume responsibility for providing the information to Ms. R. about contraception and methods so that she could make an informed decision. Others may disagree and call this an "uninformed decision," depending on their view of contraception and adolescents.

8. The range of decisions possible includes no contraception to supporting the patient's choice. In addition to the potential for unwanted pregnancy, forcing or coercing the patient to accept a method she does not want may lead to intolera-

ble side effects or nonuse, and support of patient choice when not harmful might ensure best use of the contraceptive method.

9. What would you have done in this situation if you were the nurse?
10. What did you learn about yourself and your decision-making abilities that will help you in future similar situations?

Informed Consent—Sterilization of Mentally Retarded

You are a bilingual nurse working in the labor room and caring for a non-English-speaking, fourteen-year-old having her first baby. The young girl is mentally retarded and has lived in a variety of foster homes. When it becomes apparent that a Cesarean section is needed to deliver a viable infant, the physician decides to do a tubal ligation "for her own good." You are called to translate the physician's decision on the need for a Cesarean section to the legal guardian so that permission can be obtained. As you begin, the physician tells you to avoid the topic of sterilization and that he will find some "reason for having to tie her tubes" once he opens the abdomen. The consent for surgery includes a general statement covering "procedures deemed necessary" by the physician.

In addition to applying the guidelines, please consider the following questions:

1. Would you, the nurse, proceed to translate what the physician tells you to do, and on what basis did you make your decision?
2. What are your own beliefs about sterilization of the mentally retarded, young women, and anyone without proper informed consent?
3. What value system do you think the physician is operating under? Can you support his value system if in conflict with your own?
4. What value system do you think the young girl and her legal guardian operate under, and might there be conflicts between these and yours or the physician's?
5. Would you refuse to become involved in this situation, or would you tell the legal guardian of the physician's entire plan before requesting consent?

Vasectomy

B. L. is a twenty-eight-year-old male who comes to the family planning facility requesting a vasectomy. He and his wife are the parents of two children and have decided for personal and economic reasons that their family size is complete. As the nurse counselor discusses with them the variety of contraceptive methods available, as well as the permanency of vasectomy, they appear well versed about these and continue steadfast in their desire for vasectomy.

Please consider the following questions while applying the guidelines.

1. What decisions need to be made by the nurse counselor and the physician? Are there ethical components to these decisions? Please identify.

2. As the nurse counselor, do you support this couple's request for sterilization, and would you sign the permit form as a witness? Please give the rationale for your actions.
3. Identity your own values/beliefs regarding sterilization, freedom of choice, and responsibility for informed consent.
4. What value systems might be operant in this couple?
5. Would any of your responses to the preceding questions be altered if:
   B. L. were eighteen, or thirty-five, or fifty years of age?
   The couple were not married?
   One of the partners were of far lower than average intelligence?
   The couple were on welfare?

Please give reasons for your responses to each of these questions.

=Case #8

Hospital Policy—No Contraception

Mrs. S. delivered her second child, a healthy male infant, three days ago. The nurse who has been caring for her and her infant is now helping them get ready for discharge from the hospital. As she is dressing the infant, Mrs. S. quietly whispers to her, "Can you help me get some birth control pills? Nobody seems to want to answer my questions and I can't manage having another baby next year!" The nurse appears sympathetic but responds, "I'm sorry, Mrs. S., but the hospital policies will not allow us to discuss the subject of birth control."

Using the guidelines, please consider the following questions:

1. Would you respond the same as the nurse did? Why, or why not?
2. What alternative choices did/does the patient have to get proper contraceptive information? What responsibility does the nurse have to give these suggestions?
3. How would you respond if you were the nurse and personally used the pills?
4. Is the hospital responsible for meeting the needs of its patients, or should patients have the responsibility to choose a hospital that provides birth control information?
5. What if there were no other hospitals available to this woman for a variety of reasons? Would this change any of your responses to her request?

NOTES AND REFERENCES

1. We use birth control here in the broadest sense of population control. Joseph Fletcher has pointed out that technically, only abortion is birth control. Other methods of population control are conception control or postnatal infanticide. *The Ethics of Genetic Control* (New York: Doubleday & Company, Inc., 1974), pp. 46–47.

2. John T. Noonan, *Contraception, A History of Its Treatment by The Catholic Theologians and Canonists* (Cambridge, Mass.: Harvard University Press, 1965), pp. 18–29, 85–86. Julia and Harry Abrahamson, *Who Shall Live? Man's Control Over Birth and Death* (New York: Hill & Wang, 1970), p. 9. Michael Tooley says the destruction of weak

or deformed babies was required but exposure of healthy children was less common. This latter was less a moral matter than a need for a population to maintain a large army. "Infanticide: A Philosophical Perspective," *Encyclopedia of Bioethics* 2:742–751. The Encyclopedia is cited hereafter as *EB*. See also, David Landy, "Death I: Anthropological Perspectives," *EB* 1:221–229.

3. Lloyd deMause, ed., *The History of Childhood* (New York: The Psychohistory Press, 1974), p. 25, "Hilarion to Alis," 1 B.C.

4. Op. cit., pp. 159–186.

5. Fletcher, op. cit., p. 85, sees quality-of-life (QOL) ethics in constant tension with sanctity-of-life or quantity-of-life ethics.

6. Noonan, op. cit., pp. 86–87. Walter O. Spitzer and Carlyle L. Saylor, eds., *Birth Control and the Christian, A Protestant Symposium on the Control of Human Reproduction* (Wheaton, Ill.: Tyndale House Publishers, 1969) p. xxvi. The respect for life does not ordinarily extend to war, capital punishment, and other forms of justified homicide. These are called by other names than murder. See Fletcher, op. cit., p. 83. On the current scene, Vatican II called for "responsible parenthood," which might mean birth control. Anthony Kosnik and others, *Human Sexuality: New Directions in American Catholic Thought* (New York: Paulist Press, 1977), pp. 111–114.

7. "Other Ideas & Trends," *The New York Times* (6 May 1979), E 11. Plato's *Republic* V, 460ff, and Aristotle's *Politics* VII, 16, 1335. Anne J. Davis and Mila A. Aroskar, *Ethical Dilemmas and Nursing Practice* (New York: Appleton-Century-Crofts, 1978), pp. 89–90, 93. Abrahamsons, op. cit., p. 14. Carl Djerassi, citing 1978 data, lists abortion as third after the pill (second) and prolonged lactation. Sterilization is fourth and condoms a close fifth. *The Politics of Contraception* (New York: W. W. Norton, 1979), p. 8.

8. James J. Nagle, *Heredity and Human Affairs* (St. Louis: The C. V. Mosby Company 1974), p. 112.

9. Charles F. Westoff and Elise F. Jones, "Contraception and Sterilization in the United States, 1965–1975," *Family Planning Perspectives* no. 4 (July/Aug. 1977), 9:153–157. Perspectives is cited hereafter as *FPP*. John Scanzoni, "A Sociological Perspective on Abortion and Sterilization," pp. 314–326, in Spitzer and Saylor, op. cit.

10. Nagle, op. cit., pp. 108–109. Noonan, op. cit., pp. 474–475. Ross L. Willows, "The Intrauterine Contraceptive Device," pp. 216–217, in Spitzer and Saylor, op. cit. Leroy Augenstein, *Come, Let Us Play God* (New York: Harper & Row, Publishers, 1969), pp. 67–68. David M. Feldman, *Marital Relations, Birth Control and Abortion in Jewish Law* (New York: Schocken Books, Inc., 1978), pp. 233–234. Djerassi, op. cit., pp. 19–21.

11. "Ubi dubium ibi libertas," ("where there is doubt there is liberty,") is presented as a hallowed moral axiom by Daniel Maguire, "The Freedom to Die," pp. 171–180, in *Bioethics*, ed. by Thomas A. Shannon (New York: Paulist Press, 1976).

12. Thomas J. Higgins says flatly that positive contraception is always wrong. Positive contraception is the interference by artificial means to prevent the union of sperm and ovum. This is a foul perversion, he says, because Natural Law forbids us to destroy the primary end (purpose) of a faculty such as an organ of the body. *Man as Man, The Science and Art of Ethics*, rev. ed. (Beverly Hills, Calif.: Bruce, a division of Benziger Bruce & Clencoe, Inc., 1958), pp. 392–401. Edwin F. Healy also insists contraception is wrong, except for the rhythm method for approved reasons. *Medical Ethics* (Chicago: Loyola University Press, 1956), pp. 156–162. Kosnik and others, pp. 111–114, suggest responsible parenthood may require contraception.

The risks involved in using an IUD might raise an ethical issue for some. It has been noted that the risks are less than those involved in crossing a busy street. The recall of the Dalkon Shield is a reminder, however, that continued vigilance is necessary even in crossing a busy street if one expects to cross safely. "Moratorium on Dalkon Shield Lifted by FDA," *The Hastings Center Report*, no. 3 (June 1975), 7:2. The Report is cited hereafter as *HCR*. Inadequate testing may also increase risks beyond tolerable levels. The ethics of profits versus human welfare are, of course, a widespread concern in modern life. Carol Levine, in "An Act of Greed," *HCR*, no. 3 (June 1979), 9:43–44, quotes the charge that in the marketing of thalidomide, the company suppressed negative reports on its side effects. Levine is reviewing *Suffer the Children: The Story of Thalidomide* by the Insight Team of the Sunday Times of London (New York: Viking Press, Inc., 1979). The issue of costs versus benefits is a part of many of the ethical issues discussed in this book.

13. Westoff and Jones, op. cit. Nagle, op. cit., pp. 104–108. Norman E. Himes notes that the first published description in 1564 was of a linen sheath that the Italian anatomist Gabrielle Fallopius claimed to have invented. *Medical History of Contraception* (New York: Gamut Press, 1963), pp. 59–78, 186–206. John T. Noonan, Jr., "Contraception," *EB* 1:204–216. Emily Taft Douglas, *Margaret Sanger, Pioneer of the Future* (New York: Holt, Rinehart and Winston, 1970), p. 69. Julius Preuss, *Biblical and Talmudic Medicine*, trans. and ed. by Fred Rosner (New York: Sanhedrin Press, 1978), original, 1911. Djerassi, op. cit., pp. 14–18.

14. Nagle, op. cit., pp. 104–108. Noonan, *History*, op. cit., pp. 9–10. Himes, op. cit., p. 54. Djerassi, op. cit., pp. 7–9.

15. The availability of effective techniques influences attitudes. Contrarily, Robert M. Veatch notes that in a 1957 survey, one third of the Catholic obstetricians and gynecologists believed rhythm to be the most reliable method of contraception while 2 percent of non-Catholic physicians held this view. Scientific "knowledge" is heavily influenced by other values. *Value-Freedom in Science and Technology* (Missoula, Montana: Scholars Press, 1976), p. 159.

16. "Levirate Law," *The Interpreter's Dictionary of the Bible* **3** (1962), p. 116. See also, Lansing Hicks, "Onan," ibid., p. 602.

17. The 1975 Catholic "Declaration on Certain Questions Concerning Sexual Ethics" reiterated a severe condemnation of masturbation and homosexuality. See Rosemary Radford Ruether, "Time Makes Ancient Good Uncouth: The Catholic Report on Sexuality," *The Christian Century*, no. 25 (3–10 Aug. 1977), **44**:682–685. This American report looks at both of these sexual activities with more tolerance. Kosnik and others, op. cit. For example, on p. 15, they interpret the story of Onan as an attempt to steal his brother's inheritance. Masturbation is discussed on pp. 219–229; homosexuality on pp. 186–218. The report describes (pp. 198–199) the medieval awe of semen, the "precious fluid," as almost human. Ova were unknown and the role of women virtually ignored. The "almost human" helps us understand how the Church could view contraception and masturbation as murder. It is, of course, only in modern times that we have learned or acknowledged that 95 percent of American males and 70 percent of American females masturbate. Each male ejaculate contains 200 to 300 million sperm, so on the basis of this medieval view, each time a man ejaculates without impregnating a woman, he commits murder 200 to 300 million times.

18. Feldman, op. cit., numerous references. Louis M. Epstein, *Sex Laws and Customs in Judaism* (New York: KTAV Publishing House, 1967), pp. 144–147. Noonan, *History*, op. cit., pp. 34–35. Spitzer and Saylor, op. cit., numerous references. Veatch, op. cit., p. 196. The obligation to one's dead brother is now forbidden by the Church, says Bernard Häring, "The Encyclical Crisis," pp. 54–60, in *The Debate on Birth Control*, ed. by Andrew Bauer (New York: Hawthorn Books, Inc., 1969). Israel R. Margolis suggests that it is up to men and women to decide on having a child rather than its being a decision of synagogue or church or state. He does not list "acceptable" reasons. Presumably, they could decide on economic or any other grounds. "A Reform Rabbi's View," pp. 30–33, in vol. 1, *Abortion in a Changing World*, ed. by Robert E. Hall (New York: Columbia University Press, 1970).

19. Augustine was in agreement with Roman law and the pagan philosophies of the Stoics and the Neo-Pythagoreans at this point. He was a loyal citizen of Rome in opposition to the invading barbarian Goths. He was an ex-Manichee, opposed to his old religion and their ideas, as well as similar ideas among the Gnostics. Kosnik and others, p. 112, claim the Catholic Church's insistence on procreation goes back to the Stoics rather than to the Bible.

20. It is, of course, the essential factor in the rhythm method (see following). A 1965 statement from the Greek Orthodox Church in North and South America said abstinence is the only permissible form of birth control. All others are immoral. Veatch, *Value Freedom*, op. cit., p. 194. Stanley R. Harakas notes that Orthodoxy holds mixed views. Some agree that only abstinence is acceptable. Others accept other forms of contraception. "Eastern Orthodox Christianity," *EB* 1:347–356. In India, Mahatma Gandhi pro-

posed abstinence, as did Malthus (see later) who combined it with late marriage as the solution to the population explosion. The combination has helped stabilize population growth in Ireland and mainland China. See Douglas, op. cit., pp. 65, 232. Djerassi, op. cit., pp. 183–213.

21. Veatch reports an interesting incident in which a doctor examined a sexually active twelve-year-old girl. He never even thought of prescribing contraceptives. "She's so young . . .'' *Case Studies in Medical Ethics* (Cambridge, Mass.: Harvard University Press, 1977), pp. 191–192. It is reminiscent of a teenage subculture sexual attitude that "it's OK if it's spontaneous," that is, as long as one hasn't planned or prepared with contraceptives. This takes literally the ban on contraceptives while quite ignoring the ban on extra- or premarital coitus. David F. Busby claims that many girls report the risk of pregnancy as part of the excitement of sex. He does not indicate the male attitude on this. See his "Rape, Incest and Multiple Illegitimacy as Indicators for Therapeutic Abortion," pp. 301–309, in Spitzer and Saylor, op. cit. The Abrahamsons, op. cit., pp. 54–60, say the facts indicate the fear of pregnancy, venereal disease, and detection do not stop premarital sexual activity. The authors cite studies showing that from 25 percent to 60 percent of teen-age marriages involve pregnancy at the time of marriage. This is, of course, in addition to millions of children born out of wedlock and abortions by women pregnant outside of marriage. Augenstein, op. cit., p. 78, suggests that if a moral code is based only on fear of pregnancy, it is time for a change. He adds his admiration for large numbers of people who do not engage in premarital or extramarital sexual intercourse. Fletcher, op. cit., p. 78. Douglas notes that it is not male promiscuity that bothers. The condom was exempt from obscenity laws because it prevented disease. She sees this as representative of male promiscuity. Although birth control was heavily opposed, prostitution was strong and wide open. Op. cit., pp. 101ff. Virginia Adams and Tom Ferrell cite a study of sexually active teen-agers who received contraceptive assistance with no marked increase in sexual activity. "Ideas & Trends: Patterns of 'Promiscuity,' " *The New York Times* (7 Jan. 1979), E 7. J. Mayone Sty-

cos, "Desexing Birth Control," *FPP*, no. 6 (Nov./Dec. 1977), **9**:286–292. In 1972, the United States Supreme Court refused to review a lower court decision that a Massachusetts law denying contraceptives to the unmarried was unconstitutional. The American College of Obstetricians and Gynecologists executive board statement of policy (May 1971) suggests involving parents when possible, but says minors should not be denied effective methods of contraception.

22. This and the following paragraphs draw most heavily on Noonan's historical survey, *History*, op. cit. He notes, p. 3, the problem of rationally dissecting the doctrine of contraception without caricaturing it. John Rock faced this difficulty in discussing the charge that the pill sterilizes. *The Time Has Come* (New York: Alfred A. Knopf, Inc., 1963), pp. 172–174. See also, *The Regulation of Birth, Encyclical Letter of Pope Paul VI, 'Humanae Vitae' 1968* (London: Catholic Truth Society, 1968). Bauer, op. cit. Daniel J. Callahan, ed., *The Catholic Case for Contraception* (London: Arlington Books, 1969). Bernard Häring, *Ethics of Manipulation* (New York: The Seabury Press, 1975). Maurice J. Moore, *Death of Dogma?* (Chicago: Community and Family Study Center, 1973). Ruether, op. cit. Spitzer and Saylor, op. cit. Veatch, both volumes, op. cit.

23. Present evidence is that animals engage in nonprocreative sexual activity such as copulation outside the species, homosexuality, self-stimulation. As we move up the evolutionary scale, sexual activity among animals becomes as varied as among people. Kosnik and others, op. cit., p. 57.

24. In 1958, a Catholic spokesman listed murder, adultery, and contraception as eternal wrongs. Natural Law is seen as eternal and unchanging. Rock, op. cit., p. 54.

25. Paul Ramsey, *Ethics at the Edge of Life* (New Haven: Yale University Press, 1979), p. 13. Douglas, op. cit., p. 261. The law violated Catholic principles of jurisprudence. Rock, op. cit., p. 113. Cardinal Cushing said that Catholics don't need the law in order to be faithful to their own beliefs or to impose their beliefs on others. Baruch Brody, *Abortion and the Sanctity of Human Life: A Philosophical View* (Cambridge, Mass.: MIT Press, 1975), p. 152.

26. Augenstein, op. cit., p. 75. Rock, op.

cit., pp. 108, 193–203. Sanger's birth control clinic in the 1920s included clients who were Protestant, Catholic, and Jewish in percentages equivalent to their population in the area. Douglas, op. cit., p. 185, 258–261. The practice of birth control today is nearly identical for Catholics and non-Catholics. Charles F. Westoff and Elise F. Jones, "The Secularization of U.S. Catholic Birth Control Practices," *FPP*, no. 5 (Sept./Oct. 1977), **9**:203–207.

27. Alan Ryan, "Two Kinds of Morality: Causalism or Taboo," *HCR*, no. 5 (Oct. 1975), **5**:5.

28. Harmon L. Smith, *Ethics and the New Medicine* (Nasville, Tenn.: Abingdon Press 1970), p. 83. Kosnik and others, op. cit., pp. 65–66.

29. For the liberal Catholic view, see Ruether, op. cit., and Kosnik and others, op. cit. Callahan, op. cit., also represents a more liberal view. He includes views favoring "Humanae Vitae" but emphasizes that his book is the case *for* contraception. Veatch, *Value-Freedom*, op. cit., pp. 169–170, notes that the stereotype of Catholic versus non-Catholic breaks down when cultural values are considered rather than religious affiliation. He cites a non-Catholic residency program in obstetrics that had no instruction in family planning and saw no need for it. A 1964 study showed twelve non-Catholic medical schools teaching rhythm as the preferred method. He also reports enthusiasm for birth control by many Catholics. Rock, op. cit., pp. 31ff, agrees that the issue is the larger cultural view for which the Catholic Church is scape-goated, with the active encouragement of several Catholic spokesmen. He suggests that responsible parenthood is the goal for all. Pope Pius XII stated this goal in 1951 in his address to Catholic midwives.

30. "The Pastoral Constitution of the Church in the Modern World" reinforces the understanding that marriage is valid even when there are no offspring. Smith, op. cit., p. 63. Rock, op. cit., p. 31. The two ends of marriage, procreation and unity, were reiterated ten years later in "The Declaration on Certain Questions Concerning Sexual Ethics." This was a statement by the Sacred Congregation for the Doctrine of the Faith. Tom F. Driver, "A Stride Toward Sanity," *Christianity & Crisis*, no. 17 (31 Oct. 1971), **37**:243–246. Kosnik and others, op. cit., pp. 50–52. Some Eastern Orthodox also accept two ends for marriage, but others insist that procreation is the only purpose. Harakas, op. cit., pp. 353–354.

31. David M. Kennedy, *Birth Control in America, The Career of Margaret Sanger* (New Haven: Yale University Press, 1970), pp. 154–171. Alan F. Guttmacher notes that Reform Judaism spoke in favor of contraception in 1931, and Conservative Judaism, in 1934. Orthodox Judaism holds a more reserved view. Preface, pp. ix–xxx, in Himes, op. cit.

32. Rock, op. cit., pp. 179–183. Kosnik and others, op. cit., p. 46, suggests rhythm was already approved by Pius XI in "Casti Connubii" in 1930. Djerassi, op. cit., pp. 9–10.

33. Margaret Nofziger, *A Cooperative Method of Natural Birth Control*, 2nd ed. (Summertown, Tenn.: The Book Publishing Co., 1978). This is the source of the 99 percent effective figure. The author offers to take in any unwanted babies born with the natural method. She suggests that a man's love might be expressed by his willingness to refrain from lovemaking during the unsafe period; hence, the use of the word *cooperative* in the title.

34. Nagle, op. cit., p. 108.

35. Op. cit., p. 169. In contrast, Fletcher calls the pill a sterilizer. Op. cit., p. 47. Rock, op. cit., pp. 171–174, reports that in 1958, Pope Pius XII called the pill a sterilizer. Rock is aware that the Catholic Church condemns temporary sterilization, too. He notes that this quickly sinks into absurdity, for in abstinence, both the man and the woman are temporarily sterile. A woman is temporarily sterile while she is pregnant, but this is not taken as an argument against pregnancy. Feldman, op. cit., pp. 246–247, reports acceptance of the pill in Jewish law for it does not involve the improper emission of semen and it preserves the coital act. This presumably would be the case also with the new nasal spray which alters sexual functioning but does not interfere with natural coitus. Anne C. Roark, "In Science," *The Chronicle of Higher Education*, no. 7 (15 Oct. 1979), **19**:15.

36. Djerassi, op. cit., p. 8, lists 50–80 million users world wide. It was approved for nuns in the Congo, who were in danger of rape. Rock, op. cit., pp. 176–177. The risk of using the pill has had considerable publicity. The ethics of excessive publicity might be considered. Similar attention is not paid to

the American maternal death rate or deaths caused by beverage alcohol or smoking. The ethics of prescribing a dangerous drug might be considered. Nagle claims that there are an estimated three deaths per year per 100,000 users from pulmonary embolism attributable to the pill in excess of the normal. This is compared to 25 deaths per 100,000 from pregnancies, exclusive of illegal abortions. Still, the risk is there, so the use of the pill should be monitored by health care givers familiar with the patient's medical history and with awareness of continuing research data. Nagle, op. cit., p. 111. We see here the same caution noted in n. 12. In the Third World, deaths from pregnancy may run as high as 250 per 100,000. However, there are those who claim the pill, or specific pills, have been marketed without adequate research in the rush for profits, a rush that may have withheld negative information. "Birth Control Pills: Health versus Profits," *Dollars and Sense* (Spring 1976), pp. 10–11. Since 1970, the Food and Drug Administration has required that informational brochures accompany sales of the pill. Directions, reactions, side effects, and hazards are to be explained in plain language. Djerassi, op. cit., pp. 36–41. Some similar problems of risks and benefits, and adequate testing, appear in relation to other contraceptives as well. See Carol Levine, "Depo-Provera and Contraceptive Risk: A Case Study of Values in Conflict," *HCR*, no. 4 (Aug. 1979), **9**:8–11. Allan Rosenfield, "Depo-Provera: Contraceptive Risk?," *HCR*, no. 2 (Ap. 1980), **10**:4.

37. Kosnik, op. cit., p. 48, 116–123. Thomas A. Shannon points out that although certain acts and practices have been absolutely prohibited, there have been no infallible declarations on morality. *Bioethics* (New York: The Paulist Press, 1976), p. 6. The official teaching continues in the form of papal announcements.

38. "The Encyclical Crisis," op. cit., p. 44.

39. Moore, op. cit.

40. The contrast, of course, is overdrawn. As indicated previously, there were a number of methods available. Perhaps the negative reaction came because of the expectation, encouraged by the majority opinion of the birth control commission, that the Pope would rule in favor of the pill on the bases that it regulates a natural function and what many see as an obvious need to limit reproduction. This, of course, is speculation.

41. Ruether, op. cit., p. 685. Kosnik, op. cit., p. 49.

42. Douglas, op. cit., frequently notes Sanger's early opposition from the churches and medical doctors and also cites the British report (p. 159) that clergy and doctors had the smallest families of all professional groups. Contraception was available to the rich, but not to the poor, a charge currently repeated in discussions on abortion. Pp. 68–69, 158, 225. Kennedy, op. cit. *Margaret Sanger, An Autobiography* (New York: Dover Publications, Inc., 1971, original 1938). Alice L. Fleming, *Contraception, Abortion, Pregnancy* (Nashville, Tenn.: Thomas Nelson, Inc., 1974), p. 15. Lloyd A. Kalland, "Views and Positions of the Christian Church—An Historical Review," pp. 417–464, in Spitzer and Saylor, op. cit. Linda Gordon, "The Politics of Birth Control, 1920–1940: The Impact of the Professionals," *International Journal of Health Services*, no. 2 (1975), **5**:253–277. Fletcher, op. cit., p. 77.

43. Noonan, *History*, op. cit., p. 471. Häring, "The Encyclical Crisis," op. cit., p. 55. Fletcher, op. cit., p. 44, claims no technology is against nature. If it were, it would not work. See also his *Morals and Medicine* (Princeton: Princeton University Press, 1954). It is not our purpose here to do a complete critique of Natural Law ethics. We note its continuing presence among us. Some believe that people have been manipulating nature from the beginning. We have been "playing God" since our earliest ancestors. Sherwood L. Washburn, "Tools and Human Evolution," *Scientific American*, no. 3 (Sept. 1960), **203**:2–15. Dorothy Dinnerstein, *The Mermaid and the Minotaur* (New York: Harper & Row, Publishers, 1976). Israel R. Margolis, op. cit., p. 33, suggests that we are creative partners with God so we can "build our families purposefully and joyfully, not accidentally and reluctantly." In relation to Natural Law, he notes the well-known seasonal "heat" of animal sexual desire in contrast to human love without regard to time or season. There is no natural law requiring sexual intercourse to produce a conception or a birth. Eric D'Arcy, "Natural Law," *EB* **3**:1131–1137.

44. Edward A. Murphy, "Eugenics, an Ethical Analysis," *Mayo Clinic Proceedings*

(1978), **53**:655–664. Daniel Callahan, "The Moral Career of Genetic Engineering," *HCR*, no. 2 (Apr. 1979), **9**:9, 21.

45. See n. 43 and Ruether, op. cit., p. 682. Rock, op. cit., pp. 52–62. Higgins, op. cit., p. 398, includes as part of his Natural Law argument against contraception the "fact" that if a woman continues to use contraceptives, it will endanger her health, because the female body is intended by nature to absorb sperm and get an increase in vitality from the bearer of life. Thus, if the female body is sexually starved (sic) of sperm after being sexually excited, both physical and emotional disorders result. The publication date for this interesting statement is 1958. Of the several fascinating facets of this primitive thinking, one of the more intriguing is the "fact" that with oral contraceptives (first marketed in 1960), the IUD, and several other forms of modern contraception, the 200 to 300 million sperm per male ejaculate *are* deposited in the female body during intercourse. In 1923, Dr. Marie Stopes made a claim similar to Higgins. She approved of contraception but objected to the condom. Djerassi, op. cit., pp. 14–15.

The "neither natural nor law" phraseology is Fletcher's op. cit., p. 37. As far back as 1832, Dr. Charles Knowlton published one of the earliest books on contraception, *The Fruits of Philosophy*. He agreed that family limitation is unnatural, as is shaving, cutting fingernails, and the whole of civilization itself. In 1876, his book was the basis of the test case that led an English court to rule contraceptive information is not obscene. Douglas, op. cit., pp. 68–69.

Shannon, op. cit., p. 5, claims that circumstances have always been a part of Roman Catholic ethics.

46. The *Code for Nurses with Interpretive Statements* says that respect for human dignity and uniqueness includes self-determination of clients whenever possible. (Kansas City: American Nurses' Association, 1976), p. 4. See also Lucie Young Kelly, "The Patient's Right to Know," *Nursing Outlook*, no. 1 (Jan. 1976), **24**:26–30. "The Pregnant Patient's Bill of Rights," *Journal of Nurse-Midwifery* no. 4 (Winter 1975), **20**:29–30. George J. Annas, *The Rights of Hospital Patients* (New York: Avon Books, 1975). In 1958, the ban on prescribing contraceptives was lifted in New York City hospitals. Catholic patients and professionals would be free to follow their church beliefs and others would also be free to follow their consciences. Frederick S. Jaffe, "Knowledge, Perception, and Change: Notes on a Fragment of Social History," *The Mount Sinai Journal of Medicine*, no. 4 (July/Aug. 1975), **42**:286–299.

47. Ramsey, op. cit., pp. 80–93, discusses variant Catholic views, which include "Catholic Hospital Ethics: The Report of the Commission on Ethical and Religious Directives for Catholic Hospitals of the Catholic Theological Society of America." See *The Linacre Quarterly*, no. 4 (Nov. 1972), **39**:246–248. He also discusses the legal situation of Catholic health personnel and hospitals. Numbers of laws contain a "conscience clause" so people will not have to participate in a procedure such as sterilization or abortion when it is against their conscience. He notes the difficulty of maintaining the *practice* of this "right" of health personnel. The Church amendment, sponsored by Senator Frank Church in 1973, frees hospitals sponsored by religious groups from being required to perform procedures against their religious beliefs. Public hospitals have been successfully sued and required to provide services such as sterilization.

48. Paul Ramsey, *Fabricated Man* (New Haven: Yale University Press, 1977), p. 43. Häring, *Ethics of Manipulation*, op. cit., pp. 94–96. Kosnik and others, op. cit., pp. 111–114, 140–143.

49. John W. Ratcliffe, "Power, Politics, and Fertility: the Anomaly of Kerala," *HCR*, no. 1 (Feb. 1977), **7**:34–42.

50. Harry Commoner, director of the Center for Biology of Natural Systems at Washington University, St. Louis, quoted in "Ecologist's Proposal," *The Christian Century*, no. 35 (1 Nov. 1978), **45**:1032–1033.

51. Donald H. Bauma, "The Population Explosion: World and Local Alternatives," pp. 328–339, Spitzer and Saylor, op. cit.

52. There is, however, a traditional Catholic form of argument that depends on the "common consent of mankind." Kosnik and others, op. cit., p. 57. John Ladd, "Ethics I: The Tasks of Ethics," *EB* **1**:400–407.

53. Anne C. Roark, "In Science," *The Chronicle of Higher Education*, no. 1 (4 Sept. 1979), **19**:21. Rock, op. cit., p. 9. Harakas, op. cit., p. 354. Douglas A. Walrath, "Surprising Futures," *Your Church*, no. 5 (Sept./Oct.

1978), **24**:30ff. Augenstein, op. cit., pp. 56ff. Noonan, *History*, op. cit., p. 475. The population buildup is not a matter of opinion but historical data. So is world hunger. The interpretations of these matters, however, vary considerably. Some say birth control is not the answer. We must use our technology to more evenly distribute present food supplies while developing new sources such as the oceans. In the meanwhile, an estimated ten thousand people starve to death every day. They may be fortunate because many who do not die are condemned to an incredibly low quality of life. As cited in the previous chapter, there is an ethical issue in this for both the promoters and the objectors to birth control. See the Abrahamsons, op. cit., p. 3. Mainland China was noted earlier (n. 20) for encouraging late marriage to hold down its population, which has reached one billion. More recently, the government has proposed taxing people with too many children. One child will be encouraged but three will be discouraged. The aim is to cut the birthrate from twelve per thousand to five per thousand by 1985 and achieve ZPG by 2000. "China to use tax for birth control," *Des Moines Sunday Register* (12 Aug. 1979), 6 A. H. Tristram Engelhardt, Jr., "Bioethics in the People's Republic of China," *HCR*, no. 2 (Ap. 1980), **10**:7–10.

54. LeRoy Walters has noted that between 1900 and 1970 the average life expectancy of people aged sixty-five had increased by only one and a half years. The enormous increase in life expectancies has come in the increased survival rates of children. "In Search of Health," *The Christian Century*, no. 34 (25 Oct. 1978), **45**:1014–1015.

55. In Kerala, Ratcliffe, op. cit., reports that Hindus led the population in adopting contraception. See also, Drew Christiansen, "Human Rights in India: Ethics and Compulsory Population Control," *HCR*, no. 1 (Feb. 1977), **7**:30–33, and Allan Rosenfield, "The Ethics of Supervising Family Planning in Developing Nations," ibid., pp. 25–29. Veatch, *Case Studies*, op. cit., pp. 185–189. At this writing, India continues in a state of flux. The Nazis are often cited for their compulsory sterilization program of unwanted groups. They banned abortion, however, so their policies were mixed. George H. Kieffer, *Bioethics* (Reading, Mass.: Addison-Wesley Publishing Co., Inc., 1979), pp. 195, 171. Djerassi, op. cit., pp. 21–22, 128–130, 147–151.

56. Gaylin, Thompson, Neville, and Bayles, "Sterilization of the Retarded," *HCR* no. 3 (June 1978), **8**:28–41. We note here again the rights of patients, health personnel, and hospitals. Freedom to *have* the procedure is limited because of the limited numbers of hospitals and doctors doing the procedure plus limits on age, consent, and government regulations. In the case of retarded or mentally incompetent people, we risk patients being sterilized against their will. Alternately, patients might ask for procedures and be refused because it is against hospital policy, or against the conscience of health personnel, or because the very government regulations designed to protect them are now used to deny their own request. See notes 46 and 47. Harakas, op. cit., p. 355. "Sterilization Upheld For Retard Women," *Progress*, no. 2 (Summer 1979), 22:3. Rosalind Pollack Petchesky, "Reproduction, Ethics, and Public Policy: The Federal Sterilization Regulations," *HCR*, no. 5 (Oct. 1979), **9**:29–41.

57. Kosnik and others, op. cit., pp. 128–136, 296–298. Karen Labacqz, "Sterilization: Ethical Aspects," *EB* **4**:1609–1613, points out that the bar on mutilation involves the principle of totality, which says that an organ must be preserved unless its removal is to save a life. Spitzer and Saylor, op. cit., p. xxv, and Robert P. Meyer, "New Testament Text Bearing on the Problem of the Control of Human Reproduction," pp. 25–47, in Spitzer and Saylor. Veatch, *Case Studies*, op. cit., p. 3. Ruether, op. cit., p. 683.

58. *Fabricated Man*, op. cit., p. 42. His use of the term "massive assault" for the pill is not, of course, acceptable to those who see the pill as simply regulating the menstrual cycle. His "less serious invasion of nature," however, resembles the "one shot" sin described in reference to the case cited by Veatch.

59. Veatch, *Case Studies*, op. cit., pp. 181, 191. Feldman, op. cit., pp. 124, 240ff. In the Bible, Deuteronomy 23:1 says, "He whose testicles are crushed or whose male member is cut off shall not enter the assembly of the Lord." This is interpreted as opposition to sterilization for the male. We noted earlier the greater freedom allowed women in contraception, in contrast to men. Of course, most would argue that a vasectomy is hardly

the equivalent of crushing testicles or cutting off the male member. Some interpreters of the biblical text do get carried away.

60. "If You're Sure, Sterilization," *New York Times* (24 July 1977), 18 E. Harold M. Schmech, Jr., "More in U.S. Rely on Sterilization," *New York Times* (25 Mar. 1974). In 1976, 1,200,000 Americans chose voluntary sterilization. Joseph E. Davis, "Message from the President," *Association for Voluntary Sterilization* (New York: AVS, 1977). Charles F. Westhoff and James McCarthy, "Sterilization in the United States," *FPP*, no. 3 (May/June 1979), **11**:147–152. We note once again the rights of health care personnel to be free of coercion while not imposing their beliefs on patients. By official teaching, neither Catholic personnel nor hospitals would be involved in sterilization except as a secondary effect, where the initiating operation would be something else, such as removing a cancerous womb. With the increasing number of sterilizations, this conflict may increase. See Smith, op. cit., p. 33. Kosnik and others op. cit., pp. 296–298. "Ethical and Religious Directives for Catholic Health Facilities, United States Catholic Conference, 1971," *EB* **4**:1755–1757.

61. The Abrahamsons, op. cit., pp. 64, 88. The authors report that in this country, at least, the number of unwanted children equals the number of births in excess of a stable population, that is, if only wanted children were conceived or born, the population would stabilize without coercion. Fletcher, op. cit., p. 77, claims that over 40 percent of our reproduction is unplanned. See Bauma, op. cit., p. 333. Augenstein, op. cit., pp. 65, 73, says population increases must be reduced by 2 percent, which happens to be the same percentage as children born with birth defects, so, prevent birth defects. He also relays the tongue-in-cheek suggestion of giving everyone a car down to the age of twelve. The death rate would control the population. Pro-life forces, of course, see abortion as killing so the death rate keeps down the population. Henrietta H. Marshall reports that unwanted fertility dropped "from one in five births a decade ago, to one in twelve by the mid-1970s." "Letter from the Chair," *Within Our Reach*, annual report, 1977 (New York: Planned Parenthood Federation of America, 1978), pp. 3–6. The complications of ethics might be il-

lustrated here by Eugene B. Borowitz' observation that Jews have achieved ZPG. "Judaism in America Today," *The Christian Century*, no. 36 (8 Nov. 1978), **45**:1066–1070. Feldman, op. cit., p. 304, thinks it would be as reckless to overbreed as to refrain from procreation, but the Jewish people as a group do not suffer from overpopulation for their ranks have been depleted by the mass murders of the past.

62. Cited by Helen Edey in her release on behalf of AVS, 708 Third Ave., New York, N.Y. The AVS is the former Human Betterment Foundation. Lebacqz, op. cit., p. 1612. Founded in 1937, it expanded to an International Project of the AVS in 1972. Kieffer, op. cit., p. 198. In 1973, the Supreme Court held unconstitutional a Massachusett's hospital's denial of a request for voluntary sterilization. Fletcher, op. cit., p. 184.

63. The Department of Health, Education and Welfare has established guidelines to protect competent adults from coercion such as the threat to cut off welfare payments. For minors and incompetents, HEW guidelines called for a review board. As noted in the previous chapter, a federal judge subsequently prohibited sterilization for the latter group, with or without a review board. See Veatch, *Case Studies*, op. cit., pp. 184–185.

64. Op. cit., pp. 30–32. The doctor might, of course, be a simple case of "anatomy is destiny" thinking hidden behind the concern for the future. John Scanzoni, op. cit., pp. 319–320. Ralph Thomlinson, *Population Dynamics* (New York: Random House, 1965), p. 201.

65. Kalland, op. cit., p. 440. Djerassi, op. cit., pp. 42–49. Ruether, op. cit., pp. 682–683. Kosnik and others, op. cit., p. 41, notes that women "were of no real value" and "most theological thinking took place in monasteries." Kieffer, op. cit., p. 140, points out that the majority of genetic counselors are men but most of the counselees are women. We will look at this type of problem further in Chapter Seven.

66. Miriam Manisoff, *Family Planning: A Teaching Guide for Nurses*, 4th ed. (New York: Planned Parenthood—World Population, 1973). *Obstetric, Gynecologic, and Neonatal Nursing Functions and Standards* (Chicago: Nurses Association of the American College of Obstetricians and Gynecologists, 1974), pp.

29–31. Miriam Manisoff, "The Family Planning Nurse-Practitioner: Concepts and Results of Training," *American Journal of Public Health*, no. 1 (Jan. 1976), **66**:62–64. Mary R. Zabarenko and Patricia K. Betnarz, "A Selected Annotated Bibliography on Midwives and Family Planning, Part II," *Journal of Nurse-Midwifery*, no. 3 (Fall 1977), **22**:32–38.

67. Miriam T. Manisoff, "Psychosocial and Cultural Factors in Family Planning," pp. 227–228, in Joy Clausen and others, *Maternity Nursing Today*, 2nd ed. (New York: McGraw Hill Book Company, 1977).

68. Barbara L. Tate, *The Nurse's Dilemma: Ethical Considerations in Nursing Practice* (Geneva: International Council of Nurses, 1977), pp. 10–12; 38–39. T. James Trussell and others "Efficacy Information in Contraceptive Counseling: Those Little White Lies," *AJPH*, no. 8 (Aug. 1976), **66**:761–767. Julia L. Tanis, "Recognizing the Reasons for Contraceptive Nonuse and Abuse," *MCN*, no. 6 (Nov./Dec. 1977), **2**:364–369.

69. See Robert A. Hatcher and others, *Contraceptive Technology 1978–1979*, 9th ed. (New York: Irvington Publishers, Inc., 1978), for information and overview of current knowledge on all methods of contraception. Linda K. Huxall, "Today's Pill and the Individual Woman," *MCN*, no. 6 (Nov./Dec. 1977),

2:359–363. Sr. Natalie Elder, "Natural Family Planning: The Ovulation Method," *Journal of Nurse-Midwifery*, **23**:25–30. Shirley Okrent, "Family Life Education in a Family Planning Clinic," *Bulletin of the American College of Nurse-Midwives* (1970), **15**:78–85.

70. Nancy F. Woods, *Human Sexuality in Health and Illness*, 2nd ed. (St. Louis: The C.V. Mosby Company, 1979), pp. 95–106; 228. Ramona T. Mercer, ed., *Perspectives on Adolescent Health Care* (Philadephia: J. B. Lippincott Company, 1979). See also, Sol Gordon, "What Adolescents Want to Know," *AJN*, no. 3 (Mar. 1971), **71**:535, and H. J. Osofsky and J. D. Osofsky, "Let's Be Sensible About Sex Education," *AJN*, no. 3 (Mar. 1971), **71**:532.

71. Leah L. Curtin, "The Nurse as Advocate: A Philosophical Foundation for Nursing," *Advances in Nursing Science*, no. 3 (Apr. 1979), **1**:1–10.

72. Tate, op. cit., pp. 34–35; 10–11. U.S. Catholic Conference, "Ethical and Religious Directions for Catholic Health Facilities, 1971," in *EB* **4**:1755–1757. Note especially statements 18 and 19.

73. Note the situation of Ms. Tuma, RN, discussed in Sr. A. Teresa Stanley, "Is It Ethical to Give Hope to a Dying Person?" *Nursing Clinics of North America*, no. 1 (May 1979), **14**:69–80.

ADDITIONAL BIBLIOGRAPHY

Phillips Cutright, "Illegitimacy: Myths, Causes and Cures," *FPP*, no. 1 (Jan. 1971), **3**:25–48.

Stephanie Mills, *The Joy of Birth Control*, 2nd ed. (Atlanta: Emory University Family Planning Program, 1977).

Karen Robb Stewart, *Adolescent Sexuality and Teenage Pregnancy: A Selected, Anno-*

tated Bibliography with Summary Forwards (Chapel Hill: University of North Carolina, 1977).

Student Committee on Sexuality at Syracuse University, *Sex in a Plain Brown Wrapper*, 2nd ed. (Philadelphia: Planned Parenthood of Southeastern Pennsylvania, 1976).

Chapter 4

Abortion As an Ethical Issue

INTRODUCTION

Probably no ethical issue on the current American scene is as volatile as abortion.[1] Pro-life and pro-choice forces seem locked in a seemingly endless struggle. At times the battle breaks into physical violence. More often it proceeds through court proceeding after court proceeding, legislative hall after legislative hall.[2]

Three Considerations

The legislative and court proceedings reflect the heavy legal overtones of the abortion issue. In 1973, the Supreme Court decided (seven to two) against laws restricting abortions in general but left the way open for restrictions under some circumstances.[3] We will come back to this in a moment. Two prior considerations are the questions of when life begins and its related theological question of "ensoulment."

A Series of Questions: Interweaving all three elements—law, life, soul—is one part of the broad issue of rights. In this case, the question of rights develops into a series of questions. Does the fetus have rights? If not, why not? If so, what are they? Do pregnant women have rights? This last question gives rise to further ones. How did she get pregnant (rape, voluntarily, accidentally, by choice)? Do third parties have rights? Included here are such people as the father, the doctor who is asked to perform an abortion, the nurse who is assisting her, the one(s) paying the bill (who may be the taxpayer), society (perhaps in the form of the state with its concern for health, welfare, good order), the church or religious group.

Three Perspectives

It was noted earlier that there is a tendency to divide the contraceptive issue between the religious groups of Catholic and Protestant.[4] A more accurate perspective might be the distinction between liberal and conservative, a spectrum that includes Jews, Christians, religious, secular, and so on.[5] We repeat that caution here, aware that according to one estimate (undocumented) one half of the pro-life movement draws its support from the Catholic Church. The same source, however, notes that among women getting abortions, the percentage of Catholics parallels the percentage of Catholics among the population studied.[6] This was noted earlier for contraception. This is reminiscent of Garrett Hardin who notes that men make the laws and women do what they need to do.[7]

One might see here three main positions on abortion. There are those who are against it under any circumstances (a very small minority as we shall see). Others are for complete freedom of choice by the pregnant woman. To our knowledge, no significant number of people or any significant group has declared officially that women must get abortions, although the idea comes up for some circumstances. In general, the first position might preclude the rights of the pregnant woman. The second position might preclude the rights of others.[8]

The third position is, of course, somewhere between the two extremes. Judith Jarvis Thomson in her "A Defense of Abortion" does not argue for abortion under any circumstances whatsoever.[9] The Catholic Church does not argue against abortion regardless of circumstances. The distinction between rules ethics and situational ethics is blurred here because both of these "rulists" take the situation into account. This blurring is characteristic of the broad middle ground as well as for the two extremes.

HISTORY

Historically, abortion has been around for a very long time.[10] A Chinese document suggested mercury as an abortifacient 4,500 years ago. The Ebers papyrus of Egypt gave directions for abortions about 1500 B.C. This longevity in itself does not make abortion right, or wrong. It does alert us that the contrasting views outlined here have been around for some time. We do not expect to solve the conflict, any more than the Supreme Court did, but perhaps we can contribute to some deeper understanding.

Ancient Law Codes

An Assyrian law from 1200–1400 B.C. punished a woman for self-induced abortion by death without burial. The latter meant her spirit wandered on earth and she would not rest in peace. Impalement without burial was decreed even if she died from the abortion. Accidental miscarriage might come if a pregnant woman was struck by another. Punishment varied, depending on the social status of the woman and whether her husbancd had any sons. In general, if the result of the blow was only a miscarriage, the striker was fined. If the struck woman died, the striker paid with his life, or his wife or daughter was put to death. If the struck woman was a commoner or a slave, there might be one fine for the fetus[11] and double that fine if the woman died. This is also reflected in the more ancient Law Code of Hammurabi, about 1700 B.C., which some biblical scholars see as background for the Hebrew Scriptures, where there is one reference to abortion.[12]

Biblical Reference

The single biblical reference to abortion is in Exodus 21:22–23. If two men in a fight accidentally hit a woman and cause a miscarriage, the one hitting her will be fined if that is all that happens. However, if harm follows, "you shall give life for life." This capital punishment suggests that "harm" means the death of the woman. Hence, the fetus may be seen as "not life." Yet, there is a wrong here, for the husband gets the fine payment. This assumes the husband did not do the striking. It also assumes the fetus is his property. The woman is not considered. She apparently has no property rights in the fetus. Her health is not at issue, only her death.[13]

An important change is found in the translation of this verse into Greek (about 250 B.C.) when a distinction is made between an unformed fetus (just a fine) and a formed fetus (life for life must be given). We do not know whether the change is a mere accident of translation or if it reflects the views of Greek philosophers such as Aristotle. Although both he and Plato, as noted in Chapter Three, advocated abortion as a means of holding down the population, this view of the fetus became important. Aristotle believed that prior to quickening (forty days for the male and ninety days for the female, in his view), the human fetus had only a vegetable or animal soul. The human (rational) soul came with quickening. The translation of Exodus 21 into Greek may reflect this Aristotelian thought. Because Christians usually used the Greek translation of the Bible (called the Septuagint), the translation had a major influence in Christianity.[14]

Talmudic Reference

Later, the Jewish Talmud allowed for dismembering a fetus to save the life of the mother (Mishna, Oholot, 7:6).[15] The Talmud teaches that prior to birth, the fetus is part of the pregnant woman, like an arm or a leg. This same perspective is found in Greek and Roman law.[16] Connery states that early Roman law contained no penal statute against abortion. He believes that there was no problem until the first century B.C. Because the Hippocratic oath (400 B.C.) pledges the physician not to give an abortifacient, it would seem the issue was, of interest then or there would have been no need for the directive. At any rate, it was so common in the first century A.D. that Seneca paid tribute to his mother for not aborting him.[17]

Objections to Abortion

The objection to abortion by Roman writers concerned the frequent deaths of noble women and the lack of children among them because of abortions. From an earlier day, the father had complete power in the family, including the power to kill his children[18] and to order his wife to get an abortion. However, if a wife got an abortion without his permission, the husband had grounds for a divorce.

The first laws against abortion came during the reign of the Emperor Hadrian (A.D. 135). They were designed to protect the husband's property rights. A woman convicted of abortion could be exiled. The fetus was not considered a "life" so the woman was not guilty of homicide. Parenthetically, it should be noted that Roman law gave inheritance rights to a fetus. If the husband died while his wife was pregnant, the resultant child was considered an heir to the estate. Later, in the second century A.D., the principle developed that the fetus was seen as a child already born when that was to its advantage.[19]

Some insist on the continuity of early Christianity with Judaism while also insisting Christianity was against abortion from the beginning because abortion was seen as murder. The Jewish perspective here is found in the Septuagint Bible and in the works of the important Jewish philosopher Philo. Philo declared abortion after the formation of the fetus to be murder. Palestinian Judaism (the Pharisees; the Talmud) continued to see life beginning at birth.[20] The Christian New Testament contains no teaching on abortion, although some derive a teaching from the concern of life. Some early Christian writers wrote against abortion, arguing against the charges by anti-Christians that Christians were cannibals. The charges stemmed from the eucharist in which Christians symbolically ate the body and drank the blood of Jesus in the form of bread and wine. Presumably, the charge could be refuted by accusing the Romans of infanticide and abortion.[21] The background to the conflict is that Christianity was an illegal religion until A.D. 317.

WHEN IS LIFE, LIFE?

The ambiguity of the question, when is life, life,[22] continued throughout much of our history to the present day. A major part of that ambiguity turns on the question of when life begins. One view claims that life began with the creation, or that first fusion of molecules in the primordial ooze. That is to say, life began only once. Since then, there has been continuity of life. In our concern with abortion, that means life continues from the sperm and the egg to the fertilized egg and, hence, to the fetus and the newborn, and on and on. This leads to the suggestion that the whole question of when life begins is a non-question, a smokescreen put up by pro-life forces to stop all abortion.[23]

One protestant ethicist claims that modern medicine has answered the age-old question. Life begins with fertilization of the egg, according to modern science.[24] A Catholic scholar claims that one cannot talk about abortion without talking philosophy.[25] He might not agree that medical science has nothing to do with it, but for sure, the issue of when life begins is a philosophical question, not only a scientific one.

Quickening

The chief philosopher here is Aristotle, whose views on quickening and the soul were noted previously. Quickening as the beginning of life has had widespread acceptance. In America, prior to the late nineteenth century, abortion was common in the first trimester. Abortifacients and services were advertised in newspapers and magazines, including religious publications.[26] The 1973 Supreme Court decision was a return to this common law, with modifications for the second and third trimesters.

The third trimester is usually seen as the time of true viability, the ability of the fetus or newborn to live outside the uterus. The Supreme Court ruling saw this as the time when abortion would be permitted only to save the life of the mother.[27] It was noted earlier that the Talmud allows abortion to save the life of the pregnant woman. This growing concern with the woman's life is also reflected in the ruling, noted in Chapter Three, that a rabbi allowed a woman to take a sterilizing potion when her labor was very difficult. In other words, her life and health were more important than being fruitful and multiplying.

Birth

Although the Talmud allowed ("required," says Feldman) dismemberment of a fetus to save a woman in labor, if the head was born, this extreme measure was no longer allowed. This reflects a fairly widespread view that life begins when the person is born (Plato).[28] Sometimes this is explained in terms of taking the first breath. (Stoics)[29] This is based on the idea that when God created man, He breathed into him the breath of life (Genesis 2:7).

Life seen as beginning at birth was the common view in the Roman Empire and is reflected in the Roman laws. The Stoic philosophers held this view. Augustine's view on contraception appears to have developed in opposition to the philosophies of his day, philosophies which he adhered to and then repudiated. In the early centuries of Christianty's rise to power, Stoicism was one of the main competitors for the loyalties of the intellectuals and the ruling classes. It is perhaps not surprising that Christian writers tried to show the superiority of their philosophy over the others.

Christianity rose to power with Constantine in A.D. 325. One view of the resultant cooperation was that the beliefs of those Christians who were against contraception and abortion made common cause with the Empire's growing need for troops for its armies. This represents an early form of the opposition to Margaret Sanger's work. She was accused of genocide (before the word was coined) because she opened her first birth control clinic in a Jewish neighborhood (at the request of the women of that neighborhood). After World War I, governments opposed her work because they wanted to replenish their populations after the slaughters of the war.[30]

A Soul Is Not for Walking On

Some people treat the abortion question only as a matter of life.[31] Traditionally the fetus has not been seen as only alive or not alive. The question has turned on the presence of a soul.[32] Aristotle's concept of the human soul being given at quickening had wide influence. The technical term here is *ensoulment.* His view is still present today. Alternate views tend to coincide with the question of when does life begin. Our English *soul* is the Greek *psyche* and the Hebrew word *ruah.* It is the latter word that is found in Genesis 2:7, so the breath that God breathed into the first man might be translated as the *soul.*

Traducianist: The traducianist view is that the soul is transmitted from the parent. Because ancient medicine saw the male as providing the vital force, which women merely passively received, this soul was seen as coming with the semen. It was not until 1827 that Karl Ernest von Baer discovered ova. Ferdinand Keber observed the union of a spermatozoa with an ovum in 1853. The merger of chromosomes was observed by Oscar Hertwig in 1875.[33]

The so-called *vital life force* in the male seed is still part of the thinking of some ethicists, as noted earlier. Interestingly enough, it relates directly to the view voiced by Hardin that life is continuous. It also relates to the objection to any kind of birth control that constitutes wrongful emission of seed (sperm). Although some Christian writers have suggested that the life of the sperm and the egg must be taken seriously, to our knowledge, no one has suggested that all 200 to 300 million sperm in every male ejaculate must be baptized, or even the 100,000 to one million oocytes in the female infant, or even the 390 that are actually ovulated in the average female's lifetime.[34]

Creationist: The creationist view is that each soul is newly created. This might be interpreted as ensoulment at birth, or at quickening. It is more commonly related to conception.[35] In times past, this has led to the belief that the products of natural miscarriages (estimates range from 20 percent to 50 percent

of all pregnancies) must be baptized. In more recent times, it has been found that many natural miscarriages occur very early in the pregnancy cycle, so early, in fact, that women often miscarry without even realizing they were pregnant. That may include a fertilized egg that does not attach. The problem of baptism for these souls has not yet been solved.[36]

Others: One suggestion has been that ensoulment, and hence life, comes at the time of implantation or at the blastocyst stage of the zygote development. This alleviates the baptismal problem. It also may be the position of the Catholic scholar John T. Noonan. He suggests that three main reasons have been advanced for abortion. These are to save the life of the mother, to spare a rape victim, and to prevent a defective child being born. He sees medical science as eliminating the first problem. Better drug control will eliminate the third reason. The second is handled by the now standard practice of sterilizing the uterus at once to destroy spermatozoa, or if there has been a delay for several days, uterine curettage will take care of the matter. Because Noonan objects to abortion, this presumably means he does not see these sterilizing and curettage procedures as abortifacient. It would seem he agrees with some kind of later ensoulment.[37] Thomas Aquinas thought there was no human being at all during the first few weeks of pregnancy.[38]

It is important to note here that the Catholic Church has urged its people to act as if ensoulment takes place or that life begins with conception. However, the Church has never officially ruled on this. The pope has not declared it *ex cathedra dogma,* and the official Council Vatican II, refused to legislate on this. A 1974 declaration on abortion also "passed" on this question. So it remains open for future modification, perhaps in Noonan's direction.[39]

THE LAW

The overlap between ethical and legal concerns[40] has been noted previously. The history of laws and religious teaching about abortion have paralleled that of contraception. Just as contraception has been frequently called murder, so has abortion. Contraception has achieved greater acceptance. When the Protestant-inspired laws against contraceptive information or materials were declared unconstitutional, there was no reaction comparable to that against the Supreme Court's ruling on the Protestant-inspired abortion laws. Whether abortion, already widely accepted, will also someday win more complete acceptance remains to be seen.[41] By 1976, nearly two thirds of the world population lived in countries with liberalized abortion laws, compared to one third in 1971, a rather rapid spread of acceptance. Estimates of worldwide abortions range from 25 million to 50 million per year.[42]

History: James C. Mohr,[43] in his history of abortion in the United States, notes that the state laws struck down in 1973 were largely generated between 1825 and 1870. He claims that the laws were pushed through by doctors who had graduated from medical schools. He suggests that the move put the "irregulars" out of business. These were people who learned medicine as apprentices, by accident or necessity on the frontiers, by informal training in "folk medicine." Some of these practicioners were women.[44] Some of the irregulars provided abortion services. Some of the regulars did, too, but it was frowned upon. The Hippocratic oath was the ideological standard for many regulars. When the laws were pushed through, it was on the grounds that abortion was dangerous to the health of women. The laws generally, however, punished the one performing the operation rather than the woman. It was also noted that Catholics had large families but the birthrate was declining for white Anglo-Saxon Protestants (WASPS). The appeal was thus a religious and racist one—to stop WASP women from aborting so as to keep America from being overwhelmed by Catholics, many of whom were from southern and eastern Europe.[45]

Present: It took fifty years but, by 1870, most of the states had laws against abortion, frequently based on concern for women's health.[46] None of the laws were concerned with the men who got the women pregnant. In their decision against the abortion laws that had accumulated by 1973, the Supreme Court justices took note that it is now more dangerous to women's health to have a baby than to have an abortion.[47] Thus, earlier reasoning was set aside, except that the danger of an abortion increases in the second and third trimesters. So the Court left the states the option of protecting maternal health in the latter two thirds of pregnancy, but in the first trimester, the United States was returned to a pre-1870 or, rather, pre-1825 status, in which a woman in the first trimester of pregnancy was free to get an abortion if she wanted one.[48]

The Court stated that no answer was being given to when does life begin, a question that theologians, philosophers, and medical people had been unable to answer to everyone's satisfaction. The response from these several quarters and from the pro-life groups was soon in coming. The most obvious implication has been noted earlier, that in effect the Court was going with viability for the beginning of life.[49] However, it put a higher valuation on a woman's life, for even in the third trimester, abortion was acceptable if necessary to save the woman's life.

The Court reinstated early American common law, which was taken over in part from English common law. The Protestant-inspired abortion banning movement in England took place about 1800.[50] England's new liberal abortion law went into effect in 1967. The United States Supreme Court decision reflects both philosophical and religious concepts. The quickening and ensoulment ideas of Aristotle may be part of this, but not his view that the male is superior to the female and hence ensouled fifty days earlier. The views of the Stoic, Jewish, and Roman laws that life begins with separation from the mother or with the first breath are also reflected here. The Talmud's concern with the life of the mother is included as well.[51]

ATTITUDES

It sounds harsh to say that historically Christianity has had no concern with the life or health of women. Perhaps it is an overstatement. Thomas Aquinas saw women as God's mistake. Sex was evil and because women remind men of sex, then women entice men to sex, so women are evil. The fetus is seen as either fully or potentially human, so abortion is wrong. Extreme views were that if a pregnancy was going to kill a woman, there was nothing to be done about it, because it is woman's nature to have children. That view is extended to contraception in that if too many children are killing a woman, she will just have to die. These views were carried over into Protestantism with the Protestant Reformation, and in no sense were they limited to one Christian group.[52]

On the one hand, it is important to note that prior to the rise of modern antiseptic practice, abortion was dangerous. So was childbirth. So the problem was not one of concern for the safety of the women, except that if an abortion killed a woman, she was no longer in a position to produce more children, important for the state's armies, if nothing else. So abortion was a crime against the state.

In fairness too, we must rush to underline that the change in attitude toward abortion in the present time is not limited to one religious group. Maintaining older views is not limited to one religious group. Neither change or maintenance is limited to religious groups either, but is widespread in the secular world as well.[53] It might be helpful to look at some of the changes.

Effect of Technology

Much of the current discussion in medical ethics comes from the rise of new technologies. This is true in abortion, as in many other medical procedures. Instead of the sterilizing potions mentioned in the Talmud and in Roman law (which apparently killed as often as they aborted), there now are saline solutions and oxytocic drugs. Instead of kicking his wife in the stomach to cause an abortion as a priest was accused of doing in the third century,[54] a man can take his wife to get an antiseptic abortion. She can take herself there without the fear that an abortion is grounds for divorce, at least as such. And the ten-minute aspiration method surely is an improvement over all the ancient suggestions for abortifacients, not to mention the back alley knitting needles.[55]

The new technology gives rise to the question, "Now that we can, should we?" For many, the answer is yes. For many others, the answer is no. The no-sayers tend to turn on the issue as previously outlined, that the fetus is a person or at least potentially so. Thus an abortion is killing a human being and it is murder.[56] Although this is substantially the position of the Roman Catholic Church, and hence the frequent identification of the Church with the pro-life movement, the dominant teachings of the Church allow for at least two exceptions.[57]

Conditional Pro-Life: The traditional example is a cancerous uterus. If the doctor removes the uterus while the woman is pregnant, he has, in fact, performed an abortion. That is acceptable in Catholic teaching because of the law of double or secondary effect. Technically speaking, the intention was the removal of the uterus. The abortion was an unintended (supposedly), though necessary, secondary factor in the operation.

The second exception is an ectopic pregnancy, which occurs at the rate of one to every seventy-eight uterine pregnancies, according to a 1975 study. This exception came after a long debate. Both fetus and the pregnant woman will die in such a case. Traditionally, when the health or the life of the woman is at risk, she just has to take her chances. In the ectopic pregnancy, the abortion is allowable. This is not, however, officially an exception. Rather, it was decided that the fallopian tube was pathological, so the tube could be removed. Salpingectomy is common even in Catholic hospitals.[58]

The long-standing objection to exceptions is what is known as the wedge argument. If you allow one exception, you have the wedge in the argument that may be used to allow other exceptions, and eventually everything is an exception. It's also called the slippery slope argument. The same argument is used against contraception. If you make one exception in the use of contraceptives, you have opened the door to complete and absolute promiscuity. Opponents to this kind of thinking point out that it hasn't happened. It has also been noted that traditional arguments are rationalistic. Abstractions remove the issues far from real life. While the academicians debate, the lives of real people are affected. One suggestion is that we be more human and humane.[59]

Conditioned Pro-Choice: Those who say yes to abortion may deny that the fetus is a person, or a human being. Hence, abortion is not murder and is allowable at will. More often, people say yes to some abortions, perhaps even most, but not all. The exception agreed on by most yes-sayers is that abortion should not be done for trivial reasons.[60] The difficulty here is that one person's trivia may be someone else's life and death.[61] It is often alleged that mere financial difficulty is hardly a reason for abortion. If the children one has are starving while living in a slum, a pregnant woman might want an abortion whether someone else thinks finances are trivial or not. The Roman writers who objected to abortion noted its prevalence among the nobility. In Western culture today, it is widely known that the rich can and have almost always been able to get an abortion. The rich get richer and the poor get children.[62]

Abortion for sex selection has been discussed at some length in the ethical literature on abortion. Amniocentesis not only reveals many genetic defects. It also tells the sex of the fetus. This may be important for sex-linked defects, say where the male has it but the female is normal or a carrier. However, some abortions are done because the parents want a boy rather than a girl, or vice versa. A report from China concerned one hundred women. Amniocentesis showed fifty-three pregnant with male fetuses and forty-seven with female fetuses. One male was aborted and twenty-nine females were aborted. Some see this as an abuse of amniocentesis. Some see abortion for this reason as a trivial reason.[63] For ZPG, it would be a tremendous advantage not to have to keep having children until you got the girl you wanted. It would also be less expensive than raising additional children. Others say we should take what we get and not try to control such things.

Maybe, Sometimes

As noted earlier, the Supreme Court allowed abortion even in the third trimester to save the life of the woman. Saving life is the most common exception in all laws restricting abortion. It is the most common exception in the thinking of people who allow abortion under some circumstances. Another exception is pregnancy that results from rape or incest, and a third exception is the possibility of a defective child. Although Noonan says these three are no longer problems, some people continue to see abortions for these reasons as permissible, and necessary.[64]

Those who allow abortion in the event of a pregnancy caused by rape may claim that the trauma of rape is bad enough. There is no need to punish the victim of criminal assault by forcing her to have a child against her will. They point out that traditionally it is the criminal, rather than the victim, who is punished. Rape continues to be the major exception to this double indemnity.[65]

The potential for a defective child is a special case also. We noted in the chapter on genetics Bently Glass' dictum that "every child has the right to be normal." We noted there, too, that amniocentesis now makes possible the discovery of this kind of problem more surely than mere statistical probability. One might be concerned with the child born of rape for the psychological burden under which it will live in a society that still looks down upon illegitimate children. However, the child born with genetic problems may suffer physically as well as psychologically. The child without mental development may not be aware of the latter.[66]

How much physical and other kinds of pain and suffering do we allow before we decide that a fetus with genetic defects can be aborted? Pro-life forces say that is not for us to decide. Pro-choice forces say that *not* to decide is to decide on a life of suffering for someone else.[67] Very commonly, the abortion decision is again made on a continuum. A Tay-Sachs victim has at most a few years, filled with rapidly decreasing mental awareness and much pain. A Down's syndrome fetus carries an unknown quality. Once born, the child might be only mildly affected, or grossly so. In something like Huntington's chorea, symptoms do not appear for thirty or forty years, but they are excruciating when they do arrive. Judgments in these cases are likely to be made, not on the basis of when someone thinks ensoulment takes place, but on a more practical level such as the health of the mother, the number of other children already present, the family finances, and a genuine concern for the future life of the affected fetus. We are once more concerned with quality of life. Pro-choice forces claim too often the antiabortion arguments stop with the sanctity of life in the uterus and give no consideration to the quality of life after birth.[68]

Who Is to Say?

The whole history of abortion might be seen in the light of the question, Who is to say? While the men make the laws, the women do what is necessary. Hardin points to the Rif tribe in which the men declared no abortion under any circumstances. The women go to market on women's day. On that day, the men stay away. On that day, the woman who wants to do so, can get contraceptives or an abortion. A woman shared with Hardin her experience in getting an abortion in Catholic Italy. It was easy. More than three million abortions were performed in Italy in 1968. These were all illegal, of course.[69]

It has been suggested that no woman should have to bear a child she does not want and no child should have to be born unwanted.[70] Many pro-life people are not only against abortion but against contraception as well.[71] The major exceptions are abstinence and the rhythm method. Presumably, abstinence is the only guarantee against pregnancy. Once pregnant, pro-life arguments say a woman must bear the unwanted child. The more liberal pro-lifers may allow exceptions, as noted, for the life of the woman. The humanity or potential humanity of the fetus is not set aside, but the woman's right to life is seen as a higher priority. Pro-choice forces tend to give the woman's life priority as well as her decision, which may rest on any one of the reasons cited.

An organization called Birthright was founded by Louise Summerhill in 1968. Its creed is, "The right of every mother to give birth; the right of every child to be born." The concern here is to encourage women to carry their pregnancy to term. Birthright offers financial and medical assistance as well as counseling. Although Birthright is nonsectarian, numbers of religious groups also offer assistance programs. A coordinating agency for such groups is Alternatives to Abortion.[72] Pro-choice proponents do not all agree on a "right" to give birth. They do agree on the woman's right to choose, which right she cannot legally exercise if the law does not allow abortions. The family and society also have rights.

Missing in all of this is the male who provided the sperm. Does he have any rights? In Roman times, the male was all-powerful. Until very recent times, and still in many ways, the male of the species controls the laws, the ethical codes, the medical practice, and most other factors involved in abortion. The principal change is that large families are no longer an asset, so he may want the abortion as much as the woman. Throughout history, men who started an illegitimate pregnancy have often been willing to have the woman get an abortion as well. Suppose the male does not want an abortion? The law has now changed in the direction of women's rights, so a woman may get an abortion without her husband's permission. He may know nothing about it. He may object and be overruled.[73]

In some areas, a minor may not get an abortion without her parent(s)' permission, so not all women are free to make their own decision legally.[74] This is also true for women too poor to go through the legal process. Obviously, if one cannot pay for the service, one is not free to make a choice, unless it is done illegally or by home remedies. Pro-choice forces see this as an old concept—the one too poor to afford an abortion is often refused assistance. For those on welfare, it is estimated that abortion services cost government and the taxpayer a small fraction of welfare costs.[75]

The Population Explosion

Discussed earlier were governments that have allowed abortion to control population, in contrast to governments that wanted unrestricted population growth. One might see here an encouragement to abortion, although as far as we know no government actually forces any individual woman to have an abortion.[76] The service is there if she wants to use it. On the other hand, numerous governments legally try to stop women from having abortions. Eastern European governments have practiced an on-and-off policy of free abortions and restricted abortions. Such a policy appears to be a matter of manpower needs.

One source says the number of abortions in Eastern European countries is getting out of hand and is an embarrassment. He does not say why. One suspects the embarrassment is his rather than the state's. Romania had a permissive law and reduced its birthrate from 35.1 to 13.7 per thousand. Then in 1966, it restricted abortions and the number of legal abortions dropped to less than one fifth, from 1,115,000 in 1965 to 206,000 a year later. The birth rate went up to 27 per thousand. Between 1965 and 1972, the maternal death rate from abortion (illegal) increased eight times.

Japan is perhaps the most well-known international example of a country that has reduced its birthrate. The law is not really permissive, but it is interpreted in a pro-choice fashion. Japan's birthrate was reduced from 30 to 19 per thousand between 1948 and 1969. Russia provided free abortions in 1920, applied a fee in 1924, restricted the procedure in 1935 and 1936, and then liberalized the law in 1955. Currently, abortions exceed live births in Russia, as well as in Japan, Italy, Portugal, and Uruguay.[77]

Legal and illegal abortions throughout the world are variously estimated at from 25 to 50 million every year. It is one of the most widely used forms of both control in the world. A recent report notes abortion had dropped to third place, after sterilization and the pill. One in four pregnancies is terminated by abortion. In this country, it is the second most common operation after tonsilectomy.[78] Whether women get abortions for medical reasons or for practical reasons is not known. It would appear that the practical necessities of life often carry more weight than the theoretical reasons advanced by government, religion, or even husbands.

Summary of the Issues

Abortion raises the basic issue of when life begins and the closely related theological concern of ensoulment. Under the general category of consent is the question of who decides. Is it the pregnant woman? Or do others such as the male partner, the doctor, or society decide? And on what grounds is the decision made? The fetus cannot make a decision. Does the mother or someone else have a right to make the decision for the fetus for or against abortion? The continuing concern for the sanctity of life remains in tension with concern for the quality of life. Usually, the sanctity of life, sheer existence, applies to the fetus. Quality of life applies to everybody. Freedom of choice applies at first glance to the decision for or against abortion. It also applies to health personnel who may or may not be willing to participate in the procedure.

Pro-life forces, often identified with the Catholic Church but including many others as well, in some sense see the fetus as alive or potentially so, as human or potentially so. Thus, abortion is seen as murder just as contraception was for centuries. Pro-choice forces insist the woman has a right to control her own body, whether it is a matter of her life or health or some practical reason such as finances. The concept of life or potential life may or may not enter into the decision-making process.

NURSES AND ABORTION

Nurses are involved in the ethical issues surrounding abortion as individuals as well as in their professional roles and responsibilities. Not all nurses choose to work in settings where abortions are performed. Whether nurses are exposed to caring for abortion patients or not, surveys have supported the idea that nurses hold certain values on the abortion issue.[79] Whether nurses are pro-life, pro-choice, or hold conditional or situational positions, what they believe about abortion can potentially affect how they relate to women/couples who choose to have or not have an abortion. It is important for nurses to understand their personal position on abortion in order to practice in an ethical manner with due consideration of the client's right to self-determination. Statement One of the *Code for Nurses* gives direction to all nurses who come in contact with patients having an abortion. It reads, "the nurse provides services with respect for human dignity and the uniqueness of the client, unrestricted by considerations of social or economic status, personal attributes, or *the nature of the health problems."*[80] It is suggested that readers keep this in mind as they progress through this chapter.

The Nurse As a Person

Nurses as individuals represent a cross section of the American population with varying value systems, beliefs, and religious foundations, which may influence their stand on the abortion issue. Abortion has been a subject of heated debate, especially in the last few years, and nurses have been actively involved in these debates on all sides of the issue.[81] It would appear reasonable to assume that few, if any, individuals remain totally neutral when abortion is discussed.

Uustal[82] and others[83] write of the need for nurses to clarify what values and beliefs they hold dear as individuals so that their behaviors with clients are consistent with their beliefs. We add that values clarification is also a valuable process for nurses so that they may avoid the unconscious imposition of their own values/beliefs on their clients. Because of the emotional nature of the abortion issue, one's personal value position may be clouded in an actual encounter with an abortion situation. This fact supports the need for understanding one's basic beliefs about abortion before becoming involved in actual patient care situations or choosing not to become involved.

As individuals, nurses develop their position on abortion from a variety of sources. One's religion may be the dominant factor. As noted earlier, there are a variety of religious interpretations of the rightness or wrongness of abortion, and an individual nurse may wholeheartedly adopt the church's teachings on the subject of abortion. Others may develop their value position on abortion from personal experience, either negative or positive, with abortion or caring for patients who are aborting. The nurse is often left as the sole care giver during saline abortion procedures, and repeated exposure to the products of conception may help to shape the nurse's view of the procedure. Whatever the individual nurse's personal beliefs about abortion, it is important to recognize that these may directly influence his/her ability to care for those patients.

The Nurse As Professional

The profession of nursing is a person-centered one; that is, all of the nurse's daily tasks have some relationship to the primary goal of the profession to provide health and illness services for other human beings. The nurse is also the person in most extended time contact with individual patients, and as such may develop the most intimate of professional-client relationships. By virtue of the nature of the nurse-patient relationship, what nurses value as people and which of these values are integrated into their daily practice can influence the quality of care given to other people.[84]

Roles: Today's numerous conversations on patients' rights and responsibilities bring a new focus on the role of nurses and their rights and responsibilities as well. The roles that nurses assume in the area of abortion are basically two: counselor and care giver. Although one may assume that nurses who are opposed to abortion on any grounds would not choose to work in a setting where abortions are performed, these nurses may become accidentally involved in the care process.

Nurses may choose to work in a variety of settings where abortions are discussed or performed. Some of these settings include counseling or screening centers in outpatient hospital departments, private clinics, abortion centers apart from hospitals, or in hospital obstetric and gynecologic units. The nurse who elects to work with abortion patients most likely has some idea of what her own views on abortion are, and for the most part will be accepting of abortion as a choice for pregnant women. There are, however, many reasons that nurses choose a given job (money, location, availability, work hours), so that nurses who do not support abortion as a choice for women may also be working in settings that provide abortion services.

One must be careful to note that personal acceptance of abortion is *not* a prerequisite for professional practice in an abortion unit. Many nurses give a higher priority to the patient's right to self-determination and can appropriately care for the woman who has elected an abortion, even though the nurse does not personally support abortion. Nurses who most strongly support the woman's right to choose an abortion are the most desirable staff members in abortion units.[85]

Attitudes: One of the more crucial problems for nursing is when an individual nurse chooses to work in a setting where abortions are performed without realizing her own negative view of the procedure. Often these nurses treat the abortion patient with disdain and contempt, totally against the guidelines in the *Code for Nurses*. Another problem with nurses displaying hostility and other negative attitudes toward women requesting abortions is that the probability is increased the woman will seek out another source of care, often an illegal or untrained abortionist.[86] These are difficult situations involving peer evaluation/action and the issue of quality of care being given, including the preservation of health.

One reason for nurses' negative attitudes or treatment of abortion patients, in addition to pro-life stances, is the nurses' views that abortion is a medical procedure appropriate only when clearly related to a health impairment.[87] It would seem that this stance denies social, economic, or psychological justification of the procedure. A survey of nurses in Hawaii[88] identified three major reasons for nurses not participating in abortions. These included religion and conscience, ethical stance associated with feelings about the purpose of nursing, and social view of abortion as murder. And yet, a survey of nurses in 1976[89] reported that 54 percent of nurses surveyed responded that to deny care for a postabortion patient is a violation of the *Code for Nurses*, and 44 percent said it was not. It would appear that the abortion issue is one area in which the nurse's personal moral code can be in direct conflict with the professional code of ethics, and may, rightly or wrongly, take precedence in the patient care situation.

Guidelines: In May 1972, the Nurses Association of the American College of Obstetricians and Gynecologists issued the following statement, "Principles and Guidelines on Abortion,"[90] for its members. These guidelines speak to the issue of the nurse's responsibilities in caring for the woman who has elected an abortion, and are offered for

consideration by all nurses as another example of a professional code of ethics.

1. Nurses have the responsibility to provide nursing care for the abortion patient.

2. Nurses have the right to refuse to assist in the performance of abortions and/or sterilization procedures in keeping with their moral, ethical, and/or religious beliefs, except in an emergency when a patient's life is clearly endangered, in which case the questioned moral issue should be disregarded. This refusal should not jeopardize the nurse's employment nor should they be subjected to harassment or embarrassment because of their refusal.

3. Nurses, in dealing with such patients, should not impose their views on patients or personnel.

4. Nurses have the right to expect their employers to describe to them the hospital's policies and practices regarding abortion and sterilization.

5. Nurses have the obligation to inform their employers of their attitudes and beliefs regarding abortion and sterilization.

Conscience Clauses/Coercion

Nurses also have certain rights when dealing with the abortion issue. A number of laws contain a "conscience clause" so that health professionals will not have to participate in a procedure such as abortion or sterilization when it is against their conscience. Ramsey notes, however, the difficulty of putting these conscience clauses into practice and thus supporting the rights of health personnel not to participate.[91]

Numerous examples can be cited of nurses who were discriminated against because of their negative stand on abortion and refusal to care for patients undergoing an abortion procedure. These range from the nurse-anesthetist in training who was refused further cases when she said she could not morally give anesthesia to a patient having an abortion to the nurse working in the operating suite with many other nurses who was abruptly transferred to night shift in psychiatry for refusal to circulate for an abortion procedure. Another form of discrimination may occur with nursing and medical students being "forced" to participate in "educational experiences" such as abortion in order to graduate.

A possible explanation for this type of forced participation in abortion procedures is the lack of clarity on the issue of abortion as a right and whether there exists an obligation on the part of hospitals to provide abortion services, for which trained personnel such as doctors and nurses are needed. Ramsey notes that a general obligation to provide abortion services cannot be made consistent with freedom of conscientious refusal.[92] However, if abortion is a rightful option of pregnant women and no services exist in a given community, what responsibility does the hospital in that community have to provide this medical service? Should public hospitals be required to provide this service if the private hospitals in the community refuse? And what about requiring support of abortion as a prerequisite to admission to obstetrical residency programs?

Many questions can be raised, but answers are unclear on the issue of liberty of conscience and how it might be effectively enforced. Nurses are often caught in the middle of debates on this issue and may be forced into unpleasant working situations by virtue of their moral position and adherence to the professional code of ethics. It is suggested that nurses request information about the employer's stand on abortion prior to employment, and possibly avoid employment in settings that support practices contrary to the nurse's personal or professional code of ethics.

The Nurse as Counselor

Nurses are often the first health professional to interview the pregnant woman who may wish to discuss the possibility of abortion. The counseling role is vital to the health and well-being of these pregnant women, and how the nurse handles this difficult role may influence the woman's choice of termination or continuation of pregnancy. It may also influence the woman's ability to accept her decision, once made.

The first decision involved in counseling is whether to proceed with the pregnancy or to terminate. Who decides and how the decision is made are involved in this process. Some women come to the nurse seeking to investigate the option of abortion but not convinced they will choose that option. Others come for details on how to procure the abortion they have already decided they want. Whatever stage of decision making the pregnant women are in, they may also be in a state of mental, emotional, and moral confusion. According to recent Center for Disease Control statistics on abortion (1976),[93] the majority of abortions were done on unmarried women (75.4 percent) who may need additional counseling as well.

Approach: Suggestions on the approach to counseling are numerous and begin with the nurse creating an atmsophere of safety and acceptance. Mace[94] lists the following steps in abortion counseling, which encompass a variety of authors' ideas.[95] First, encourage the woman to tell her story and get facts straight while the nurse listens attentively and sympathetically. Next, encourage the woman to express her emotions and then help her examine her feelings. The nurse then provides facts about the abortion procedure, cutting bureaucratic tape when possible, and helps the woman move toward decision making. The woman is encouraged to consider the various options available to her (pregnancy, adoption, abortion) and explore with the nurse the expected consequences of each option. The final step in keeping with the professional code of ethics is encouraging the woman to take responsibility for her own life and to act as an autonomous person in accord with her own value system. In summary, the nurse provides preabortion counseling with the goal of offering information, supporting and guiding the woman in the decision-making process, with greatest emphasis on respecting the woman's right to decide for herself which action she will take.

Nurses need to be aware of their limitations in the counseling process and should try to recognize those women who might benefit by referral to social service or psychiatry. Likewise, nurses often note that inclusion of "significant others" in the counseling process may be of benefit to the pregnant woman.

The counseling sessions often include informal teaching on basic reproduction, physiology, and contraception related to the individual's sexual patterns and preferences. In addition, the counselor explains the abortion procedure. Continuity of care giver (usually the nurse), when possible, from the counseling stage through the procedure is also a supportive way of providing total care for the abortion patient. Nurses are well prepared for this type of role if they choose to work with abortion patients. The combination of medical knowledge, social awareness, and feminine understanding by female professional nurses allows them to offer a unique contribution to the total care of women electing an abortion.[96]

The Nurse As Care Giver

Nurses who provide direct care services to a woman having an abortion may be involved in taking the history and performing the screening physical exam, sizing the pregnancy, assisting the physician during the actual procedure, and/or caring for the patient during postprocedure. Whatever the responsibilities accepted, nurses can benefit from a regular evaluation of their moral and ethical stance on abortion so they stay in touch with how their personal position may potentially affect their ability to carry out their professional responsibilities to patients.

Dilemmas: One of the most difficult situations that nurses who support abortion as a choice face is when they are expected to dispose of the products of conception from a saline procedure. Caring for a viable fetus is discussed in Chapter Five. The emphasis here is on the dilemmas of a nurse possibly not being able to medicate patients according to their need because of a physician's negative attitude on abortion and refusal to write the orders for medication, or of a nurse being left with the delivery of the fetus. Many hospital personnel do not believe it necessary to move a woman delivering a sixteen- to twenty-week fetus to a delivery room, so she is often forced to deliver in the bed—a difficult and untidy procedure at best. Nurses working in labor and delivery units are accustomed to assisting with normal births and participating in the joy of the occasion. Having to attend to aborting women in the same setting and often at the same time and facing neonatal death is a most trying situation for the nurse, even if she is supportive of abortion as an option. Many institutions are beginning to recognize the importance of having separate facilities for women who are aborting and those recovering from postabortion. This is one possible solution to the nurse's dilemma with saline procedures, but the nurse must reckon with feelings of caring for stillbirths.

Postabortion care also poses some particular problems for nurses. If the patient is placed in the usual postpartum unit for her recovery, she is close to many mothers with their babies. This situation may be unfair not only to patients, but to nurses as well. It is sometimes difficult to deal with the mixture of feelings as the nurse moves from family units with infants to family units without infants. The postabortion patient is often perceived as more demanding of the nurse's attention. If some nurses are unable to give that attention, the patient will feel ignored. Special counseling needs are also evident, but many nurses may not receive the support and training needed to provide for these needs. Guidelines for approaching counseling, given earlier in this chapter, are pertinent here, also.

The Nurse As Accidental Participant

Nurses who choose for various reasons to not participate in abortion counseling or procedures may become accidental participants. Sometimes nurses are required to cover a specific unit because of staff shortages, and these units may include care of the abortion patients. If this is a common rationale used for assigning a nonsupportive nurse to care for abortion patients, the nurses involved might do well to change their place of employment. Another accidental involvement results from the unpredictability of delivery from saline procedures. Some labor room nurses would not willingly work with abortion patients and choose certain shifts to avoid this possibility (usually evenings or nights). Occasionally the pregnancies terminate on the wrong shift.

The point of mentioning these accidental

exposures to abortion is that nurses who have expressed negative views of abortion may not provide the most supportive nursing care to women having an abortion. The conflict of being forced to work in a setting in which they do not wish to be and holding a pro-life position on abortion may interfere with the nurse's ability to care for the patients without being negativistic or punitive. It is suggested that these nurses be helped to deal with their feelings and sort out the conflict of personal and professional values.[97] It is also hoped that these accidental exposures to abortion will be kept to a minimum in any setting for the good of patient care as well as for the morale of the hospital staff.

CASE STUDIES

A sampling of cases involving nurses and abortion is included here for study and reflection. The Guidelines are suggested as the framework for approaching these cases, and the first case will be partially analyzed to demonstrate use of these Guidelines.

Case #9

Postabortion Counseling

Ms. L. is the nurse assigned to interview and counsel postabortion patients regarding birth control methods before their discharge from the abortion unit of a local hospital. In the course of her daily rounds, she introduces herself to Ms. P., a twenty-two-year-old woman, who seems in good spirits and who is looking forward to going home shortly. During the progress of the interview, the nurse asks Ms. P. which method of birth control she has considered using at the present time. Ms. P. quickly responds that she does not intend to use any method of birth control, and goes on to explain that "I don't have sex that often. Besides, if I get pregnant, I'll just have another abortion if I'm not ready to have kids." The nurse decides to continue the discussion and begins to explain the potential danger to Ms. P.'s health if she has repeated elective abortions. She goes on to state, "and in addition, this hospital strongly recommends that every patient consider using a method of birth control other than abortion." Ms. P. listens patiently, then responds that she doesn't like to use birth control, and she just won't plan on having sex again until she is ready to have a baby. Then the patient turns her back to the nurse and continues to prepare her suitcase for home.

Analysis

1. a. There is current disagreement in the literature as to whether cervical damage results from repeated, forced dilation during first trimester abortion. Consequently, one needs to separate data given to patients on this issue based on fact versus one's personal or professional belief.
   b. The decisions that need to be made are whether Ms. P. intends to use a method of birth control and, if so, which one is most appropriate for her in consideration of her physiological status, sexual patterns, and personal preferences.
   c. The ethical components of the decisions include the patient's right to self-determination in choice of contraceptive method, whether abortion or something else.
   d. It would appear that Ms. P., the nurse, and possibly the hospital are those most involved in the decisions to be made (possible inclusion of future sexual partners?)
2. Further data that may help in this situation include more information on the nurse's responsibility to the institution to make sure postabortion patients accept a method of contraception, what the nurse's values are in regard to birth

control methods and abortion as a choice, and the extent of Ms. P.'s knowledge of reproductive physiology, her own sexual behaviors, and her understanding of other birth control methods.

3. The ethical issues of informed consent, freedom of choice, quality of life, and rights of health professional, hospital, and Ms. P. are central to this case.

4. The first, third, and fourth statements of the ANA *Code for Nurses* may be helpful to the nurse involved in this situation. Interpretive Statements 1.1, 1.4, 1.5, 3.1, and 4.2 seem particularly relevant in this case.

5. The nurse's value system would appear to accept abortion as a choice for women, but not under all possible conditions (used as a method of birth control). The nurse also appears to value her role of providing information about other methods of contraception though one might question her approach to the counseling session. Ms. P. appears accepting of abortion as a method of birth control, even if it means repeated abortions. She also wishes to maintain her right to choose no other form of birth control and to have sex, though unmarried, and accept the risk of pregnancy. Though information is scanty, the hospital appears to accept the responsibility to provide abortion services but asks for patients' choice of contraception other than abortion before discharge.

6. The value conflicts in this situation are between the nurse and patient on the issue of the use of abortion as a method of birth control, between the patient and the hospital on the issue of choosing an alternative method of birth control, and possibly between the nurse and the hospital on the issue of the patient's needing to choose a birth control method before discharge. Because the nurse used "hospital" in her rationale to the patient, it is difficult to know if she did not want to be associated with this policy or merely thought this would add strength to her statement.

7. It would appear that the patient is the most logical one to make the decision on the method of birth control to be used. There is no way anyone else can "use" the birth control for her.

8. Possible decisions or actions range from the nurse's acceptance of the patient's decision to the nurse's insistence that the patient choose a method, at least "for the record." The nurse could call on institutional power and threaten the patient with loss of care in the future, or could approach the patient with information regarding birth control without requiring a choice. Many actions are possible, and which is chosen will, to some extent, determine the ethical nature of the choice.

9. What action(s) would you take as the nurse, and why?

10. What have been your experiences in this type of situation, and what have you learned from analysis of the situation that may be helpful to you in future situations of this kind?

Case #10

Request for Abortion

Mrs. J. has been referred to the nurse-counselor for discussion of her unplanned pregnancy. She is currently ten weeks pregnant. As the nurse begins her questioning about plans for this pregnancy, she notes that Mrs. J. appears angry or tense. She asks Mrs. J. about this apparent anger, and Mrs. J. blurts out that her husband wants this baby but she doesn't. Then she says that she doesn't wish to discuss this any further, and just wants to hurry and finish the necessary details so she can get an abortion and "get this whole mess over with." The nurse accepts Mrs. J's desire to rush although she feels the need to ask her if she has considered the option of carrying this pregnancy to term. Mrs. J. glares at the nurse and retorts, "Oh my God! Not you, too. Everyone is trying to convince me to have this baby, and I'm the one who has to carry it!"

In addition to applying the Guidelines, please consider the following questions:

1. How might you have responded to Mrs. J's request to hurry through the counseling? Relate your reasons for this response to your personal and professional beliefs/values about counseling and abortion.
2. How might you respond to Mrs. J's interpretation that the nurse is trying to convince her to carry this pregnancy to term? Explain your reasons for responding in this manner.
3. What factors might you consider in counseling Mrs. J. that will help to ensure support for self-determination as well as informed consent? (These might include how much information to give on options, when and where one draws the line on information and coercion, and so on.)

Case #11

Referral for Abortion Counseling

Mrs. L., age thirty, has been followed in the Family Planning Clinic sporadically for the past five years. She has used a variety of methods for short periods of time, including foam, diaphragm, and the "pill." During her current visit she states that she thinks she is pregnant. Physical and pelvic examination findings reveal a pregnancy of ten to twelve weeks' gestation, confirmed by pregnancy testing. Mrs. L. requests termination of the pregnancy, and the nurse-practitioner attempts to determine if this is the decision of the moment or if Mrs. L. has talked about this decision before coming to the clinic. Because the nurse-practitioner does not support abortion as an option in controlling family size, she refers Mrs. L. to a colleague of hers who will proceed with the abortion counseling and scheduling of appropriate tests and appointments. Mrs. L. has to wait a half hour to be seen by this colleague, and complains to other patients in the waiting room that the clinic ought not to employ nurses who do not believe in abortion, because they won't give the care needed.

In addition to applying the Guidelines, consider the following questions:

1. Do you think Mrs. L. is justified in her complaint that nurses who do not believe in abortion should not be employed in a family planning clinic? State the rationale for your answer.
2. On what basis would you decide whether the nurse-practitioner functioned in an ethical manner in caring for Mrs. L. and in making the referral to a colleague?
3. How would you respond to a patient you were caring for if she made a decision in direct conflict with your personal value system? Under what circumstances would you continue to provide nursing care?

NOTES AND REFERENCES

1. Generally speaking, we use the term *abortion* to mean induced abortion or therapeutic abortion, and the term *miscarriage* for "natural" abortion. See André E. Hellegers, "Abortion: Medical Aspects," pp. 1–5, *Encyclopedia of Bioethics*, ed. by Warren T. Reich (New York: The Free Press, 1978). The Encyclopedia is cited hereafter as *EB*. We note here that the difficulty in being objective about this subject is in one sense obvious. In some cases, it is a subtle difficulty as in the titles of abortion studies that call abortion an agonizing, or a terrible choice or decision. Women are supposed to have psychological trauma about abortion, say some male authors. The facts are difficult to determine. One survey suggests that 74 percent of the women having abortions had no serious physical or psychological consequences. Jerome W. Kummer reports postpartum psychosis as 2 percent, but it was difficult to find any incidence of postabortion psychosis. Some studies show 1 percent to 2 percent of abortion clients have prolonged guilt or depression. If this is accurate, one could assume that the decision was not so agonizing. In contrast, Dr. and Mrs. J. C. Willke cite studies showing guilt in from 9 percent to 88 percent of the women studied. *Handbook on Abortion* (Cincinnati: Hiltz Publishing Co., 1972), pp. 41–46. See John A. Scanzoni, "A Sociological Perspective on Abortion and Sterilization," pp. 312–326, in *Birth Control and the Christian*, ed. by Spitzer and Saylor (Wheaton, Ill.: Tyndale House Publishers, 1969), p. 317. Anne J. Davis and Mila A. Aroskar, *Ethical Dilemmas and Nursing Practice* (New York: Appleton-Century-Crofts, 1978), p. 91. Jan Wojcik, *Muted Consent* (West Lafayette, Ind.: Purdue University Press, 1978), pp. 55–56. Kummer, "A Psychiatrist's View," pp. 96–105, in vol. 1, *Abortion in a Changing World*, ed. by Robert E. Hall (New York: Columbia University Press, 1970). George H. Kieffer, *Bioethics* (Reading, Mass.: Addison-Wesley Publishing Co., Inc., 1979), pp. 157–175.

2. Susan Fraker and others, "Abortion Under Attack," *Newsweek*, XLL, no. 23 (5 June 1978), 36–37, 39–42, 47, and condensed as "The War Against Abortion," *Reader's Digest*, no. 667 (Sept. 1978), **113**:179–182. It is important to note that the legal issue is different from the ethical. The two concerns overlap, but they are distinct. For example, such Catholic thinkers as Callahan, Drinan, and Wassmer called for abolition of laws on abortion in our pluralistic society. This doesn't necessarily mean they approve of abortion. See Joel Feinberg, "Introduction," pp. 1–9, in *The Problem of Abortion* (New York: Wadsworth Publishing Co., Inc., 1973), p. 6. See Daniel J. Callahan, *Abortion: Law, Choice, and Morality* (New York: Macmillan Publishing Co., Inc., 1970), p. 493. Robert F. Drinan, "Abortion and the Law," pp. 51–68, in *Who Shall Live?*, ed. by Kenneth Vaux (Philadelphia: Fortress Press, 1970). Bernard H. Baumrin, "Toward Unraveling the Abortion Problem," pp. 109–112, in *Bioethics and Human Rights*, ed. by Elsie L. and Bertram Bandman (Boston: Little, Brown and Company, 1978).

3. *Roe* v. *Wade*, and *Doe* v. *Bolton* (22 Jan. 1973) "The 1973 Supreme Court Decisions on State Abortion Laws: Excerpts from Opinion in *Roe* v. *Wade*," Feinberg, op. cit., pp. 180–188.

4. Although we reject the division, we are aware of Kurt Baier's observation that the Catholic opposition to abortion is by common consent the most fully worked out and most carefully reasoned case. In addition, Catholic leaders do not make a narrow sectarian appeal, but claim moral convictions common to our pluralistic society. For the broad appeal and careful reasoning, see, for example, Edwin F. Healy, *Medical Ethics* (Chicago: Loyola University Press, 1956). Baier, "Preface," pp. xv–xviii, in Susan Taft Nicholson, "Abortion and the Roman Catholic Church," *Journal of Religious Ethics Studies in Religious Ethics* II (1978), pp. xvi–xvii. What that means here is that Catholic thought appears again and again as consistently representing one side of the abortion concern. This is, of course, the official position, one with which not all Catholics agree. Nicholson, p. 97, claims Catholic condemnation of certain therapeutic abortions cannot claim the support of secular morality and is inconsistent with Catholic moral theology in other

aspects. Eastern Orthodoxy is generally against abortion because life is the gift of God. Stanley S. Harakas, "Eastern Orthodox Christianity," *EB* 1:347–355. George Grabbe, "Abortion: The Orthodox View," St. Nectarios Educational Series, no. 62, offprint. We thank Dr. Constantine Tsirpanlis for sharing this reference.

Margaret Steinfels introduces a series, "Is Abortion a Religious Issue?" The articles are a response to the Hyde Amendment (1977) which withheld Medicaid funds for abortion except when the woman's life was in danger, there was a grave threat to the women's health, or pregnancy resulted from rape or incest. Kieffer, op. cit., p. 162, noted that 1978 statistics show a 98 percent drop in Medicaid abortions. A lawsuit was filed, claiming the Hyde Amendment unconstitutional because it was based on religious beliefs. The article writers saw religion involved, but answered the question negatively. *The Hastings Center Report* (hereafter *HCR*), no. 4 (Aug. 1978), **8**:12–17. Daniel Lewis and Caroline Herron, "Lines Harden in the Battle Over Abortions," *New York Times* (28 Jan. 1979), p. 2 E. Richard Lincoln and others, "The Court, the Congress and the President: Turning Back the Clock on the Pregnant Poor," *Family Planning Perspectives*, no. 5 (Sept./Oct. 1977), **9**:207–214. From a traditional Jewish perspective, it is a matter of religion because man was created in the image of God. Fred Rosner, "Induced Abortion, Jewish Law and Jewish Morality," *Man and Medicine*, no. 3 (Spring 1976), **1**:213–224. Traditional Christianity has certainly seen it as a religious, that is, moral issue. In 1975 the National Conference of Catholic Bishops issued a "Pastoral Plan for Pro-Life Activities." The bishops call for public and political opposition to abortion (Fraker, op. cit., p. 39). This action would be strange indeed if abortion were not a religious issue, at least for the bishops. The bishops' involvement was resented by several hundred Protestant and Jewish teachers and writers of religious ethics. They supported abortion rights, against the Hyde Amendment, in "A Call to Concern," *Christianity and Crisis*, no. 15 (3 Oct. 1977) **37**:222. The Religious Coalition for Abortion Rights (RCAR) consists of twenty-seven religious and ethical groups. " 'Pro-Choice' Abortion View Given," *The United Methodist Reporter*, no. 8 (2 Feb. 1979), **7**:3. For these

groups, it is a religious issue. R. F. R. Gardiner says keeping religious views out of the abortion question is naive, if not dishonest. *Abortion: The Personal Dilemma* (Old Tappan, N.J.: Spire Books, 1974), p. 76.

In early 1980, Federal District Court Judge John Dooling, Jr., ruled the Hyde Amendment unconstitutional on the basis of the First and Fifth Amendments but not on religious grounds. "Medicaid Abortions: Federal Court Overturns Hyde Amendment," *HCR*, no. 2 (Ap 1980), **10**:2. "Abortion Ruling Brings Commendation," *The Interpreter*, no. 3 (Mar 1980), **24**:38. In July, 1980, the Supreme Court ruled 5–4 that the Hyde Amendment *is* constitutional. The Court refused to consider religious grounds. Justice Harry Blackmun (United Methodist) and Justice William J. Brennan (Roman Catholic) voted with the minority, against the Hyde Amendment. Joyce Hopkins, "Views Mixed on Abortion Ruling," *The United Methodist Reporter*, no. 17 (11 July 80), **8**:1. *The Bioethics Letter*, no 7 (15 July 80), **1**:3 (hereafter TBL).

5. Note that these are general terms, not necessarily equivalent to political or economic conservatives and liberals. See Tom L. Beauchamp and Leroy Walters, *Contemporary Issues in Bioethics* (Encino, Calif.: Dickenson Publishing Co., Inc., 1978), p. 188. Note, too, the interrelatedness of the contraception and abortion issues. Roman Catholic Gregory Baum thinks Catholics opposed to abortion should favor sexual education and birth control. "Abortion: An Ecumenical Dilemma," pp. 24–34, in *Bioethics*, ed. by Thomas A. Shannon (New York: Paulist Press, 1976), p. 31. This is a major change, for traditionally the Catholic Church has linked contraception and abortion as both being murder.

6. Fraker, op. cit. Garrett Hardin, *Mandatory Motherhood, The True Meaning of the "Right to Life"* (Boston: Beacon Press, 1974), pp. 6–7, notes that on the one hand a list of sixty-three groups calling for reform of abortion laws in 1972 included many Protestant churches, but not the Catholic Church. On the other hand, the only Catholic member of the Supreme Court, William J. Brennan, voted with the majority to remove laws against abortion. Hardin also notes a June 1972 Gallup poll in which 65 percent of the Protestants and 56 percent of the Catholics agreed

that the abortion decision is to be made solely by a woman and her physician. In some polls the percentages are even higher. In Roman Catholic Chile, 27 percent of the women in a 1965 study admitted to having an abortion, and in France, a 1961 study showed abortions equal in number to live births. A report said there were 3 million abortions in 1968 in Catholic Italy. These figures, of course, only underline practice while laws and church teaching remain opposed to abortion. See Hardin, op. cit., pp. 32–33. Callahan, op. cit., pp. 163–170. Harold Rosen, "A Case Study in Social Hypocrisy," pp. 299–321, in *Abortion in America*, ed. by Rosen (Boston: Beacon Press, 1967). Carl Djerassi, *The Politics of Contraception* (New York: W. W. Norton, 1979), pp. 22–30, 43. *Medicolegal News*, no. 1 (Feb. 1980), **8**:14. Note also that a liberal attitude among Protestants is a late development, and major Protestant theologians such as Barth, Bonhoeffer, and Thielicke can still be quoted as against abortion. Earlier Protestants such as Luther (1483–1546) and Calvin (1497–1560) were against it. See Drinan, op. cit., p. 54. Paul Ramsey, *Ethics at the Edge of Life* (New Haven: Yale University Press, 1978). Harold O. J. Brown, "Abortion on Demand? Why Protestants Should Oppose the Present U.S. Legal Situation on Abortion," leaflet (Dover, N.J.: Clergy Concerned for Life, n.d.) Dr. and Mrs. J. C. Willke, op. cit., p. 31, quote 1971 and 1972 studies that suggest 80 percent of the population do not favor elective abortion.

7. Hardin, op. cit., p. 32. John T. Noonan, Jr., says that laws made by men are *not* "misogyny" (hatred of women) "as though a conspiracy against womankind had designed the punishment of the risk of pregnancy as a condition of coitus." He also calls pregnancy "the price of natural intercourse" and sees abortion as sadistic or masochistic. "Introduction," *The Morality of Abortion* (Cambridge: Harvard University Press, 1970), pp. xv–xvi. Some agree with him that pregnancy is punishment. This punishment concept may reflect the view that sex is sinful and pregnancy is the price or penance for sin. Others would disagree on both points. Pro-choice proponents might note the punishment is indeed the price men have forced women to pay, by denying contraceptive or abortion knowledge and practice. It is noteworthy that Noonan does not talk about males paying any price, being punished for having sex, or getting someone pregnant. David Mace makes Hardin's point also when he notes that all through the centuries, abortion has continued, even when it was called illegal and immoral. The theories about abortion were developed by men, usually celibate priests, who paid nothing at all for pregnancy and stood to gain. If men had unwanted pregnancies, they would have made different laws. Women faced reality but, as noted in Chapter Three, women were not usually consulted in the development of ethical thought. As more and more women enter the field of ethics, one might expect changes in the rules on abortion, though not necessarily. See Mace, *Abortion* (Nashville, Tenn.: Abingdon Press, 1972), p. 59. William B. Kiesewetter, "Christian Ethics, the Physician and Abortion," pp. 560–566, in Spitzer and Saylor, op. cit. Hardin, op. cit., p. 33. Callahan claims that consistent surveys (unidentified) show women less approving of permissive abortion than are men. "Abortion: Some Ethical Issues," pp. 13–24, in Shannon, op. cit. Kieffer, op. cit., pp. 171–172, points out that 100 percent of the primitive cultures that bar abortion are run by men. Of those that permit abortion, 71 percent are run by women (matrilineal).

8. *If* a pregnant woman with freedom of choice chooses abortion, that choice may violate the rights of the fetus *if* one agrees the fetus has rights. It might also preclude the rights of a husband or potential father, or potential grandparents, or others. The rights of society might go either way, depending on one's point of view. There appears to be some agreement that neither the husband nor anyone else has a right to force a woman to have an abortion, though the Roman husband had this power and it still happens in practice. There are exceptions. See J. M. Finnis, "Abortion VI: Legal Aspects," **EB** 1:26–32. Some claim that women have no *right* to an abortion, such as the Protestant writer John G. McEllhenney. He agrees abortion might be a tragic necessity under limited circumstances, however. *Cutting the Monkey Rope* (Valley Forge: Judson Press, 1973), p. 103. In contrast, the APHA, the National Abortion Rights Action League (NARAL), and others insist women *do* have a right to abortion, and further, that all economic barriers to this

should be removed. "Policy Statements Adopted by the Governing Council of the American Public Health Association, October 18, 1978," *The American Journal of Public Health*, no. 3 (Mar. 1979), **69**:296–313. See further later.

9. *Ethical Issues in Modern Medicine*, ed. by Robert Hunt and John Arras (Palo Alto, Calif: Mayfield Publishing Co., 1977), pp. 140–158.

10. M. S. Guttmacher, "The Legal Status of Therapeutic Abortions," pp. 175–186, Rosen, op. cit., p. 175. George Devereux claims "abortion is an absolutely universal phenomenon." He cannot even imagine a social system without it. "A Typological Study of Abortion in 350 Primitive, Ancient and Pre-industrial Societies," pp. 97–152, in Rosen, op. cit.

11. We use *fetus* throughout in the general sense, aware of technical distinctions. These include conception (the egg is fertilized by the sperm) and the formation of the single-cell zygote. This multiplies to sixteen cells (multicell zygote) in three days. The *conceptus* is this period from fertilization to *implantation* or *nidation* (Latin *nidus* means nest) in seven to fourteen days. The implantation period is also called the blastocyst stage (Greek *blastos* means root or bud; Latin *cyst* from Greek *kystis* means bladder or swelling; Greek *kyein* means to be pregnant), or trophoblast stage (Greek *trophe* means nourishment). The embryo is the development from implantation to the eighth week, the beginning of detectable brain waves. Organs, limb buds, and face begin in the fourth to fifth weeks. Technically, *fetus* (Latin for pregnant) covers the period from eight weeks to term, but fetus is also used for the entire process from conception to birth. See Feinberg, "Introduction," op. cit., pp. 2–3. Beauchamp and Walters, op. cit., p. 188. André Hellegers, "Fetal Development," pp. 194–198, in Beauchamp and Walters. Mace, op. cit., pp. 36–37.

12. James B. Pritchard, *Ancient Near Eastern Texts Relating to the Old Testament*, 2nd ed. (Princeton: Princeton University Press, 1955), pp. 163, 175, 181, 184–185. D. Winton Thomas, *Documents from Old Testament Times* (New York: Harper & Row, Publishers, 1961), pp. 34–35. John Connery, *Abortion: The Development of the Roman Catholic Perspective* (Chicago: Loyola University Press, 1977),

p. 11. Bruce K. Waltke, "Old Testament Texts Bearing on the Problem of the Control of Human Reproduction," pp. 6–23, in Spitzer and Saylor, op. cit.

13. Waltke, op. cit., originally interpreted the silence of the Old Testament as an argument in favor of abortion. The verse does also because the fetus is not life, or does not have a soul. However, the fine and the biblical idea that offspring come from God means the fetus has great value. This Protestant view is opposed by another Protestant who argues from the same verse that there is a soul present from conception. He interprets the "harm" as the death of the fetus or the mother, whereas "no harm" is interpreted as meaning the delivery of a healthy child. John Warwick Montgomery, "The Christian View of the Fetus," pp. 67–89, in Spitzer and Saylor, op. cit. Waltke has since shifted to the view that the fetus is human and should be protected. "Reflections from the Old Testament on Abortion," *Journal of the Evangelical Theological Society*, no. 1 (Winter 1976), **19**:3–13. Connery, op. cit., pp. 16–20, interprets the text as opposed to abortion.

14. Feldman, op. cit., pp. 257–259, 266, 269. The Talmud sees the forty days as the time the fetus changes from mere fluid and forms a human embryo. The Christian theologian Augustine acknowledges this also. Aristotle discusses abortion in his *Politics* VII, 16, 1335. The Plato reference is to *The Republic* V, 460ff. Devereux, op. cit., p. 140, notes that the Greek philosopher Zeno (c. 336–264 B.C.), founder of the Stoic School, did not believe the unborn child had a soul at all. In contrast, the Pythagoreans believed ensoulment was at conception. Davis and Aroskar, op. cit., p. 93. Feldman, op. cit., p. 268. The Eastern Roman (Byzantine Christian) Emperor Justinian, in his law code (A.D. c. 550) exempted from penalty abortions prior to forty days and legalized quickening at forty days for both male and female, but the male-female distinction was still around for centuries. Guttmacher, op. cit.

15. Maimonides (A.D. 1135–1204), the Spanish rabbi and philosopher, interpreted this under the law of self-defense. See Rabbi Arnold E. Cohen, "A Jewish View Toward Therapeutic Abortion and the Related Problems of Artificial Insemination and Contraception," pp. 166–173, in Rosen, op. cit.

16. This is also the position of some liberal pro-choice people today. See Smith, op. cit., p. 40. Joseph Fletcher, *Morals and Medicine* (Princeton: Princeton University Press, 1954), pp. 150–152. Israel R. Margolis carries the Jewish view a step further when he notes that if a fetus dies during birth or even during the first thirty days of infancy, no funeral is held and no Kaddish (memorial prayer for the dead) need be said, for it is as though this child never lived. "A Reform Rabbi's View," pp. 30–33, vol. I, Hall, op. cit.

17. Connery, op. cit., and Noonan, "An Almost Absolute Value in History," in *The Morality of Abortion*, op. cit., p. 7. The Seneca statement is also ascribed to Pliny in the same period. Hippocrates gave a woman directions for an abortion. Immanuel Jakobovitz notes that the ban on abortion may be a Christian addition to the text (Ambrosian manuscript). The pagan version of the Oath (Urbinas manuscript) limits the ban to the use of pessaries. *Jewish Medical Ethics* (New York: The Philosophical Library, 1959), p. 172.

18. This power was eliminated by the Emperor Hadrian in A.D. 135. Hebrew parents had a similar power over their children (Deuteronomy 21:18ff). Later rabbinic interpretation by A.D 200, made this life and death power inoperable (M. San. 8:1ff; B. San. 71a). See David Novak, "A Call to Concern: A Response," *Sh'ma*, no. 144 (23 Dec. 1977), 8:214–215.

19. Noonan, "Introduction," op. cit., pp. ix–xi, notes the increase in legal rights for the fetus in our own day, even as abortion becomes more common. Some of the cases are documented by Thomas F. Lambert, Jr., "The Legal Rights of the Fetus," pp. 369–414, in Spitzer and Saylor, op. cit. Prior to 1946 in the United States, the general rule was no liability for harm done to a fetus, in contrast to the biblical and ancient Near Eastern rule. Since then, numerous cases have upheld liability. This includes harm, such as brain damage, done by doctors. Augenstein, op. cit., p. 117, comments on a state law by which a child after birth can sue for damages going back to the end of the first trimester, but a name and burial are not required for a fetus prior to the end of the second trimester. We might see this legal movement as a return to the Bible and the ancient Near Eastern tradi-

tion but, in the light of the move to legal abortion, it is more of a return to Roman law. Feldman, op. cit., pp. 253–254, compares similarities in the legal status of the fetus in Roman and Jewish law. However, in his opinion, this "could hardly be sufficient for determining the morality of" abortion.

We noted earlier the concept of "wrongful life," as part of our study of genetic and birth defects. In this context, the issue relates to abortion, or, rather, the failure to abort a defective or an illegitimate fetus. Although no one has *successfully* sued parents for failure to abort, it appears to be only a matter of time before this happens. Lambert, op. cit., pp. 397–400, and Philip Reilly, *Genetics, Law and Social Policy* (Cambridge, Mass.: Harvard University Press, 1977), pp. 169–175.

20. Feldman, op. cit., pp. 255, 269. Noonan, "An Almost . . . ," op. cit., p. 18, notes that the distinction between the formed and unformed fetus was eliminated by A.D. 450 and abortion from conception was seen as wrong. Nicholson claims the distinction was not eliminated from canon law until 1918 though excommunication for abortion at any stage of gestation was decreed in 1869, op. cit., p. 14. Feldman, op. cit., p. 269. Actually the issue bounced around among the theologians throughout the centuries, as seen in Noonan's survey and that of Connery, op. cit. The distinction was specifically reintroduced by Gratian (A.D. 1140). Pope Innocent III (A.D. 1216) ruled that a monk was guilty of homicide if the fetus had quickened. While playing with his mistress, the monk had accidentally caused her to miscarry. It is of interest that the problem is the miscarriage. If he was guilty of homicide, he would be suspended from his priestly functions. Apparently it was no problem for a monk to have a mistress and get her pregnant, although Kosnik and others report three years' penance for clerics guilty of fornication. *Human Sexuality* (New York: Paulist Press, 1977). Similarly, Pope Sixtus V excommunicated prostitutes who aborted. Being a prostitute was apparently no problem. Both Connery and Noonan claim that the early Christians were in agreement against abortion. If they were, it was the only thing the early Christians agreed upon, judging by the long record of their disputes.

21. Noonan, op. cit., p. 11, quotes a church

father who wrote that Christians do not hide their fornications by abortion as the Romans, so that shows the Christians respect life and could not be guilty of cannibalism. Connery, op. cit., p. 37.

22. Technically, this is the question of the ontological (being) status. See Beauchamp and Walters, op. cit., pp. 188–189. A common way of phrasing this concern is the humanity or personhood of the fetus. Is it human, or a person? Does it become human at birth, or does it become human earlier, for example, at quickening, or the embryo stage, or at implantation, or fertilization, or some other point such as the forty days? The conservative position tends to place this early at conception or, possibly, implantation. Nicholson, op. cit., pp. 3–12, claims that if the fetus were not human at all, the Catholic Church would still say that abortion is evil. The background is hostility toward sex and sexual pleasure for women. Celibacy is the ideal. Sex is evil and only excusable when for the production of offspring, out of duty to the human race. So contraception and abortion leave one without an excuse for sex. The sin is not the killing of a human being but having intercourse without procreation. It is sexual sin that is being condemned. Note again, however, the monk who was not condemned for having a mistress and sex, but would be condemned if the miscarriage was of a formed fetus. Pope Paul declared again in 1976 the absolute immorality of nonprocreative sex. About one hundred years ago, other voices spoke in favor of sexual pleasure and, more recently, Vatican II spoke in favor of sexual love as having value for marriage. Kosnik and others, op. cit., pp. 48–52.

This attitude toward sex dominated Protestant traditions also until recent times. Feldman, op. cit., pp. 81–105, contrasts this Christian rejection of sexual pleasure with the attitudes of Judaism. God created sex, so it is good. The Hebrew Scriptures encourage men and women within the marriage bond to enjoy the gift of God. Feldman points out two additional factors in the Christian position. A woman cannot have an abortion for that would relieve her of the pain of childbirth to which she is assigned by the curse of Eve. (For Judaism, this is a negative commandment that does not have to be fulfilled.) Similarly, the original sin of Adam and Eve is the reason the fetus must be baptized at all costs. The woman who aborts sends the ensouled infant to hell. Because she is already baptized, canon law is more concerned for the soul of the fetus than for the life of the woman. Feldman, op. cit., p. 270.

Pro-life advocates, the Willkes, suggest we accept our human sexuality joyfully but also responsibly, op. cit., p. 132. That's a position with which many Catholics and people of all religions, or none, would heartily agree.

23. Lisa H. Newton, "No Right at All? An Interpretation of the Abortion Issue," pp. 113–118 in Bandman and Bandman, op. cit. Hardin, op. cit., p. 48. Cyril C. Means, discussion in "Abortion and Animation," vol. 2, Hall, op. cit., p. 10. Fletcher, op. cit., p. 143, makes a similar point and adds that life is a process rather than an event. Even the fertilization of an ovum by a sperm takes two hours. So the "moment of conception" is an old wives' tale. Roger D. Masters asks if sperm and unfertilized eggs have a right to life. In theory, they could be used to create offspring. "Is Contract an Adequate Basis for Medical Care?", HCR, no. 6 (Dec. 1975), 5:24–28. Reality, of course, makes his rhetorical question absurd. Kosnik and others, op. cit., pp. 198–199, report the superstitious awe of semen in the past. Virginia Held notes the arbitrariness of moral concern and legal protection for zygotes but not for the billions of sperm wasted every day through masturbation. "Abortion and Rights to Life," pp. 103–108 in Bandman and Bandman, op. cit. She is not arguing for protection of sperm but for women's right to an abortion.

24. Paul Ramsey, "Points in Deciding about Abortion," pp. 60–100, in Noonan, op. cit., p. 67. Ramsey relates the genetic origin of the individual to the beginning of life in conception. His position here is similar to Noonan's, op. cit., p. 57, who claims that "a being with a human genetic code is a man." Yet he is willing for a rape victim to have a D and C, so at least on occasion he is willing to have the "man" go to its "death." Sissela Bok and others note that if the fertilizd ovum is a "man" in the full sense, logically, we should make monumental efforts to save all natural miscarriages. We should also give proper burial to all we do not save. In view of the inconsistency, she suggests this view of humanity was adopted to oppose abortion rather

than from real belief in the human rights of the first few cells after conception. "Ethical Problems of Abortion," pp. 35–61, in Shannon, op. cit. Held, op. cit., p. 104. Newton, op. cit., p. 113. Fletcher, op. cit., p. 140. Hellegers, op. cit., p. 198, claims that it is not a function of science to prove or disprove where in the conception to birth process human life begins. Several cultures, such as the Chinese and Korean, count a child as nine months or a year old at the time of birth. For them, life begins at conception. This, however, has not stopped abortion in these cultures. Beverly Harrison notes that anyone who ignores the difference between the scientific and the moral paradigms (models, patterns), is committing the naturalistic fallacy in moral argument. The fallacy is Natural Law, whatever "is" is right; that is, it "ought" to be. If "is" equals "ought," we would ban all health care and do what comes naturally. "Continuing the Discussion, How to Argue about Abortion: II," *Christianity and Crisis*, no. 21 (26 Dec. 1977), **37**:311–313. Charles E. Curran, "Abortion V: Contemporary Debate in Philosophical and Religious Ethics," *EB* **1**:17–26.

25. Daniel J. Callahan, "Abortion: The New Ruling, 4," pp. 194–196, in Feinberg, op. cit. Callahan sees the Court decision as deciding life begins with viability. In contrast to the ethicists, but in line with Noonan's *practice*, biologist Alan S. Parkes sees conception as beginning with implantation. Thus, the IUD is not an abortifacient. "The Future of Fertility Control," pp. 205–212, in *Biological Aspects of Social Problems*, ed. by Parkes and J. E. Meade (New York: Plenum Publishing Corporation, 1965).

26. James C. Mohr, *Abortion in America* (New York: Oxford University Press, Inc., 1978). Hardin, op. cit., pp. 1, 46–47.

27. This standard of permission is widely represented in other countries, and in the proposals of the American Law Institute (1962), the American Medical Association (1967), and the American College of Obstetricians and Gynecologists (1968). See Lambert, op. cit., pp. 402, 404, 410.

28. This concept also appears in law. A Pennsylvania judge ruled that feticide was not murder. A man was accused of murdering his wife who was nine months pregnant. The ruling was that he would be tried for only one murder because the fetus did not have an existence independent of its mother, that is, with the umbilical cord tied and cut. "Feticide Ruling," *The Christian Century*, no. 17 (10 May 1978), **95**:496.

Feldman, op. cit., pp. 254–255, 275, "the fetus is not a person." Yet (p. 257), abortion "diminishes God's image." A conservative Protestant volume reflects the variety in Protestant belief but in general holds that an infant is a human being from the moment of birth. The authors also believe that the fetus is not merely a mass of cells but a potential life, so the Christian physician will see abortion only for greater values sanctioned by Scripture. These include individual health, family welfare, and social responsibility. "A Protestant Affirmation of the Control of Human Reproduction," pp. xxiii–xxxi, Spitzer and Saylor, op. cit. The Supreme Court noted the view of life beginning with live birth and related it to the Stoics, the Jews (not unanimous), and large segments of Protestantism. Feinberg, op. cit., p. 185. It is also the view of Shinto, the traditional religion of Japan. See Davis and Aroskar, op. cit., p. 95. Callahan, *Abortion: Law, Choice and Morality*, op. cit., p. 258. Thomas A. Wassmer, discussion in "Abortion and Animation," vol. 2, Hall, op. cit., p. 3.

The "abortion only for greater value" concept contrasts with the view that in the first trimester the fetus is only a piece of tissue and its removal is no more a moral issue than an appendectomy. See Thomás S. Szasz, "The Ethics of Abortion," *The Humanist* (1966), **26**:148.

29. The Wilkes, op. cit., p. 3, wonder about a live birth in an abortion procedure. They don't understand why the doctor tried to save the baby. One explanation is that for many people life begins at birth or with the first breath. Gardiner, op. cit., p. 112. See Wassmer, op. cit., p. 3. Newton, op. cit., p. 115, notes that Anaximenes thought the air was holy. The soul entered the body with the first breath of air.

30. Hardin, op. cit., pp. 82–83, notes that the Nazis outlawed abortion as one of their first official acts. The ban was kept throughout their regime. Kieffer, op. cit., p. 171. See also, Bok, op. cit., p. 56. Mohr, op. cit., p. 250, and Fletcher, op. cit., p. 139, note, as a motive in nineteenth-century antiabortion legislation, a concern to maintain population

growth, a situation that has changed considerably to today's concern with the population explosion. Rosner sees an exception to the present situation. He thinks Jewish women should not have abortions. They should have their babies and give them to Israel, which needs Jews. Op. cit., pp. 215, 222. Some pro-life proponents urge women to have their babies and give them to couples who want to adopt children. Gregory Baum, op. cit., p. 31, looks at the inconsistency of abortion foes who are not bothered by death in war. He thinks their real problem is sexual morality. The same point is made by Gordon C. Zahn, "A Religious Pacifist Looks at Abortion," pp. 63–70, in Shannon, op. cit., and Fletcher, op. cit., p. 83. The Willkes not only protest abortion but also injustice in general and particularly the billions spent on bombs, op. cit., p. 132.

31. Malcolm Forbes, *The Sayings of Chairman Malcolm* (New York: Harper & Row, Publishers, 1978), p. 106.

32. Paul K. Jewett, "The Relationship of the Soul to the Fetus," pp. 49–66, Spitzer and Saylor, op. cit. Theoretically, the concept of a soul should be no problem to people who do not believe in one, or to those who base their ethics or values on nonreligious considerations. However, ensoulment often parallels "when life begins," so the concept continues to influence quite secular decisions. See Aristotle and also Paul Ramsey's report, op. cit., pp. 60–62, that even the Supreme Court recognizes secular humanism as religion. In contrast, Roger Wertheimer believes the religious position gets its believability from independent secular considerations. Religion is an expression of these, and talk of a soul is irrelevant. See his "Understanding the Abortion Argument," pp. 33–51 in Feinberg, op. cit.

33. Noonan, op. cit., p. 38. Means, op. cit., p. 10. Kosnik and others, op. cit., pp. 198–199. Montgomery, op. cit., p. 78, ascribes the traducianist view to Augustine, the traditional Roman Catholic theologian, and to Martin Luther, the Protestant Reformer (1483–1546). James B. Nelson, "Abortion: Protestant Perspectives," *EB* 1:13–17. Other sources claim Augustine believed in late ensoulment (Fletcher, op. cit., p. 136), which suggests a creationist view. Tertullian believed the soul came into existence with the body as a biolog-

ical transmission from Adam through our ancestors. Harmon L. Smith, *Ethics and the New Medicine* (Nashville, Tenn.: Abingdon Press, 1970), p. 27.

34. Noonan, op. cit., pp. 55–56. Hardin, op. cit., pp. 72–73. Held, op. cit., p. 106.

35. See n. 24. Creationism has been ascribed to Clement of Alexandria, Pelagius (who was opposed by Augustine and judged a heretic), Peter Lombard (an early Protestant), the Catholic Thomas Aquinas, the Protestant John Calvin (1509–1564) and followers, and the Roman Catholic magisterium. Montgomery, op. cit., p. 76. Nelson, op. cit., p. 14. Fletcher, op. cit., p. 136. Some religious groups, such as the Mormons, think of souls as existing in heaven waiting for a body to enter. The Babylonian Talmud (Nitdah 13) suggests The Messiah will not come until the souls of the unborn are born. This suggests yet a different view than the traducianist or creationist. Among the Ainu, the white Japanese, the father is believed to give the child its soul within twelve days after birth. McEllhenney, op. cit., p. 95. The Greek philosopher Heraclitus thought the soul was infused at puberty. See Wassmer, op. cit., p. 3. This may be reflected in the lack of children's rights throughout history; that is, pre-adults are not really or fully human.

36. The problem has not been solved either for the fertilized egg that seven days after fertilization divides into identical twins. In 4 percent of cases, the division takes place after implantation. Gardiner, op. cit., p. 109. Does such a twin have half a soul? Because scientifically we can now divide the fertilized ovum to form twins, this could give us the power to divide a soul in half or create a new soul if ensoulment comes at this time or earlier.

Canon 747 of the Roman Catholic *Codex Juris Canonici* (1917) says a living aborted fetus must be baptized unconditionally if alive, conditionally if in doubt, but regardless of age "even though it be aborted immediately after conception." See Marvin Kohl, "Abortion and the Argument from Innocence," pp. 28–32, in Feinberg, op. cit. Means, op. cit., p. 11. Smith, op. cit., p. 29. Healy, op. cit., pp. 355–373. One of the problems here is determining if there is any life left in the fetus (zygote, blastocyst, conceptus, embryo). When in doubt, baptize. Technically, this answers the problem of miscarriages. They must be baptized. The problem of detection remains staggering and amusing. At one time, a special baptismal syringe was in vogue. It could be used to squirt baptismal water into the uterus. It was especially important in the death of a pregnant woman.

37. Noonan, op. cit., pp. xi–xii. He cites no source for his information about standard practice in rape cases. He is wrong when he says the casuistry (the solving of special cases of right and wrong; Latin *casus* means case) of theologians and the common sense of lawmakers agree that the mother could not be required to prefer the child's life to her own. Over and over again, this is exactly what both have insisted upon. In fact, both have insisted for centuries that she must sacrifice her own life even when there was no reasonable chance of giving birth.

In the legal sense, he is right about the D and C being nonabortifacient. Because the fertilized ovum, if there is one, is still in the fallopian tube, abortion, technically, has not taken place. Of course, removing the lining of the uterus prevents implantation, so this procedure might be seen as a contraceptive measure. This is banned by his and other religious groups, as noted in Chapter Three (see especially the discussion of IUD action). See Hellegers, op. cit., p. 195, and *Encyclopedia*, op. cit., p. 3. Healy, however, op. cit., pp. 275–278, says Catholic ethics allow douches for up to sixteen hours after rape. The semen can be killed as an aggressor, but not a fertilized ovum. He does not comment on this deprivation of "the vital life force."

38. Kohl, op. cit., p. 30. Aquinas (died A.D. 1274) is cited as believing in ensoulment after three months (he said different things at different times). See Davis and Aroskar, op. cit., p. 94. Rabbi Meir Abulafia (d. 1244) said the soul enters at conception, but the embryo is not a person until it is born, so the time of ensoulment is irrelevant to abortion. Feldman, op. cit., pp. 273, 275.

39. Vatican II in 1965, for the first time, says Noonan, op. cit., p. 46, made a distinction between contraception and abortion. Prior views, as in Pope Pius XI's "Casti Connubii" encyclical in 1930, associated contraception and abortion without distinction. Now only abortion would be murder, pre-

sumably. The line was drawn sharply between the sperm-egg stage and the fertilized egg stage, but no decree was made on when life begins. See Connery, op. cit., p. 308. Still, Paul VI's "Humanae Vitae" reaffirmed the immorality of contraception, so the distinction is not firm. We are reminded here of Nicholson's point that the real sin of abortion is that it makes the parents sexual sinners. She notes the various views of the time of ensoulment. One place this appears is in penalties for abortion: penance for one year if fetal development is less than forty days, and ten years (the penalty for murder) if animation had taken place. It was not until 1917 that canon law dropped all references to the distinction between an ensouled and an unensouled fetus. Op. cit., p. 14.

40. The Supreme Court noted that state abortion laws may have come from a Victorian social concern to discourage illicit sexual conduct, but the law before them was not so based nor have courts taken this argument seriously. Feinberg, op. cit., p. 181. This argument is common. The suggestion that available abortion will encourage illicit sex was also presented as an argument against contraception. No available evidence supports this view; yet it remains part of the thinking of many people. Once again, abortion appears wrong as a coverup for sexual sin. Nelson, op. cit., p. 14.

41. "Acceptance" and legality do not necessarily mean everyone gets an abortion who wants one. Davis and Aroskar, op. cit., p. 92, note that in 1976 an estimated 700,000 women wanted abortions and could not get them. They cite reluctant doctors and hospitals as the cause. Catholic hospitals are not allowed to offer the procedure. Only 27 percent of all general, non-Catholic hospitals provide this service. The Alan Guttmacher Institute puts the figure of unobtainable abortions at between 150,000 and 650,000. *Annual Report 1976*, p. 16. A 1977 figure of unobtainable abortions is 550,000, or 30 percent of those who wanted abortions. Jacqueline D. Forrest, Christopher Tietze, and Ellen Sullivan, "Abortion in the United States, 1976–1977," *Family Planning Perspectives*, no. 5 (Sept./Oct. 1978), 10:271–279.

We repeat here our earlier observation that acceptance, legality, and morality are overlapping but differing concepts. Frequency of practice does not necessarily mean that the practice is right, or wrong.

42. "UN Study Shows Liberal Abortion Laws Have Spread Worldwide," *HCR*, no. 2 (Apr. 1976), **6**:2. The Helms Amendment (1973) restricts the use of U.S. foreign aid funds for abortions. Donald P. Warwick, "Foreign Aid for Abortion," *HCR*, no. 2 (Ap. 1980), **10**:30–37.

43. Mohr, op. cit. See also, Finnis, op. cit.

44. Devereaux, op. cit., pp. 136–138, notes that in many cultures, the midwife also performed abortions and in general functioned in family planning. Some cultures have specialists in abortion, which Mohr also notes. This country, of course, has had such specialists for most of its history, but for the past one hundred years they have been illegal for the most part.

45. Nelson, op. cit., pp. 14–15, says Americans wanted population growth to fulfill America's manifest destiny as God's new Israel.

46. Rosen, "Introduction," pp. xv–xix, op. cit., notes (p. xvii) the interesting fact that the best medicine of that day would be quackery today.

47. The Court noted, however, that in the *second* trimester the health of the mother could again be a concern for state regulation. Childbirth is eight times more dangerous than early abortion, says Hardin, op. cit., p. 12. The Willkes, op. cit., p. 66, say abortion is twice as likely to kill the mother as childbirth at any stage of pregnancy. The study they cite reflects second and third trimester abortions. Christopher Tietze reports that for 1972–1975, only abortions of sixteen or more weeks' gestation were more dangerous than childibrth in the United States. "Induced Abortion: 1977 Supplement," *Reports on Population/Family Planning*, no. 14, 2nd ed., Supplement (Dec. 1977), p. 14.

48. In 1976, 89.4 percent of the 988,267 recorded abortions in the United States were performed in the first twelve weeks of gestation. *Center for Disease Control, Abortion Surveillance, 1976* (USDHEW, PHS no. 78–8205).

49. Rosen, op. cit., p. xvii, quotes state court cases of 1872 and 1923, which recognized life in the embryo but denied the embryo was a living child or a human being.

Muslim law has life beginning after 120 days when the fetus is recognizable as a human. Abortion is permissible in this first 120 days according to the Grand Mufti of Jordan. See Isam R. Naser, "Abortion in the Near East," pp. 267–273, in Hall, op. cit. However, Muslim scholars in Turkey object to abortion from conception. Nusret H. Fisek, "Discussion," in Hall, op. cit., p. 353.

50. Scanzoni, op. cit., p. 322.

51. Some Jewish interpreters view this in broad terms to include psychological and social reasons, whereas others adhere strictly to the saving of physical life. Some Jews believe life begins with conception. See Cohen, op. cit., pp. 171ff.

52. Martin Luther said, "If a woman grows weary and at last dies from childbearing, it matters not. Let her only die from bearing; she is there to do it." *Margaret Sanger, An Autobiography* (New York: Dover Publications, Inc., 1971), p. 210. A conservative Protestant study, Spitzer and Saylor, op. cit., has only one woman, a geneticist, among twenty-eight contributors. Of 284 contributors to the prestigious *Encyclopedia of Bioethics*, op. cit., thirty-two, or 11 percent, are women. Daniel J. Callahan says the "Catholic position does not genuinely allow consideration of the woman's welfare . . ." See *Abortion . . .*, op. cit., p. 409. There was a concern in medieval Christianity for the woman's soul. If she were baptized, death released her from this "vale of tears" and her soul went to Paradise. If her fetus were baptized, it too went to Heaven. But if it were unbaptized, its soul went to Limbo or to Hell.

53. In 1962, the ALI published a *Modern Penal Code*. This did not authorize abortion on demand and, in fact, unjustified abortion was listed as a crime. The Code allowed abortion for the traditional three reasons (physical or mental health, defective fetus, felonious intercourse) and required a licensed physician in a licensed hospital with two licensed physicians certifying the need, all occurring before viability. The AMA endorsed this in June, 1967, as did the American Psychiatric Association. England's new law was in October 1967. Here abortion was extended to social concerns and allowed for such things as family size, housing, strain on the mother, and so on. The ACOG also included concern

for the patient's total environment, but it followed the ALI recommendations and rejected abortion on demand (1968). The American Civil Liberties Union in 1968 suggested the removal of all laws on abortion, as did the American Public Health Association (APHA), The Physicians Forum, and Planned Parenthood–World Population. In 1969, the General Federation of Women's Clubs endorsed a statement similar to that of the ALI. In 1970, the AMA suggested abortion should be the decision of patient and physician, which might be interpreted as abortion on demand (Rosner, op. cit., p. 216). In 1973 (reaffirmed 1978), the APHA said abortion is a personal health service and should be available regardless of ability to pay. "Abortion Funding," *The Nation's Health*, no. 9 (Sept. 1978), **8:**8, and *The American Journal of Public Health*, op. cit., vol. 69, p. 310. The 1977 Statement of the ACOG neither condemns nor approves abortion but calls for a balanced approach. The final decision should be the physician's, in consultation with the patient. The welfare of the client and adequate facilities are major concerns, as is also the freedom not to perform abortions. This joint concern for patient and freedom is endorsed by The Nurses Association of ACOG, The American College of Nurse-Midwives, and The American Nurses Association. See ACOG Statement of Policy: Statement on Abortion," June 1974; "The NAACOG Statement on Abortions and Sterilizations," 3 May, 1972; "ACNM Statement on Abortion," January 1971; "ANA Division on Maternal and Child Health Nursing Practice: Statement on Abortion," 12 June, 1978. See also, Noonan, op. cit., p. xiv; Lambert, op. cit., pp. 402–405; Donald H. Bouma, "Abortion in a Changing Social Context," pp. 525–531, in Spitzer and Saylor, op. cit. Harry and Julia Abramson, *Who Shall Live?* (New York: Hill and Wang, 1970), pp. 99–104.

54. Noonan, op. cit., p. 14. Connery, op. cit., p. 43. The priest Navatus was accused of parricide by Cyprian (A.D. c. 250), bishop of Carthage. There are cases in which a woman gets an abortion under coercion. The threat of being killed or beaten can be quite persuasive. So can threats to cut off financial support, which includes pressure from welfare boards as well as from husbands or male friends. Freedom of choice and informed consent remain major ethical concerns.

55. In 1976, the suction method was used in 82 percent of the recorded abortions in the United States, and D and C was used in 10 percent, saline in 6 percent, and hysterectomy and hysterotomy combined accounted for 0.2 percent.

56. One interesting argument in abortion is the so-called argument of innocence. See Kohl, op. cit., pp. 28–32. The theory is that the fetus is an innocent human being, so it is wrong to kill it. For those who do not see the fetus as a human being, there is neither innocence nor guilt, so the argument is irrelevant. If those who believe in "innocence" want to justify abortion, for example, in an ectopic pregnancy, they then try to show the fetus is guilty (not innocent) of aggression, so the woman is justified in killing her "pursuer." This was also the point of the Jewish philosopher Maimonides (see n. 15). Healy, op. cit., pp. 90–94, says Catholic doctrine does not approve this "aggressor" concept. There are those, of course, who do not believe in taking innocent life, so such mass slaughter as by war and the automobile should be banned. Still others oppose capital punishment, for the taking of human life is wrong even if the person to be killed is guilty. Conservatives and liberals on abortion are not necessarily consistent in their view of other aspects of killing.

57. Noonan, op. cit., p. 14, and Connery, op. cit., pp. 303ff, document the continuing controversy. Some statements insist that abortion is never licit, with no exceptions. The distinction that follows in the two cases is technically known as "indirect" abortion, as opposed to "direct" abortion, which is what is usually practiced in therapeutic abortion. One way around the problem, of course, is to not call these "exceptions," but to give them a different name and refuse to call them abortions at all. Hellegers, *EB* **1:**3. He puts uterine curettages in this category. He believes this procedure leads to the loss of thousands of fertilized eggs annually. Healy, op. cit., pp. 213–231.

58. In 1902, the Holy Office forbade this operation. Doctors could only wait for the tube to rupture. In 1944, Bouscaren claimed placental cells eroded the tubal wall prior to

rupture so the tube is weakened. Removal of the tube was justified. The death of the tubal fetus was indirect killing. See Nicholson, op. cit., pp. 19, 30. Hellegers, ibid. Healy, op. cit., pp. 94–101, 220–231. *TBL*, no. 8 (15 Aug. 80), **1**:2.

59. James M. Gustafson, "A Protestant Ethical Approach," pp. 101–122, in Noonan, op. cit., p. 105. Smith, op. cit., p. 34. Bouma, op. cit., p. 526. Feldman, op. cit., pp. 265, 282–291, emphasizes a humane concern for the woman in Judaism. Some branches of Judaism emphasize this more than others.

60. A 1966 survey showed 71 percent approval of abortion for the woman's health, 56 percent in rape cases, and 55 percent for defective fetus, but only 21 percent for low income, 18 percent if unmarried woman, and 15 percent if married but wants no more children. The survey was made by the National Opinion Research Center. There were no differences between Protestant and Catholic respondents. Bouma, op. cit., p. 530. Interestingly, in Catholic moral doctrine, one is required to use only ordinary means to preserve life. Among extraordinary means are excessive expense, pain, or other inconvenience. Nicholson, op. cit., p. 83, interprets this to mean that abortion, or at least some categories of abortion should be licit under the latter conditions. Our point, of course, still holds: one person's excessive is another person's trivia. Stanley Budner reports that in a large but unrepresentative sample of abortion patients, 60 percent were not using contraceptives; 77 percent knew about the pill, IUD, and diaphragm, but only 37 percent ever used them, even if irregularly. In another sample, 32 percent said it was too much bother to contracept. "Value Conflicts and the Uses of Research: The Example of Abortion," *Man and Medicine*, no. 1 (Autumn 1975), **1**:29–41.

61. Christopher T. Reilly, "Threatened Health of Mother as an Indication for Therapeutic Abortion," pp. 169–188, in Spitzer and Saylor, op. cit. One writer is worried about abortion on demand degenerating into whim and fancy. David F. Busby, "Rape, Incest and Multiple Illegitimacy as Indications for Therapeutic Abortion," pp. 299–309, in Spitzer and Saylor, op. cit. He cites no source for his concern. In a dissenting opinion in 1973, Supreme Court Justice Byron R. White accused

his colleagues of holding that the Constitution "values the convenience, whim or caprice of the putative mother more than the life or potential life of the fetus." Hardin, op. cit., p. 28, notes that nothing is said about the putative father. Emily C. Moore asks, "Can anyone imagine an abortion 'for no reason at all'? We could have expected less 'loaded' terminology from learned men." See "Abortion: The New Ruling," HCR, no. 2 (Ap. 1973), **3**:4–7.

62. In 1968, the ACLU opposed all laws with criminal penalties for abortion. See n. 52. The four reasons cited were that the laws at the time discriminated against the poor; they infringed on a woman's liberty to decide the use of her body; they infringed on privacy; and they interfered with a physician's right to practice medicine. Hardin, op. cit., p. 39, notes the irony that because the rich pay for the children of the poor through welfare and public hospitals, the proverb may soon be reduced to ". . . and the poor get children."

Feldman, op. cit., pp. 51, 301–302, notes that poverty is not an acceptable reason for contraception in the Jewish tradition. One would assume this precludes abortion also. In Israel, one third of the country's abortions were for "social hardship." This is opposed by the ultra-conservatives. "Israeli Abortion Amendment," *The Christian Century*, no. 17 (10 May, 1978), **95**:497. Margolies, op. cit., p. 33, speaking from a Reform Judaism perspective, says it's up to men and women to decide on their own on the birth of a child. It's not up to synagogue or church or state. The laws of several countries include social needs as a reason for abortion. These include England and the Scandanavian countries. Where abortion is available on demand, one could assume that economics and/or social considerations are part of the decisions on abortion.

63. Morton A. Stenchever, "An Abuse of Prenatal Diagnosis," *Journal of the American Medical Association*, no. 4 (24 July 1972), **221**:408. See also Marc Lappé, "Choosing the Sex of Our Children," HCR, no. 1 (Feb. 1974), **4**:1–4. Kenneth Vaux, "New Moral Demands in Baby-Making," *The Interpreter*, no. 8 (Sept. 1977), **21**:36–38.

64. See n. 52. Connery, op. cit., p. 293, suggests also that abortion to save the mother's life is no longer necessary. He

ascribes this in part to safe procedures for Cesarean sections. Paul Ramsey, op. cit., p. 87, agrees. Eugene B. Linton, M.D., says abortions to save the life of the mother are only a small percentage of those performed today. "Medical Indications for Therapeutic Abortion and Sterilization," pp. 157–168, in Spitzer and Saylor, op. cit.

Saving life is often broadened to include health, including mental health. The Willkes suggest this is just an excuse for abortion, op. cit., pp. 37–40.

65. The Willkes, op. cit., pp. 33–36, cite studies showing pregnancy resulting from rape is extremely rare. Reasons are the difficulty of proving rape and of proving the pregnancy is the result of the rape. They add their belief that the unborn child should not be punished for the father's crime. We might add here that rape is a major issue in the women's movement, which has also been vociferous in support of abortion by choice.

It is common to classify rape and incest in the one category of felonious intercourse. George H. Williams makes an interesting distinction. In rape, an immediate curettage is allowed (he doesn't say who allows it). However, the woman may choose to give birth. In incest, the conceptive act of both parents is felonious, and the state should procure an abortion to avoid genetic defects. "The Sacred Condominium," pp. 146–171, in Noonan, op. cit. He doesn't say why the woman is at fault. Perhaps he assumes she participates willingly, which may not be the case. He is assuming too that the rights of the state here supersede the rights of the woman, so the state can coerce her into an abortion. Others would disagree.

66. Dr. and Mrs. J. C. Willke, pro-life advocates, believe that anyone who opposes abortion without also working for social justice is "frankly immoral." They note that the poor are neglected, mothers of handicapped children are left to fend for themselves, and pregnant schoolgirls are ostracized. They call for a society of love and concern, which includes love for defective children. Op. cit., pp. 131–132. The concern for the defective fetus poses the question, "Abortion: For the Fetus's Own Sake?" Paul F. Camenisch answers his own question with yes, maybe, but the abortion decision is often from mixed motives. HCR, no. 2 (Apr. 1976), 6:38–41. Subsequent

discussion was both pro and con. Part of it turned on the issue of whether a fetus is a person and whether nonexistence is better than a life of pain and suffering. "Correspondence," HCR, no. 4 (Aug. 1976), 6:4, 30–33. See also, Vaux, op. cit., pp. 36–38.

67. Noonan, "Introduction," op. cit., pp. xv–xvi, called abortion sadistic. Here, prochoice proponents could claim sadism on the part of those who bring defective children into the world. Fletcher, op. cit., p. 126, claims there is no such thing as a right to bring crippled children into the world. Because we can now know in advance, we have no excuse for doing so. People who do it anyway are as guilty of wrongdoing as contributing to a wrongful death (p. 189).

68. Jewett, op. cit., p. 65. Fletcher, op. cit., p. 196, calls quality of life (QOL) the number one moral imperative of mankind.

69. Hardin, op. cit., pp. 13–15, 32–33. Devereaux, op. cit., p. 137.

70. Scanzoni, op. cit., p. 324. Bouma, op. cit., p. 337. Hardin, op. cit., pp. 97–100. Abrahamsons, op. cit., pp. 64–65. Henrietta H. Marshall reports that unwanted fertility has declined from 20 percent in 1967 to 8.3 percent in 1977. "Letter from the Chair," pp. 3–6, Within Our Reach, Annual Report 1977 (New York: Planned Parenthood Federation of America, 1978). The Willkes, op. cit., pp. 47–52, suggest that unwanted/wanted is an idyllic concept. There are unwanted wives, Jews, Blacks, Catholics, Chicanoes, and so on. They suggest we try to achieve that wonderful world where all are wanted. Studies are cited to show that unwanted pregnancies become wanted babies, and one sixth of wanted pregnancies become unwanted children. Hardin, op. cit., Appendix C, cites a longitudinal study of children born in Sweden when their mothers had been refused an abortion. The incidence of delinquency and social problems was higher than that expected for that population.

71. The Willkes, op. cit., p. 134, offer family planning as a positive alternative to abortion. These pro-life proponents insist no one has the right to say how many children parents should or should not have. Planned Parenthood also takes this position of individual freedom of choice, both to have children and to have an abortion. See 1972 and 1976 Policy Statements, Planned Parenthood of

America, 810 Seventh Avenue, New York, N.Y. 10019. Margolies, op. cit., p. 33, reflects the same thought from the perspective of Reform Judaism.

72. Birthright, 699 Coxwell Avenue, Toronto, Ontario, Canada. Birthright, 18 Euclid Street, Woodbury, N.J. 08096. Alternatives to Abortion, 2608 Valleybrook Drive, Toledo, Ohio 43615. This movement is endorsed by the Willkes, op. cit., pp. 137–142. It is also supported by R. F. R. Gardner who sees himself as a Christian physician. Gardner believes in abortion for some cases. Op. cit., p. 316.

73. See n. 52. The ACOG added the need for informed consent by the woman and her husband, or herself if unmarried, and by the nearest relative if she is a minor. Mace, op. cit., pp. 65–66, notes that many men don't care, but they should care in a responsible society. Father Drinan argued for elimination of all laws on abortion except that there should be a law requiring the consent of the father, that is, the male who impregnated the woman, before permitting an abortion. Hardin, op. cit., pp. 32–33, asked the woman who easily arranged an abortion in Italy what her husband thought of it. She never told her husband. She considered him much too immature for such things. In 1976 the Supreme Court voted against spousal and parental consent for abortion. Ramsey, *Ethics at the Edge* . . . , op. cit., p. 9.

74. See the ACOG concern, n. 72. But see Ramsey, ibid. It should be added that the Court's ruling was not absolute. "Nonmature" and "noncompetent" minors are still required to have parental consent. See George J. Annas, "Abortion and the Supreme Court: Round Two," *HCR*, no. 5 (Oct. 1978), **6**:15–17. The "mature minor" is a relatively recent concept. Marguerite Mancini, "Nursing, Minors, and the Law," *AJN*, no. 1 (Jan. 1978), **78**:124, 126.

75. The legal battle see-saws back and forth. Thus, people with independent means can get an abortion. Those dependent on the government are more restricted. The pro-choice movement condemns this double standard for rich and poor. However, we can note that the feared increase in illegal abortions does not seem to have materialized as in Romania. See "After Medicaid Cut-off CDC Sees No Increase in Illegal Abortions,"

HCR, no. 2 (Apr. 1979), **9**:2–3; *HCR*, no. 4 (Aug. 1977), Mary C. Segers, "Abortion and the Supreme Court: Some Are More Equal Than Others," **77**:5–6; Sidney Callahan, "The Court and a Conflict of Principles," pp. 7–8; George J. Annas, "Let Them Eat Cake," pp. 8–9. Speaking to this issue from a moderate Jewish perspective, Sid Z. Leiman suggests "Abortion Needs Concern, Not Subsidy," *Sh'ma*, no. 144 (23 Dec. 1977), **8**:215–216.

76. H. Tristam Engelhardt, Jr., reports that in the People's Republic of China, a pregnant women who already has two children is confronted by her social group which insists she has a duty to seek abortion. She usually agrees. "Bioethics in the People's Republic of China," *HCR*, no. 2 (Apr. 1980), **10**:7–10. The 9 May 1968 statement of the ACOG firmly refused to support abortion for population control. See Reilly, op. cit., pp. 173–175. The Helms Amendment (1973) forbids the use of U.S. foreign aid funds for abortion for family planning purposes. Warwick, op. cit., pp. 30–37.

77. Mace, op. cit., pp. 70–84. Scanzoni, op. cit., pp. 316–317. Guttmacher, op. cit., p. 178. Abrahamson, op. cit., pp. 17 and 85. Hall, op. cit., Part V, "The Global Aspects of Abortion," pp. 245–359, reflects the situation through 1966–1967. Tietze, op. cit., pp. 5–6, brings the data up to mid-1977. The current report is from "Other Ideas and Trends: Abortion Statistics," *The New York Times* (Sunday, 6 May 1979), p. E 11. The figures are quoted from The Population Crisis Committee. See also, Alfred Kotasek, "Artificial Termination of Pregnancy in Czechoslovakia," *International Journal of Gynecology and Obstetrics*, no. 3 (May 1971), **9**:118–119. Djerassi, op. cit., pp. 23–30. Warwick, op. cit., pp. 30–37.

As noted earlier, population growth is influenced by any law on abortion as in Great Britain or the United States, even though population control as such may not be the aim of the law.

78. Abrahamson, op. cit., p. 14. Gail Sheehy, *Passages* (New York: E. P. Dutton & Co., Inc., 1976), p. 71. *The New York Times*, op. cit., (6 May 1979).

79. "Nursing Ethics, The Admirable Professional Standards of Nurses: A Survey Report, Part 2," *Nursing 74*, p. 53. See Ramsey, *Ethics at the Edge* . . . , op. cit., p. 45, and "Abortion Yes or No; Nurses Organize Both

Ways," *AJN*, no. 3 (March 1972), **72:**416. Also, Helen Branson, "Nurses Talk About Abortion," *AJN*, no. 1 (Jan. 1972), p. 106, and "Nurses' Feelings, a Problem Under New Abortion Law," *AJN*, no. 2 (Feb. 1971), p. 350.

80. ANA, *Code for Nurses with Interpretive Statements*, Kansas City, 1976, pp. 4–5.

81. "Catholic Nurse Legislator Files for Abortion Reform," *AJN*, no. 3 (Mar. 1971), p. 459.

82. Diane B. Uustal, "Values Clarification in Nursing: Application to Practice," *AJN*, no. 12 (Dec. 1978), p. 2058.

83. Steele and Harmon, *Values Clarification in Nursing* (New York: Appleton-Century-Crofts, 1979), Chapter One.

84. Coletta, "Values Clarification in Nursing," *AJN*, no. 12 (Dec. 1978), p. 2057.

85. Keller and Copeland, "Counseling the Abortion Patient Is More than Talk," *AJN*, no. 1 (Jan. 1972), p. 103.

86. Hendershot and Grimm, "Abortion Attitudes Among Nurses and Social Workers," *American Journal of Public Health*, no. 5, **64:** 438.

87. Ibid., p. 440.

88. Branson, op. cit., p. 50.

89. "Nursing Ethics . . . Survey," op. cit., p. 53.

90. "OB/GYN Nurse Group Takes Stand on Abortion," *AJN*, no. 7 (July 1972), p. 1311.

91. Ramsey, op. cit., pp. 49–80. Mary F. Liston, "Abortion Decisions—Impact on Nursing Practice, Maternity and Child Care," *The Jurist*, no. 2 (1973), **33:**230–236.

92. Ibid., p. 53.

93. Center for Disease Control, op. cit., p. 5.

94. Mace, op. cit., pp. 115–120.

95. Keller and Copeland, op. cit., p. 103. "Nursing Interviews Helpful at Abortion Center," *AJN*, no. 2 (Feb. 1971), p. 352, and Muriel Ryden, "An Approach to Ethical Decision-Making," *Nursing Outlook* (Nov. 1978), pp. 705–706.

96. Branson, op. cit., p. 106.

97. Davis and Aroskar, op. cit., pp. 104–106.

Chapter 5

Neonatology and Ethics

INTRODUCTION

There are three areas of concern in this chapter. One concern continues the discussion of abortion. The second moves more directly to the special or neonatal intensive care units (NNICU's).[1] The third relates to research.

This continues the issues of Chapters Two, Three, and Four. Some abortions relate to a potential birth defect child. We noted earlier the genetic studies that attempt to determine genetic and other problems in advance to allow for contraception. The most crucial ethical issues in the NNICU relate to children with birth defects. Research to prevent birth defects or help us learn more about them for therapeutic purposes may not be in accord with ethical sensibilities.

All of this points to a larger issue called the Quality of Life (QOL). Shall we follow natural law and let whatever children be born who are going to be born? And shall we then let nature take its course and if they die, they die? The concern here might be for the quality of life for those already born or for the child or the child-to-be.

Of course, merely asking such questions will be offensive to some. We continue here, too, our awareness of the liberal-conservative spectrum.[2] Stanley Scott asks, when should medical technology be used to keep an infant alive? He claims that no accepted body of principles has been developed to guide the use of this technology.[3] A reviewer protests that such a question is disturbing. The idea that there is no accepted body of principles ignores 2,400 years of tradition. The reviewer does not elaborate on that statement. The time factor coincides with the Hippocratic Oath. It includes the Christian period and much of the Jewish. A further objection is that the concern in the Scott text is to combine the doctor's role as healer with that of social executioner.[4]

VIABLE PRODUCTS OF ABORTION

In Western history, contraception, abortion, and infanticide have sometimes been linked together and labeled murder. Killing is not wrong in the Western tradition, at least for many people. Millions are killed in wartime, but it is not usually called murder. Although contraception kills or "lets die" eggs and sperm, more and more people are unwilling to call it murder. Many are unwilling to call abortion murder. Some see it as killing, but not necessarily murder.

When Does Life Begin?

By traditional Jewish law, and for many others as well, the postnatal child *is* a child.[5] Even here, however, there are various traditions. One understanding is that when the child takes its first breath, life begins. A Talmudic text, however, puts this moment during parturition, with the birth of the head. Yet other traditions, however, say that if the child dies within thirty days, no funeral is necessary and the prayers for the dead are not said.[6]

When life begins relates to abortion because, on occasion, the result of an abortion is a live child, live by the preceding definition. According to the pro-life position, outlined in Chapter Four, the fetus is alive. Usually, the fetus does not survive the abortion procedure, especially first trimester abortions. "Live" births in the second trimester are rare, but they are more common in the third.[7] This relates, of course, to the whole issue of viability as discussed in Chapter Four.

What to Do?

Our concern here is what do you do with this live birth? It is often assumed that an abortion is aimed at the death, or, if you prefer, the nonlife, of the fetus. For a defective or abnormal fetus, that may be true. It may or may not be true in other situations. If an abortion is intended to save the pregnant woman's life, for example, it does not follow that the death of the fetus is also desired. The point here is that some ethicists argue that although a woman may have some reason for terminating the pregnancy, she does not have the right to determine the death of the fetus, even though that is usually the result of an abortion.[8]

Legal Aspects

This concern for the life of the fetus as distinct from the life of the woman has been encapsulated in some laws. One of the best known is a 1976 California law. Here, a live child resulting from an abortion becomes a ward of the state. At this point, the child is to be treated medically as any other child, with proper care.[9]

In contrast, laws requiring an abortion to be performed so as to *ensure*, if possible, a live birth, have so far been struck down by the U. S. Supreme Court. Thus, legally, although a state can move to protect the living child resulting from abortion, a government cannot move to try to ensure live births from abortions. The latter are to be performed by the method most appropriate to the individual situation.[10]

Statistics on such live births are difficult to assess for accuracy.[11] Estimates range from very few to a considerable number. The statistics are of importance here because the number has presumably increased. The greater the number of abortions, the higher the number of live births. Because of the increased number of abortions throughout the world, including the United States, the number of live births has increased, making this a more common problem, though how common is not clear.

Bruce Hilton reports a case of a doctor performing an abortion. Instead of an inert fetus, he found a living, breathing, premature baby.

He took care of the mother, had the baby placed in a bassinet, and went to the cafeteria for a smoke and time to think about what he might do. When he returned, the baby was no longer breathing. He called the Institute of Society, Ethics, and the Life Sciences (Hastings Center) to ask what he should have done. A law such as California's would have given one answer. The Center did not try to answer the question but posed other questions that might bear on the decision. They asked about how much importance should be placed on the intention of the mother and on her ability to rear the child. They asked about rights, such as the right of the child to life and the rights of the five siblings. They asked about brain damage from the saline solution. And they asked about who decides or who should have been consulted.[12]

At first glance, the California law seems to offer a quick solution. Robertson, however, raised some complicating factors. The duty to care for an aborted fetus arises if it actually lives outside the uterus. Is there a legal duty to resuscitate every viable fetus when the resulting life is only a matter of minutes, hours, or a few days?[13] Perhaps we need to add the consideration of potential in the case of the defective fetus or one damaged in the abortion procedure. Again, is the commitment to life without regard to circumstances, or does the situation influence, if not determine, such decisions?

ORDINARY VERSUS EXTRAORDINARY TREATMENT

Nicholson brings up an important medical and ethical distinction, called the distinction between ordinary and extraordinary means. She notes that in 1957 Pope Pius XII said that we are normally required to use only ordinary means to preserve life and health. Ethicists do not all agree on what constitutes "ordinary." In preantiseptic days, any surgery was extraordinary. That's true also of many medical procedures that have since become routine, including the medical procedure of abortion. Catholic ethicists use "ordinary" for those medical procedures that have a reasonable hope of benefit and are without excessive expense, pain, shame, or other inconvenience. Extraordinary, of course, is the

opposite. Note that although we do not need to use "extraordinary means," we may.[14]

People, of course, vary in their interpretations. Shall we consider genetics only for certain categories but not others? Is contraception or abortion acceptable for "trivial" reasons, recognizing that one person's trivia is another's important reason? What constitutes "excessive" in the explanation? Nicholson suggests such reasoning can be applied to abortion for the sake of the fetus, that is, when the fetus is defective. She sees such abortion as justifiable, but pro-life proponents generally do not. Our concern here is with the live birth from abortion and in neonatology in general. Shall we use only ordinary means to sustain life? Who interprets when a procedure is extraordinary? We will return to this issue in dealing with the death of an adult.

As noted earlier, we now have the technology to save many natural miscarriages. Should we? So, too, we have the technology for keeping at least some, if not many, fetuses alive. Should we? It is being done for research purposes. Should we? Should we do this without regard to research but only for the sake of life—life without regard to other circumstances?

The California statute called for all reasonable steps except extraordinary means in preserving the life and health of the viable fetus that becomes a live-born person in an abortion. A *viable fetus* was defined as having the ability to increase in tissue mass, increase the number, complexity, and coordination of the basic physiological functions, and become a self-sustaining organism independent of its mother. *Live-born* was defined as having outside the womb a sustained heartbeat, umbilical pulsation, spontaneous respiration, and movement of voluntary muscles. As amended and finally passed, the law gave to the live birth from an abortion the same rights as an infant of similar medical status who is born prematurely.[15]

Formal-Equality Principle

Walters calls the preceding point the *formal-equality principle*. It does not specify exactly what treatment should be given, only that it be equal. He cites as an example a 2.2-

pound infant delivered in a hysterotomy procedure. If the NNICU would normally try to save a premature infant of the same health status, age, and weight, then this principle would require equal treatment for the abortion case. Other situations are not so clear, as with a one-pound, twenty-week-old with probable brain damage following a saline-induced abortion.[16]

Although agreeing that the California law is an effort at concern, Sissela Bok thinks that we need a law prohibiting abortions late in the pregnancy cycle. In the meanwhile, she claims such legislation as the California law is wrong. If a fetus has been severely damaged by the abortion procedure, maintaining its life may impose extraordinary suffering on it, and legally constitute battery. She suggests that medical personnel should have the same freedom of judgment they have with prematures.[17]

In practice, such judgments may be made on the spot. They may be as much intuitive as logically measurable. "Gut reactions" may or may not be based on adequate information.[18] The judgments *are* being made, not only in abortion situations, but in others as well.

SPECIAL CARE OF NEONATES

An estimated 30,000 neonates a year in the United States raises the moral question, "Is it perhaps the ultimate kindness to let the severely defective child die naturally, or more beneficently, to hasten its death?"[19] A reported 58 percent decrease in the infant death rate occurred in the United States from 1940 to 1970.[20] NNICU's played an important part in this. Another 1970 report indicated that neonatal mortality rates were about half those for hospitals without these units.[21] Yet, these units have been called horror chambers. Mechanical heroics have sacrificed the human to efficiency. "The beep of the oscillograph is becoming the voice of the new barbarism."[22]

History

How did we get to this point? We noted earlier the practice of infanticide in most world cultures, ancient and present.[23] It was

so common in ancient times that the biblical prophet Ezekiel could use it as a metaphor (Ezekiel 16:1–4). It was usual throughout the South Sea islands, Australia, and New Zealand. It was widely practiced in Japan before Commodore Perry (1854). In the Americas, some tribes practiced it and some did not. It was very common in the Swahili culture, although less so in the rest of Africa. In Madagascar, children born on "unlucky" days were killed to prevent bad luck. It was normal in China (especially female infanticide) and among the ancient Arabs who even saw it as a duty. The Arab Muhammed the Prophet, founder of the Muslim religion, forbade infanticide and allowed plural marriage as a way of caring for the excess female population.[24]

Greece, Rome: The more direct antecedents of Western culture are the ancient societies of Greece and Rome. It was customary in Greece to expose weak and deformed infants, and the state of Sparta required it by law. The Greek moralist Plutarch (A.D. c. 100) did not think it was good for the child or for the public interest to raise a child if it did not have promise of becoming vigorous and healthy. Earlier, the Greek philosopher Aristotle said deformed infants should not live. His teacher Plato wanted the destruction of both defective children and the children of inferior parents. In Rome, the weak or deformed infants were destroyed, if not by law, at least by custom. It was less common with healthy infants, though less from a moral perspective than the need to maintain a large army.[25]

Christianity: Once Christianity gained power, there was a major change in the moral perspective. The change in practice was a good deal slower. Infanticide continued as a significant factor in limiting European population growth until the nineteenth century. This was true in spite of church teachings listing infanticide as a capital offense. The reason for the ban may have been the idea of life as a gift from God, man as created in God's image, the view that humans are different in kind from other animals, the teaching that unbaptized infants go to hell, or a combination of these.[26] Of course, one could get around the last point by having the infant baptized and then exposing it, but its birth and existence would be a matter of public record.

Modern Scene

On the modern scene, Callahan reports the practice of "masked infanticide." Mothers sometimes allowed young children to die from infections, especially diarrhea, rather than having them treated. They would even refuse treatment when it was offered.[27] With the already high infant mortality rate through the centuries and in many areas today (700 per 1,000 live births in parts of Africa), such infanticide would be difficult to distinguish from natural death.

Except for the teaching on baptism, Christian belief was largely derived from Judaism. The Ten Commandments condemn murder. Philo Judaeus was a philosopher in Alexandria, Egypt, from about 20 B.C. to A.D. 50. He labeled infanticide as murder, and hence against the commandments. We noted earlier the Talmudic teaching that once the head was exposed in parturition, the infant was to be considered alive and could not be killed, even to save the life of the mother.

Summary

At first glance, infanticide is obviously murder. But it is obvious only to the mind accustomed to thinking in this way.[28] The Greco-Roman culture in which Philo lived did not think so. The Christian European culture may have officially taught that infanticide was wrong. The continuing practice suggests the rank and file may have believed differently. We have noted this contrast or conflict earlier in relation to contraception and abortion. This conflict has now grown to larger proportions with the success of modern medicine.

This success was noted in previous studies of genetics, contraception, and abortion. A high infant mortality rate removed many of the premature, weak, or defective infants from our midst. The lack of medical expertise did and still does allow many to die. In a personal encounter in the Near East, a local citizen noted that his wife had given birth seven times. Four of the babies died because his wife had no milk and could not breast feed them. In a day of canned and powdered milk and numerous commercial formulas, this seems unusual. But a remote village, only recently in regular touch with the modern world, knew little of such things and had no money to pay for them if they were known. In the more cultured West, modern nutrition and modern medical technology can keep more and more babies alive. Should we?

If We Can, Should We?

To the question, if we can, should we? comes a flat answer of yes from one direction. Following the traditional Judeo-Christian teaching that every life is precious, every possible human effort must be made to keep every baby alive that health personnel and modern medical technology possibly can. One Jewish perspective favors aggressive treatment for defective newborns, regardless of the degree of impairment. Religious law does not regard quality of life as a relevant moral factor.[29] From another perspective, Feldman notes an abortion decision that is acceptable when it is for the sake of the woman who fears a defective child. But if she requests an abortion for the sake of the child, the authorities would say no. One does not finally know for sure the child will be defective and, if it is, perhaps a handicapped life would still be better than no life at all.[30]

Still, Judaism does not slip into an absolute evaluation of life. There are higher duties such as the prohibitions against idolatry. Reich and Ost suggests that no serious moral theory holds life to be the absolute value. Neither is life the greatest good nor is death the greatest evil. Although respecting life, there are limits to one's obligation to sustain life.[31]

Vitalism

The doctrine that life is the highest good, higher than personal value, is what Joseph Fletcher calls *vitalism*. This view refuses to let someone die. It insists that a severely deformed newborn, such as a radical spina bifida, must be kept alive without regard to increasing pain or dehumanization. On the other hand, Fletcher claims that reverence for life is one thing, but making life sacrosanct is a different matter. From his Protestant Christian perspective, he suggests that Jesus did not come to bring mere life, but to bring an abundant life. He quotes Dr. Malcolm Watts of the California Medical Association as seeing the relative value of human life, rather than the absolute. In the past, medical personnel have tried to preserve, protect, repair, prolong life. Fletcher calls this "the old vitalistic, undiscriminating, sanctity-or-quantity-of-life ethics" that is now giving way to a quality-of-life ethics.[32]

Quality of Life

Paul Ramsey from his Protestant Christian perspective agrees that quality of life is directly opposed to equality of life.[33] He sees the latter as the long-standing Western standard, related to the biblical concept that God is no respecter of persons. He would not prolong the dying of neonates any more than of the aged or anyone else. If, in fact, a neonate is dying, it should be removed from the NNICU, for babies are not born to die burdened by intensive care that has no purpose except to extend their dying. He can also accept the equal nontreatment of whole categories for whom there is no hope or for whom society decides there are inadequate resources. Ramsey, as Reich and Ost, knows of no medical ethics that ever subscribed to "life-saving at all costs."[34] But he notes that defective newborns as such are not necessarily dying. Those who are should receive care.[35] Those who are not dying should receive care without regard to their condition, their social ability, their burden on the family or society, their own potential (IQ, relationship, and so on), or any pain or suffering they might have.[36] A decision to treat or not treat should be based on whether the treatment is beneficial or not to the infant. A newborn is a person who is protected by the Fourteenth Amendment and cannot legally or morally be allowed to suffer benign neglect.[37]

Others agree with Fletcher or the direction of his thinking. Duff and Campbell report that survivors of the NNICU may be healthy. Others continue to suffer from chronic cardiopulmonary disease, short-bowel syndrome, brain damage, or a myriad of congenital malformations that would previously have brought death. They note that many people are distressed by the long-term results of trying to save life at all costs and under all circumstances. One presumes that they mean the negative results just mentioned, and that on this basis, they quote Eliot Slater's suggestion that our formulation of the sanctity-of-life ethic needs to be revised if this is one of the consequences.[38]

How to Decide? If we move away from the principle of "save this life at all costs if at all possible," to where do we go? How do we assess the future quality of the life before us? Some say we assess on the basis of the humanness of this future life. Then it is a question of what is human. Some answer that it means a sufficiently high intelligence quotient. That is, because the essence of man as compared to animals is the ancient Greek philosophical concept of the rational, we judge the rational capacity or the future intellectual capacity. That's not always easy to do, as with Down's syndrome. But it is one perspective. Others say that to be human is to have the capacity for relationship. Many, if not most, of the Down's children have such capacity for relationship.[39]

Others move away from such philosophical concepts and ask simply, "Do the parents want the child?" If the baby's life is hanging in the balance in the first minutes after birth, there may not be time to ask. In some cases there is time. In some of the more famous of these cases, parents have decided not to operate or resuscitate. In some instances, medical personnel have accepted the parental decision, whereas in others, the hospital has gone to court to get an order to operate or otherwise sustain life. There does not seem to be much argument when parents decide all possible must be done to preserve the child's life, but there may be some doubts on the wisdom of such a decision.[40] These may turn on the medical prognosis or the ancient medical tradition of "do no harm."

On the basis of medical prognosis, Duff and Campbell report treatment was terminated for forty-three infants who died. They were part of a larger group of 299 deaths; that is, 256 were treated but died anyway. So we have not quite achieved the "near-utopian state" that Zuelzer suggests we have attained. One appreciates the "awesome finality" of the forty-three decisions, but 256 decisions to continue treatment did not result in life either. Occasionally, even a decision to discontinue treatment does not result in death. John Lorber has published criteria for nontreatment of spina bifida patients.[41] Part of the objection is that a child may live in spite of nontreatment and be a good deal worse off than if treatment had been provided.[42] That problem appears with other situations as well. So the decision for nontreatment on the basis of medical prognosis is not an absolute. Still, the decision is made and usually the infant dies. One basis of the decision is "first do not harm" (*primum non nocere*).

Primum Non Nocere: When Hippocrates formulated his medical oath about 400 B.C., medical science was much more limited than it is now. He suggested that if the physician could not help, at least he should "do no harm."[43] Theoretically, we treat people although aware that the treatment might cause pain, inconvenience, and expense. In ordinary treatment, it is assumed that the benefits are worth the cost. Frequently, this is obvious. An aspirin to relieve a headache is usually well worth the cost. An operation for a brain tumor is a bit more serious. If it relieves the headache and gives a reasonable extension on a normal life, one might readily agree. If it results in a permanent coma and "life" lingers for months or years, not everyone would be willing to pay that cost. Thus, one might see the brain operation as "extraordinary." The papal statement of 1957, referred to earlier, suggests, at least from a Roman Catholic perspective, that extraordinary measures need not be taken to preserve life. Pope Pius XII was referring to the machinery that keeps the aged alive.[44] McCormick applies this standard to the NNICU.[45] Questions remain. Who decides what is extraordinary? When should an infant not be treated? When should treatment be stopped? At what point does treatment start doing more harm than good to a patient?

Other Views: There are not always clear-cut answers to such questions. Sometimes, medical personnel decide within minutes after birth. Sometimes, others are involved—nurses, the hospital, clergy, other professionals, and the courts. The emphasis here is that the decision-making process is medical, ethical, and legal, as well as social and economic, familial and personal.

At the personal level, one might recall the statement attributed to Joseph Stalin that one death is a tragedy but a million deaths are a statistic. Louis Lasagna took what we might call the statistical attitude toward birth defects until his seventh child was judged to have Down's syndrome. We have noted this impingement of the personal in the abortion, contraception, and genetic issues. In this case, Lasagna moved to a positive perspective from his trained statistical neutrality.[46]

Roderic H. Phibbs reports on Pediatric Grand Rounds presented at the University of California.[47] The Rounds included the senior staff nurse, residents, and interns. In the three cases presented, and in general, decisions and judgments differed. The nurses who spend the most time with an infant not infrequently have a different judgment than the specialist who sees the child on occasion or the intern who visits frequently. Although judgments need to be made with all the information possible, we are reminded here of the constructive role of intuition. For all our sophisticated medical technology, medicine and health care remains, in some sense at least, an art as well as a science.

Although Duff and Campbell used medical prognoses as a basis for decision, they involved parents in the decision-making process. They also call for involvement of the larger public. In contrast, F. J. Ingelfinger said it is the doctor who leads the process, and the onus of decision making falls on the doctor. Lorbers' criteria for selective treatment of spina bifida infants appears objective but is based on judgment of medical prognosis.[48]

No Treatment: One way of considering the ethical perspective is in the traditional terms of euthanasia, commonly called "mercy killing."[49] To directly kill an infant is active or direct euthanasia. In neonatology, it is also involuntary from the infant's perspective.[50] To "let someone die" usually means to not use the machinery, the resuscitators, the medical technology that might keep the person alive, at least for a little while. It may be that when a decision is made to not treat, or to suspend treatment, the neonate does not die immediately. Life might linger on for days. The suffering that may take place during this time has led some to suggest that active euthanasia would be the more merciful procedure. This is, of course, what was done historically and in other cultures. Officially, our culture does not approve. It came up publicly in 1963 in Liege, Belgium, with a thalidomide baby. The mother and the doctor (for complicity) were brought to court, but were acquited.[51] More generally, the decision for "no treatment" means a passive euthanasia, which is becoming more common or, perhaps we should more accurately say, more well known in our society.[52]

Treatment: The decision to treat may also cause life to linger. Although new therapeutic techniques have increased survival, they have also delayed death. A report on hyaline membrane disease care noted this. From 1961 to 1965, only a few deaths were after seventy-two hours, and a few survived for five weeks. From 1969 to 1972, 25 percent survived the seventy-two hours, and a few survived for three weeks. In addition to the suffering of the children, the delayed deaths prolonged the anxiety of parents and increased the burden on nursing and medical staffs. Costs rose from $45,000 during 1966 to 1968 to $250,000 in 1969 to 1972.[53] One wonders if such treatment should be classified as experimentation or research.

RESEARCH

In *The Ethics of Fetal Research*, Paul Ramsey distinguishes between research involving fetal tissue from and including nonliving fetuses (even by pro-life proponent standards) and that involving living fetuses. This includes "in utero" experiments, usually in pre-abortion situations, to test drugs, and other categories of research. Included here too are the still living, previable abortus experiments, as well as work done on a delivered exteriorized fetus while the placenta is still in place. Ramsey's concern focuses on the previable or nonviable fetus for "surely we do

not mean to do experimentation on possible viable fetuses."[54]

Fetal

Research on previable fetuses should be banned or at least severely restricted in Ramsey's opinion. Because, obviously, the fetus cannot give its own informed consent to such experimentation, it is not right. Those in favor of it claim that the research is helpful, or potentially so, to others.[55] Ramsey claims it is right to experiment only if there is genuine potential for the fetus itself. He is following the model that a procedure is justifiable if it may help the patient but not if it is merely done for potential help to other patients.[56]

Neonatal

Hemphill and Freeman note that much therapy for newborns is experimental although it is not controlled research.[57] It is supposedly done for the welfare of the newborn on whom it is done, although some of them die from it. The intent passes Ramsey's standard for ethical care. The practice may not. Duff and Campbell recall an experienced nurse observing that they had lost a child "several weeks ago. Isn't it time to quit?" Again, a house officer asked if it wasn't time to turn off curiosity and turn on kindness. They saw these children, like many others, as having acquired the "right to die" when even the intent is missing.[58] Colleen McElroy objects to the curiosity that continues to order procedures on a "no treatment" infant, even if something might be learned to benefit another patient. The procedures can be needless, pointless, and cruel.[59]

Another difficulty may be one of the research controls. Can one justify withholding what has become standard therapy just to see if there is any difference in outcome? Hemphill and Freeman cite as an example the use of chloramphenicol, administered prophylactically because it has been helpful with adults and older children. The death rate increased. When controlled studies were introduced, it was found that those without this treatment were more likely to survive.[60]

It would appear that good intentions alone were not sufficient justification for a procedure. If Hemphill and Freeman are right that much therapy on newborns is in fact experimental, it may be that doing nothing may be more beneficial than doing everything we can.

How to Proceed?

There may not be any single answer to the problem. In part, that may be because of the time factor—decisions to treat or not treat, and if treat, how to treat may need to be made within moments in the neonatal period. In other cases, however, as with the chloramphenicol, there are possibilities for reflection. One such case is the report of a proposed experiment, arranged with controls. The proposed study was rejected because it involved taking experimental risks with newborns. The deliberate lowering of body temperature in order to study the most effective means of bringing the temperature back up to normal was rejected by parents, nursing staff, and peers. Further inquiry suggested that the risks were minimal, and, in fact, the lower temperatures required by the experimental protocol were already occurring in the natural setting of the delivery room. The controlled therapy then became one of using differing procedures to see which would do the most good to the newborns. This was acceptable to all three groups and, as a controlled study, made a significant contribution to neonatal treatment.[61]

THE ISSUES

Traditional health care has stressed the saving and prolonging of life, alleviating suffering, doing no harm, achieving maximum health. At times, these principles may be in conflict: to prolong life may impose suffering. Usually, this has been balanced against the good it did the patient. There are times, however, when the suffering may outweigh the good. Who decides when that point is reached—parents? physicians? health care personnel? lawyers? clergy? Jonsen suggests the really essential question is not who de-

cides but on what basis the decision should be made. What are the underlying values regarding infants, suffering, economics, handicaps, the role of the healing professions, the future of the human race?[62] Sanctity of life versus quality of life and the use of scarce resources are among the major issues in the neonatal area.

The concern with abortion asks if or when the effort should be made to save the live product of the procedure. The research "imperative" raises questions about the use of live subjects, even when the subject comes from an abortion. When medical procedures are carried out on fetuses or newborns that will not live, the procedure or research is for the benefit of someone else. Is this acceptable?[63]

NURSES, NEONATOLOGY, AND ETHICS

Nurses who work in neonatal intensive care units are the principal focus of this chapter. Nurses who work with abortion patients as well as in labor and delivery rooms, postpartum wards, and regular newborn nurseries may also face the ethical issues summarized here.[64] All can benefit by being aware of this area of bioethics. There are a variety of approaches to ethics for nurses working with neonates. The one chosen here is based on the roles nurses assume such as care giver, decision maker, and patient advocate.[65]

There are a variety of value systems among nurses. There are also differing views of what might or might not be done for neonates. Knowing how the nurse arrives at these views may help in understanding her value system and how it might conflict or coincide with others involved in care and decision making—parents, physicians, other nurses. Steele and Harmon claim that the decisions of value judgments made about the beginning or end of life should not be on an arbitrary basis. They offer guidelines for decision making. Others claim that it might be more humane if there were no set guidelines. This way, one can weigh the factors specific to an individual situation.[66] Whatever approach the nurse takes, understanding his/her own values can enhance both the care of patients and human relationships.[67] For example, it helps avoid unconscious imposition of one's personal position on another.

It may be appropriate here to add some reminders for all health professionals. The intensity of stressful conditions in NNICU's may cloud the issue of whose benefit is being considered—the neonate, the family, society, or medical science. The science of neonatal or perinatal medicine and nursing are still growing by leaps and bounds. Some neonatologists see the knowledge life-span as seven years. If this is true, in seven years what is now known and the basis for practice may no longer be appropriate. This fast-changing knowledge and technology continues to create ethical dilemmas for all personnel working in the NNICU's. It is not surprising if decision makers often feel they are working in a vacuum in such circumstances.[68]

Multidisciplinary Task Force: One way of dealing with the complexity of decision making for neonates has been the establishment of multidisciplinary ethical task forces.[69] These groups may consist of physicians, social workers, psychiatrists, clergy, lawyers, economists, anthropologists, and nurses. Sometimes, specific stellar cases are reviewed by all. However, to date, the nurse has not always been a recognized decision maker. She is often called upon for her knowledge of the infant's daily status or the parents' reactions/support of the neonate, but not for her/his opinion on what should or should not be done in treatment. This is ironic because nurses have the most extended and prolonged contact with a given neonate. They often have the most complete knowledge of his physical condition and family situation.[70]

We noted earlier Duff and Campbell's call for such multiple support as these interdisciplinary teams.[71] This focus on the complex, unusual cases may be natural enough, but it gives little attention to the day-by-day ethical decisions being made. These are not uncommonly made by physicians, with nurses left to carry them out.[72] Cechanek[73] notes how difficult it is to carry out an ethical decision with which the nurse may disagree without knowing how the decision was reached, or without any input into the decision-making

process. The daily sharing of the bases for decision making and the inclusion of nurses' input will enhance the decision. Parental participation in decisions has been noted. Their participation in the committee and daily decisions might also be encouraged when possible.

Nurses As Care Givers

By far the most common role assumed by nurses in NNICU's is that of providing direct nursing care. Nurses usually have the most contact with the individual neonates and provide for the majority of his/her needs. This caring process is central to the practice of nursing, but it also creates conflicts.[74]

Carrying Out Orders: As mentioned earlier, nurses carry out the decisions made by others, often with limited or no input into the process. For example, an infant with Down's syndrome has been admitted to the NNICU. Within hours the physician informs the nursing staff to keep the infant warm and comfortable. They are not to feed it. There will be no surgical repair of the bowel obstruction. It takes from a few days to a few weeks for such an infant to starve to death. It is the nurse who is left to care for this infant from day to day. The nurse watches as the child becomes more and more irritable and less and less responsive to any comforting. Some nurses faced with caring for such an infant report feeling like an "executioner." The physician may avoid contact with the infant and may let it be known that he doesn't wish to hear about it any more, further isolating the nurse and her feelings.

The nurse may be confused about her/his role of care giver when told not to care for the infant's total needs. Stifled in discussing feelings or the child's reactions, the nurse may become resentful of physicians and families. Some have suggested that families who decide to allow such an infant to die should take the child home with them instead of "dumping" their unpleasant decision on the nursing staff. Others, however, accept such a decision and provide the prescribed care without anger or resentment. These nurses provide the caring and comforting for the infant throughout the final days of life.[75]

Nursing Input: Again, one effective way of reducing confusion and antagonism is to have all members of the team responsible for the infant discuss the case before making a decision on whether or not to continue life support systems.[76] Cechanek notes that good communication among team members fostered during grand rounds or team conferences encourages each team member to respect one another openly and to share the dimensions of the decision to be made and their individual opinions on the matter. These discussions require courage and sensitivity from all team members as individual positions are presented, but they can lead to better decisions and less emphasis on one person being solely responsible.[77]

Concerns: Part of the problem for health professionals may be the apparent inconsistency of approach in caring for neonaates with specific disorders. Why is it that some premature infants are delivered by Cesarean section to improve chances of survival and others of the same gestational age and apparent condition are allowed to deliver vaginally and may not be offered minimal resuscitative support? Or why do some very premature infants receive all out heroics, whereas others of the same weight and apparent condition are left to their own immature forces? The case of a viable product of an induced abortion may be included here. In one instance, one is expected to care completely and assist in the heroic efforts. With the next child, one is expected to accept death as its fate without questioning or heroics. Discussion of the factors involved in the decision can clarify the issues and be helpful in providing the best care.[78]

Infants who are long-term residents of neonatal units pose special problems for nurses and others involved in their care. An emotional attachment often develops for these infants.[79] Nurses may find it increasingly difficult to support a "no treatment" decision. Another problem arises when there are limited beds available. A sick newborn with a positive prognosis needs the equipment and bed occupied by a long-term infant with an unknown or poor prognosis. Who should get the limited resources? Nurses may not be asked to participate in the decision,

but they may be aware of inconsistencies in deciding who gets the limited resources.

Emergencies: The nurse's role as caregiver involves participation in carrying out the doctor's orders to resuscitate in emergency situations. In an emergency, a physician may aggressively intervene and attempt to revive a severly anoxic infant. Under such circumstances, most nurses will assist until the infant recovers or a negative prognosis is clear. When possible, discussion of the case after the emergency can help him/her understand why the physician insisted on resuscitation. Such discussion permits input from the nurse's evaluation of the situation. Other NNICU personnel might be included in such postemergency discussion to the benefit of all concerned.

Nurses As Decision Makers

New Skills: We have commented on the lack of involvement of nurses in the daily ethical decisions made in NNICU's. However, some nurses are demanding and assuming a more active role in ethical decision making. These units, with their sophisticated technology, require highly skilled practitioners caring for the patients. Many units have recognized the utility of preparing selected nursing staff to provide the highly skilled care needed, such as intubation, umbilical vein catheterization, instituting respirators, and so on. Graduate programs in neonatal nursing have also been initiated in order to provide the highly skilled nursing specialist for NNICU's.

When to Act: Now that we have these new skills, when does the nurse use them? In emergency situations, the tendency is to act first and then evaluate if efforts should be continued. In nonemergencies nurses can try to gather data on the individual situations in order to participate in the decision-making process. Nurses may lack a firm prognosis, just as the physician does. Input from others, including the family, can improve decision making even when the prognosis is unclear.

Nurses as decision makers also face the

problem that once treatment is initiated it is difficult to stop. Laws and ethics, as well as emotional attachment to the individual, combine to make it difficult to stop treatment.[80] On the other hand, nurses have suggested that certain infants have "acquired the right to die." Continued treatment may be not only difficult but inhuman and needlessly cruel. Case Study 12 is an illustration of this. Nurses may be in a position to encourage careful thought before initiating treatment and to encourage "giving up" when chances for survival are very limited. The nurses who observe these infants for hours at a time may have a better idea of the child's potential for meaningful life than the physician who stops by occasionally.[81]

Covert Decisions: Nurses also participate in decision making on a less obvious plane. Nurses might move very quickly in response to a situation, or just the opposite. An example of the latter is included in Case Study 12 when the nurse decided to move *slowly* across the room to respond to the physician's request for equipment. Possibly she may have hoped the delay would decide the fate of the 700-gram infant, or she may have thought the physician should know where the equipment was kept. Either way, the slowness of movement could have potentially meant the difference between life and death for such a small infant. Her slowness represented the nurse's decision.

A note of caution is offered here again. Some nurses have opted for a recognized role in decision making. They may forget or not realize the toll it takes in personal emotional energy to be continually faced with life-and-death issues. Nurses in our society can often defer difficult or unwanted decisions to the physician, but the physician may not have that luxury. "Passing the buck" is itself an ethical decision, of course. It is suggested that nurses accept the decision-making role advisedly and responsibly. Another aspect of decision making of which one should be aware is that the value systems of the professionals and the parents may be divergent and in conflict. The nursing code gives priority to patients. Neonates may have value but do not have value systems. Among the adults, whose system predominates and under what circumstances may be difficult decisions.

Nurses As Advocates

The role of patient advocate is most important in the neonatal nursery because the neonate is totally unable to speak for itself. This does not automatically imply that the nurse should assume the role of advocate, but it raises the question of who is the best person to speak on behalf of the neonate.

Some nurses claim they are the ones to speak on behalf of the neonate. They support this view with the statement that they have the infant's interests in mind and are not tempted to decide on factors not immediately related to the individual neonate, such as other children in the family, costs of care, wantedness of child, or threat of malpractice. Other nurses counter with their concern that it is unrealistic to advocate a decision contrary to the parents' desires, as the nurse cannot care for all the sick neonates rejected by families. However, assuming the role of advocate does not necessarily imply making the decision on treatment so much as fairly representing the neonate's interests. Nurses can do this.[82]

Nurses and Research

Neonatal nurses are often involved in research efforts affecting infants in their care. As mentioned earlier, neonates cannot give their informed consent to participate although family consent is obtainable. Conflicts may arise if the nurse caring for the infant in a research situation senses that the infant is being kept alive purely for research purposes with little consideration of his/her right to die or not be subjected to painful and otherwise uncomfortable life-prolonging procedures. If the research requires uncomfortable or invasive treatment, should it be allowed to continue?

Another possible conflict of practice arises when anencephalic infants incapable of living are kept alive mechanically for research to explore the effects of treatments that cannot be performed on living infants. This type of research is certainly not going to help the individual infant, but it may help other infants born later. Nurses need to sort out their own stand on the research issues and discuss these with the physicians and others involved in designing and permitting research on neonates to be carried out. Participation on human investigation committees is one way for nurses to have input in the decision on fetal and neonatal research.

CASE STUDIES

The following case studies are selected to illustrate some of the more common ethical dilemmas of neonatal nursing. They are not meant to be all-inclusive. They are based on actual experiences of nurses. The cases will reflect the categorization of ethical issues by age and diagnosis of a neonatal condition. These include 1) the very premature infant, 2) the neonate with a severe congenital defect, disease, or condition with an unknown prognosis, and 3) the viable product of an induced abortion. Once again, the first case will be analyzed in some detail to assist the reader in the application of the guidelines for evaluating ethical decision making. The remaining cases are for self-study.

Case #12

Very Premature Infant

D. J. is the nurse-midwife on duty in a large tertiary care center. As she listens to the change of shift report, she is told of a patient who is aborting a twenty-one- to twenty-three-week gestation spontaneously. No one is sure of the actual length of pregnancy, but the fetus is estimated to weigh less than 500 grams (1 pound). She overhears the physician coming on duty ask if resuscitative measures are to be instituted and if the delivery should take place in the delivery room where such equipment is more readily available. The answer is to let the patient deliver in bed in the labor room. If the infant shows signs of life, call the pediatrician. As the report continues, the nurse-midwife hears the patient calling for help and runs into the room in time to catch the fetus being delivered. The physician follows and notes that the infant is gasping and has a heart rate. She, in turn, calls the pediatrician, who arrives within seconds, wraps the infant in a towel, and runs to the transitional nursery. The infant's weight is approximately 700 grams, and the doctor requests help from the nurse in resuscitating the infant. The nurse glances over at the limp infant and *slowly* responds to the pediatrician's request for help, questioning why the doctor is taking time to resuscitate. After approximately three minutes, the infant in successfully intubated, ventilated, and the color and heart rate improve along with limb motion.

Analysis

1. The basic health problem for this infant is its very immature status, with little indication of its ability to survive outside the uterus. The basic decision that needed to be made initially was whether this infant should be resuscitated. Now that ventilation has been accomplished, should it be stopped? Scientific knowledge is very limited in regard to infants of 700 grams and their ability to eventually survive without mechanical assistance. The ethical issues most evident are presented in item 3 following. The individuals directly involved in the decisions to be made are the infant (who has no voice) and the infant's parents. The health personnel—obstetrician, nurse-midwife, pediatrician, neonatal nurse—are involved to some extent in making the decision, but do not appear to be the principal participants.

2. Further information that might have been helpful in deciding whether to initiate treatment or ventilation of this infant includes the parents' wishes for this child, based on informed data *prior* to delivery. The nurse caring for this woman prior to delivery could have obtained the parents' reactions to the impending birth and

their desires concerning attempts to resuscitate, as could have the obstetrician assigned to the case. Data from the parents on the wantedness of this pregnancy might also have been helpful if known prior to delivery, providing the obstetrician or nurse-midwife considered this aspect in their decision to attempt resuscitation. Now that resuscitation has been initiated, it could be important to ask the parents' opinion/desires about continuing it. Some might feel this is wrong because the parents had no say in initiating the resuscitation, and others may feel strongly that once initiated, it is up to parents to decide or help decide on whether to continue. The parents may wish to see the infant before making such a decision, or they may not. Chances are they will want to know something about the child's prognosis—its chances for survival.

3. The ethical issues involved in this situation include the quality of life versus sanctity of life for the infant; a determination of who is best able to decide whether efforts at initiating or maintaining life should continue; and a determination of the rights of the infant, health personnel, and parents in regard to choice of life for the infant. Because the nurse and pediatrician took it upon themselves to resuscitate in the first place with limited knowledge of the situation, a problem of informed consent seems evident.

4. Sections of the ANA *Code for Nurses* of particular relevance in this case study are Statement One, especially 1.6; Statement Three, especially 3.1, and Statement Four.

5. The value systems operant in the many individuals involved in this event were quite divergent, it would seem. The nurses caring for the woman during the night apparently did not think it important to ask the mother/parents about what they would like done if the infant delivered alive. The nurse-midwife appeared to be responding to the call for help and performed the delivery as she would with any other patient. The obstetrician who made the decision to allow the patient to deliver in the labor bed might have thought that this fetus had no chance for survival and that the efforts to resuscitate would be wasted. The physician who appeared and called the pediatrician was responding to the respiratory gasping and heart rate of the fetus, with limited or no data on potential for future life. This is common in emergency situations where nurses and doctors respond with efforts to save life immediately, and then think about the consequences later. The nurse in the transitional nursery seems to have already decided that the infant was too small to merit resuscitation, as evidenced by her slow response. She could value quality of life over sanctity of life, or be convinced that such a small infant could not possibly survive, hence, why make the efforts to resuscitate? This nurse could also have witnessed too many small infants resuscitated, only to develop other conditions incompatible with life, lingering on for months at great expense, and then dying in spite of team efforts to save them, or worse yet, developing bronchial pulmonary dysplasia and turning into a respirator cripple for months, or even years. It is difficult to analyze the parents' value system because they were not included in the decision to initiate resuscitation.

6. Value conflicts are apparent in this case study between pediatrician and nursery nurse, and possibly between parents and others, although the parents have not been included in the decision process as yet.

7. There are varying ideas on who is best indicated to make the decision to initiate resuscitation, and how to decide whether to continue the ventilation support. It appears that the pediatrician has assumed the role of patient advocate. It is difficult to decide who best could fulfill this role. One might accept the parents as the decision makers on continued treatment even if they did not create the situation now requiring a decision. Others might think that the parents are too close to the situation to make such a decision and it would be easier on them if the doctor or someone else decided.

8. The actions regarding the current decision range from stopping the respirator immediately or waiting indefinitely for infant maturity or death. The *Code for Nurses* speaks to safeguarding the client and providing nursing care, but there is little to help the individual nurse know how to act in such a difficult situation as this. Who is to make a decision on the issue of resuscitation or no? No code will help the nurse deal with her individual value system and views on the quality of life for the very premature. The field of biomedical ethics implies that the nurse can analyze her own value systems and the issues present, as well as formulate a basis for action that remains somewhat consistent from case to case of this nature.
9. Do you think the nurse-midwife and neonatal nurse acted in an ethically sound manner? What is the basis for your decision? How would you have responded if you were either the nurse-midwife or neonatal nurse in this situation? On what basis did you choose an action.
10. What did you learn from this case study that may be helpful to you in future situations of this nature?

Congenital Disease[83]

Ms. D., a thirty-eight-year-old primipara, delivered her first child twelve hours ago. The baby girl has Down's syndrome in addition to severe cardiac defects incompatible with life, though surgically reparable. The nursery nurse accompanies the physician to Ms. D.'s room where he explains the infant's cardiac condition, noting that the child will probably not live long. He adds, "This is really a blessing because the child is mentally retarded. I do not think we should do anything that will keep your baby alive because she will not be able to lead a normal life. Think about it, and I will came back tomorrow for your decision." As the doctor leaves, Ms. D. tearfully asks the nurse, "Isn't there anything that can be done for my daughter? I have waited so long to have a baby of my own, I don't want to lose her." The nurse answers that surgery could correct the heart problem, but would not change the Down's condition.

The nursery nurse conveyed this information to the head nurse along with her concern that Ms. D. needed more complete information about Down's syndrome. The head nurse talked with Ms. D. and asked her if she would be interested in talking with parents of a Down's child before making her decision about surgery for her daughter. Ms. D. agreed and met with the parents that evening. The next morning, Ms. D. informed the doctor that she wanted everything done for her daughter so that she could live.

In addition to applying the Guidelines, consider the following questions:

1. What is the nursery nurse's responsibility to the patient in regard to ensuring informed consent? Did her actions speak to this responsibility?
2. What is the head nurse's responsibility to the physician, and should he have been informed of her plan to bring other parents of Down's children to Ms. D.?
3. Did the nurses respond to this situation in an ethically sound manner? What other alternative actions might have been taken by them or anyone else involved in the situation?

Viable Product of Abortion

B. D. is the nurse assigned to work on the labor ward, and her responsibilities today include caring for Mrs. P., a thirty-year-old para 3003 (three fullterm pregnancies, no prior abortions), who is in the process of aborting a sixteen-week pregnancy by a saline instillation. All goes well until Mrs. P. exclaims that the fetus is coming out. At this time the physician and nurse note that the infant is still alive, though struggling to breathe. The physician quickly clamps the cord, cuts it, and hands the fetus to the nurse with instructions to wrap the infant and carry it over to the other delivery room. When asked if the pediatrician is to be called, the physician answers, "no." B. D. does as told, and when she gets across the hall, she notes that the gasping efforts have ceased although there is still an occasional heartbeat. She is confused as to how to proceed to care for this infant, having assisted in the resuscitation of many premature infants. Just then, the physician arrives and tells her to return to the mother to care for her. He will stay with the infant.

In addition to applying the Guidelines to analyze this situation, consider the following questions:

1. Does a woman who chooses an abortion have the right (or responsibility) to choose to allow the product of that procedure to be resuscitated?
2. Should the nurse or doctor initiate resuscitative efforts without consulting the mother (or father) of the child?
3. Who is best indicated to speak on behalf of this infant?
4. If the nurse did not believe in abortion by choice, might she have been more eager to resuscitate this infant?
5. How does one know if this infant was damaged by the saline instillation during the abortion procedure?

NOTES AND REFERENCES

1. The word was coined in 1960 by Dr. Alex Schaffer, according to Clement A. Smith, "Neonatal Medicine and Quality of Life: An Historical Perspective, pp. 31–36, in *Ethics of Newborn Intensive Care*, ed. by Albert R. Jonsen and Michael J. Garland (San Francisco and Berkeley: Health Policy Program and Institute of Governmental Studies, University of California, 1976), p. 32.

2. Raymond S. Duff and A. G. M. Campbell note that parents and medical staff deciding to withhold treatment of defective newborns included various religious groups. See "Moral and Ethical Dilemmas in the Special-Care Nursery," *The New England Journal of Medicine*, no. 17 (25 Oct. 1977), **289**:890–894. *The Journal* is abbreviated hereafter as *NEJM*.

3. "Forward," pp. xiii–xv, Jonsen and Garland, op. cit. Gordon B. Avery also notes that medical science, established custom, and law do not provide the answers in these complicated cases. We are into the personal meaning and purpose of life. See "The Morality of Drastic Intervention," pp. 11–14 in *Neonatology*, ed. by Avery (Philadelphia: J. B. Lippincott Company, 1975), p. 11. Darrel W. Amundsen suggests that prolongation of life did not become part of medical practice until the time of Francis Bacon (1561–1626). This concept is not part of the Hippocratic Corpus of literature. "The Physician's Obligation to Prolong Life: A Medical Duty without Classical Roots," *The Hastings Center Report*, no. 4 (Aug. 1978), **8**:23–30. *The Report* is abbreviated hereafter as *HCR*.

4. Mildred F. Jefferson, M.D., review of Jonsen and Garland, *The Linacre Quarterly*, no. 4 (Nov. 1977), **44**:369–370. Dr. Wolf W. Zuelzer points out that "until recently the very questions we are here to ask were taboo in a society whose medical ethic has not changed since Hippocrates." "Relationship to Pediatrics," pp. 16–20, in *Ethical Dilemmas in Current Obstetric and Newborn Care*, Report of the Sixty-Fifth Ross Conference on Pediatric Research, ed. by Tom D. Moore (Columbus, Ohio: Ross Laboratories, 1973), p. 16. Breaking taboos is disturbing, so Dr. Jefferson is not the only one disturbed. Historically, according to Amundsen, op. cit., only a minority followed Hippocrates throughout the centuries. It was only with the rise of medieval guilds that one could say there was such a thing as a medical ethic.

5. This is the legal situation in this country and most of the world. John A. Robertson, "Involuntary Euthanasia of Defective Newborns: A Legal Analysis," *Stanford Law Review*, no. 2 (Jan. 1975), **27**:213–269, reprinted, pp. 335–364, in *Vulnerable Infants*, ed. by Jane L. and Lawrence H. Schwartz (New York: McGraw-Hill Book Company, 1977). See also, Paul Ramsey, *Ethics at the Edges of Life* (New Haven: Yale University Press, 1978), pp. 198–199. Ramsey interprets Jewish law (Sanhedrin 37a, Leviticus 19:16) as opposed to euthanasia. Some Jewish interpreters disagree. Marvin Kohl and Paul Kurtz, "A Plea for Beneficent Euthanasia," pp. 233–238, in *Beneficent Euthanasia*, ed. by Kohl (Buffalo, N.Y.: Prometheus Books, 1975).

6. This resembles the "delayed personhood policy" advocated by some. One suggestion is that the state withhold birth certificates and names for a time for high-risk infants, trusting in the parents to make the right decisions, as is now done in abortion decisions. See F. Raymond Marks, "The Defective Newborn: An Analytic Framework for a Policy Dialog," pp. 97–119, in Jonsen and Garland, op. cit., pp. 110–111. Joseph Fletcher, "Indicators of Humanhood: A Tentative Profile of Man," *HCR*, no. 5 (Nov. 1972), **2**:1–4. Michael Tooley has argued that the justification for abortion extends to infanticide. Newborns have no right to life, because they lack a concept of self. Thus death may be allowed, at least for a time, say a week, after

birth. "Abortion and Infanticide," *Philosophy and Public Affairs*, no. 1 (Fall 1972), **2**:37–65. Fletcher agrees. See *The Ethics of Genetic Control* (Garden City, N.Y.: Anchor Press/Doubleday, 1974), pp. 132–143, 185–186. Others disagree, noting that once the child is born and has a separate existence, it has an independent moral claim for care and support. See John Fletcher, "Abortion, Euthanasia and Care of Defective Newborns," *NEJM*, no. 2 (9 Jan. 1975), **292**:75–78. Robertson, op. cit., James M. Gustafson, "Mongolism, Parental Desires, and the Right to Life," *Perspectives in Biology and Medicine* (Summer 1973), **16**:529–557. Ramsey, op. cit., pp. 203–204.

7. Hysterotomy is most likely to result in a live birth. The saline method is usually fatal to the fetus. The safer prostaglandins (labor-inducing) that are increasingly being substituted for saline, apparently result in more live births. See Sissela Bok, Bernard N. Nathanson, David C. Nathan, and Leroy Walters, "The Unwanted Child: Caring for the Fetus Born Alive After An abortion," *HCR*, no. 5 (1976), **6**:10–15.

8. John A. Robertson, "After 'Edelin': Little Guidance," *HCR*, no. 3 (1977), **7**:15–17, 45. Bok and others, op. cit. The American College of Obstetricians and Gynecologists 1976 statement sees abortion as a resolution of a conflict between the fetus and the pregnant woman. The solution is removal of the fetus, not necessarily its death. See ACOG statement of policy as issued by the executive board of ACOG, "Further Ethical Considerations in Induced Abortion," Dec. 1977, pp. 1–4. See André E. Hellegers, "Abortion: Medical Indications," pp. 1–5, *Encyclopedia of Bioethics*, ed. by Warren T. Reich (New York: The Free Press, 1978). *The Encyclopedia* is abbreviated hereafter as *EB*.

9. A doctor was indicted in Massachusetts for the "death" of a fetus or infant during a hysterotomy. He was first convicted and later acquitted on appeal. Part of the issue was whether the fetus/infant breathed or showed other signs of life. Another issue was whether the doctor had made an effort to ensure the fetus' death before removal from the uterus. Robertson, *HCR*, **7**, op. cit.

10. Tom Farrell and Virginia Adams, "Abortion Law Further Refined," *The New York Times* (14 Jan. 1979), 22 E.

11. Walters, op. cit., pp. 13–14, offers a series of figures from New York State. Of thirty-eight live deliveries in eighteen months, one survived to the point of discharge to its mother. Life for the others ranged from less than one hour to a maximum of twenty-seven hours and five minutes. There was a live delivery ratio of 1.7 per 1,000 abortions for saline, and 8.5 per 1,000 for hysterotomies. In another statistic, the latter figure was 1.2, the overall live-delivery rate was 3 per 1,000, with prostoglandins 22 per 1,000. He extrapolated these to the United States as a whole for 1974 to get an estimate of 196 infants, of whom six or seven might have survived to grow up. Moore, op. cit., p. 45, reports forty-nine live births in 260,000 abortions in 1971. Of these forty-nine live births, forty-seven died within hours.

12. "Doctors' Ethics in Upheaval: Tough Questions from the Brave New World of Medicine," *Family Weekly* (9 Sept. 1973), reprint. Dr. Mildred Stahlman in her introduction at the Ross Conference, op. cit., p. 12, suggests that we do not have the answers but we can define the questions we need to ask.

13. Op. cit., *HCR* 7:16. George J. Annas notes that in mid-1976, in *Danforth* v. *Planned Parenthood of Missouri*, the Supreme Court ruled that a state cannot require the preservation of fetal life in an abortion until after viability. "Abortion and the Supreme Court: Round Two," *HCR*, no. 5 (1976), 6:15–17.

14. Susan Taft Nicholson, "Abortion and The Roman Catholic Church," *Journal of Religious Ethics, Studies in Religious Ethics II* (1978), p. 83. The papal statement is "The prolongation of life: address of Pius XII to an international congress of anesthesiologists," *The Pope Speaks* (1957–1958), 4:393–398. See Gerald Kelly, "Notes: the duty to preserve life," *Theological Studies* (1951), 12:550–556; and his *Medico-Moral Problems* (St. Louis: The Catholic Hospital Association, 1958), pp. 128–141. Edwin F. Healy, *Medical Ethics* (Chicago: Loyola University Press, 1956), pp. 60–90. Ethically, the principle comes from an analysis of human nature (p. 60). He notes that ordinary means may not be required where the results are not of sufficient benefit (p. 66).

Even oxygen or intravenous feeding may not be required if they merely prolong life for a brief period (p. 80). What is true for the adult patient also applies for relatives or parents in cases of coma or children (pp. 78, 80–82). However, if a normal child would receive artificial respiration (a temporary procedure), a defective child, for example, a hydrocephalic, requiring artificial respiration should have it (pp. 88–89). Yet, if a procedure, such as a stomach tube, is required as a permanent necessity, it may be regarded as extraordinary, whether the child is defective or normal (p. 89). See also Paul Ramsey, *The Patient as Person* (New Haven: Yale University Press, 1970), pp. 118–139. Anne J. Davis and Mila A. Aroskar, *Ethical Dilemmas and Nursing Practice* (New York: Appleton-Century-Crofts, 1978), pp. 114, 117. Richard A. McCormick, "The Quality of Life, The Sanctity of Life," *HCR*, no. 1 (Feb. 1978), 8:30–36. Anthony Shaw notes that "yesterday's heroic efforts are today's routine procedures." See p. 889 in his "Dilemmas of 'Informed Consent' in Children," *NEJM*, no. 17 (25 Oct. 1977), 289:885–890.

15. Bok, op. cit., p. 10.

16. Op. cit., p. 14. Paul Ramsey, *The Ethics of Fetal Research* (New Haven: Yale University Press, 1975), pp. 59–60.

17. Bok, op. cit., p. 11. In a related area, the authority to terminate life support systems has sometimes been legally left to the judgment of physicians and guardians. One case involved two children aged three and four. They had been overcome with smoke, had no cognitive or vegetative brain activity, and flat EEG readings. Respirators kept organs functioning. When these were removed, the functioning stopped. The ruling that directed this authority to physicians and guardians required consultations, including a hospital ethics committee. "Let the Doctor Decide," *The Christian Century*, no. 30 (27 Sept. 1978), 95:881. In other situations such as lifesaving operations for defective newborns and blood transfusions, courts have ruled against parental wishes. See Robert M. Veatch, *Case Studies In Medical Ethics* (Cambridge, Mass.: Harvard University Press, 1977), pp. 338–340. George J. Annas, "After Saikewicz: No-Fault Death," *HCR*, no. 3 (June 1978), 8:16–18.

18. Nathanson, op. cit., p. 12. John M. Hemphill and John M. Freeman, "Infants: Medical Aspects and Ethical Dilemmas," *EB* 2:717–724.

19. George H. Kieffer, *Bioethics: A Textbook of Issues* (Reading, Mass.: Addison-Wesley Publishing Co., Inc., 1979), p. 186. Virginia Adams and Tom Ferrell, "Ideas & Trends: Mother's Blood may Signal Fetal Defect," *The New York Times* (Sunday, 15 Apr. 1979), E 7. Again, to ask is disturbing to some. Albert R. Jonsen sees conflict with an old idea in medicine: "to save endangered life." "Introduction," pp. 1–8, in Jonsen and Garland, op. cit., p. 3. C. A. Smith, op. cit., p. 32, claims that about 1960, as more and more newborns were kept from dying, people began to think more about the QOL of their future.

20. Kieffer, op. cit., p. 186. Duff and Campbell, op. cit., p. 890. Jane V. Hunt reports not only improved survival rates but also reductions in retardation and other neurological handicaps. "Mental Development of the Survivors of Neonatal Intensive Care," pp. 39–53, in Jonsen and Garland, op. cit., p. 39. Marcia J. Kramer sees a mixed blessing involved. There's a high incidence of congenital anomalies and prematurity in the NNIC population. So, a disproportionate share of the NNICU survivors suffer impairment. "Ethical Issues in Neonatal Intensive Care: An Economic Perspective," pp. 75–93, in Jonsen and Garland, op. cit., p. 75. The numbers of course are less important than the existence of the problem, as noted by Bok, op. cit., p. 10. She sees a moral dilemma whether we are talking about one child or 10,000. Bradley E. Smith refers to the poignant moral and economic implications. Of 19,160 consecutive deliveries, the question, "not to resuscitate" only came up for thirty-eight and was a practical dilemma in only a few of these. "Resuscitation, Apgar and Outcome," pp. 54–58, in the Ross Conference report, op. cit., p. 55.

21. Duff and Campbell, op. cit., p. 890.

22. Zuelzer, op. cit., p. 18.

23. John A. Robertson is aware that non-treatment of defective infants has been going on all through "history but only recently has the medical profession openly acknowledged the scope and alleged desirability" of this. "Involuntary . . . ," op. cit., p. 213.

24. Michael Tooley, "Infanticide: A Philosophical Perspective," *EB* 2:742–751. David Landy, "Death I: Anthropological Perspective," *EB* 1:221–229. The Arab tribes were in an almost constant state of war before Mu-hammed unified them. This would, of course, kill off warriors and leave an "excess" of females. But we note also C. A. Smith's observation that neonatal mortality is greater in males. Op. cit., p. 32. The Japan reference is from Daniel J. Callahan, *Abortion: Law, Choice and Morality* (New York: Macmillan Publishing Co., Inc., 1970), p. 258. Louis Lasagna, *Life, Death, and the Doctor* (New York: Alfred A. Knopf, Inc., 1968), p. 185. Bruce K. Waltke, "Old Testament Texts," in *Birth Control and the Christian*, ed. by Spitzer and Saylor (Wheaton, Ill.: Tyndale, 1969), p. 14.

25. Tooley, op. cit., p. 742.

26. Tooley, op. cit., p. 743. John T. Noonan, Jr., *Contraception: A History of Its Treatment by the Catholic Theologians and Canonists* (Cambridge, Mass.: Harvard University Press, 1965), pp. 18–29. Thomas McKeown, *The Modern Rise of Population* (New York: Academic Press, Inc., 1976). William L. Langer, "Infanticide: A Historical Survey," *History of Childhood Quarterly: The Journal of Psychohistory* (1974), **1**:353–365.

27. Op. cit., p. 159. His reference is to Columbia. This is similar to Arthur J. Dyck's "good death," from the Latin *benemortasia*, in which he suggests that it would be merciful to withhold ordinary treatment, for example, for pneumonia in severely brain-damaged children. He is not suggesting euthanasia, he says, but a merciful retreat in the face of death's inevitability. "Beneficent Euthanasia and Benemortasia: Alternative Views of Mercy," pp. 117–129, in Kohl, op. cit., p. 126.

28. Lasagna reminds us that we scorn the civilizations that slaughtered their infants but our treatment of the retarded may be more cruel. Op. cit., p. 192.

29. Warren T. Reich and David E. Ost, "Ethical Perspective on the Care of Infants," *EB* 2:724–735.

30. David M. Feldman, discussion on "Abortion and Morality," pp. 91–116, vol. II, *Abortion in a Changing World*, ed. by Robert E. Hall (New York: Columbia University Press, 1970), pp. 97–98. Paul Ramsey also calls attention to the Jewish tradition (R. Chaim Palaggi, Chikeki Lev., I, Yoreh De'ah, no. 50) that only disinterested parties may take action leading to premature death, and that, only prayer. Others (family, medical personnel) may not even pray for death. *Ethics at the Edges of Life*, op. cit., p. 203.

31. Reich and Ost, op. cit., p. 727. The Roman Catholic concept of double effect may allow actions or omissions that lead to death because (among other reasons) it is not necessary to prolong life in extreme cases. Allowing death is not automatically evil. See H. Tristam Engelhardt, Jr., "Ethical Issues in Aiding the Death of Young Children," pp. 180–182, Kohl, op. cit., p. 190, n. 4. Joy K. Ulfema suggests inhumanity is the enemy, rather than death. "Dare to Care for the Dying," *American Journal of Nursing*, no. 1 (1976), **76**:88–90. The Journal is cited hereafter as *AJN*. Shaw, op. cit., p. 889, calls his philosophy "humane and loving," considering each case, rather than a "right to life" philosophy. Ramsey, *Patient . . . ,* op. cit., p. 137, commends the humane wisdom in traditional Roman Catholic ethics. His reference is to Kelly, op. cit.

32. Joseph Fletcher, *Ethics of Genetic Control*, op. cit., pp. 131, 156–157. Roman Catholic Richard A. McCormick rejects vitalism as idolatry. This is also true for the opposite view, a medical pessimism that kills when life seems useless. The middle course for which he opts is the Judeo-Christian attitude that life is good but as the condition for other values. See p. 174 in his "To Save or Let Die," *Journal of the American Medical Association*, no. 2 (8 July 1974), **229**:172–176. He notes further, op. cit., *HCR* **8**:1, p. 35, that sanctity of life should not be set over against quality of life. QOL decisions should be made with reverence for life as an extension of one's respect for the sanctity of life.

33. The phrase, quality of life versus equality of life, is from arthur J. Dyck, "The Value of Life: Two Contending Policies," *Harvard Magazine*, no. 5 (Jan. 1976), **78**:30–36, quoted by Ramsey, *Ethics . . . ,* op. cit., p. 265, n. 35.

34. The concept may not be in any system of professional ethicists. It is not an unknown concept, however. Dr. J. Robert Wilson notes the professional role "to preserve life at all costs." He suggests the conviction has been shaken by abortion and sterilization, not to mention increasing numbers of defective children. He notes the interesting perspective that in an earlier day, if a brain-damaged infant lived twenty-eight days, it was considered a therapeutic triumph. Its condition was rarely in the published statistics. "Relationship to Obstetrics," pp. 12–16, 70, Ross Conference, op. cit. Zuelzer, op. cit., p. 16, notes that "our unconditional commitment to the preservation of life" was no problem when death was seen as the will of God. Now he asks if we should "preserve life against nature's apparent intentions" simply because we have the gadgets to do so? He notes that morality has in the past approved cannibalism, slavery, rape, and war, but it has changed. He holds out the hope for a new morality that will allow the use of medical powers in an humane way. Joseph Fletcher notes that none at the Sixty-fifth Ross Conference "defended the sanctity doctrine, but it is still commonly and sincerely held by many segments of the public." "Moral Aspects," pp. 70–71, Ross Conference, op. cit. Robert M. Veatch says, "Except for certain interpretations by medical professionals, there has never existed an absolute obligation to prolong life." Ross Conference, op. cit., p. 91.

35. Colleen McElroy, "Caring for the Untreated Infant," *The Canadian Nurse*, no. 12 (Dec. 1975), **71**:26–30. McElroy insists upon caring and conversely she insists that the untreated child should not be a guinea pig for continuing and unnecessary procedures. Ramsey in *The Patient as Person*, op. cit., p. 153, calls this "the categorical imperative: Never abandon care! . . . Upon ceasing to try to rescue the perishing, one then is free to care for the dying." The last sentence is from an old Protestant hymn by Fanny J. Crosby (1820–1915). See also, James D. Thullen, "When you can't cure, care," *Perinatology/Neonatology*, Nov./Dec. 1977, reprint.

36. Zuelzer, op. cit., pp. 19–20, suggests this puts us "in the position of the atomic physicists who detonated the bomb first and asked the questions afterwards."

37. Ramsey, *Ethics at the Edges of Life*, op. cit., pp. 189–267. The courts tend to agree. Annas, "After Saikewicz . . . ," op. cit., p. 17.

38. Duff and Campbell, op. cit., p. 890. See Engelhardt, op. cit., on "the injury of continued existence," and life as an injury rather than a gift. This concept is comparable to that of "wrongful life" noted in our discussion of genetics. Engelhardt, "Euthanasia and Children: The Injury of Continued Existence," *The Journal of Pediatrics* (July 1973), **83**:170–171. Ramsey, *Ethics at the Edges of*

Life, op. cit., p. 207, opposes such thinking. He vigorously insists that life "is an inexplicable gift." Healy, op. cit., pp. 266–270, also insists that God alone has ownership of human life. Orthodoxy holds a similar view. Stanley H. Harakas, "Eastern Orthodox Christianity," *EB* 1:452.

39. See Joseph Fletcher, *HCR* **2**, op. cit. Fletcher, *Humanhood;* Buffalo: Prometheus Books, 1979, pp. 7–19. His indicators of humanhood include intelligence, self-awareness and control, a sense of time, relationship, communication, curiosity, and neocortical function. Ramsey, *Ethics at the Edges of Life*, op. cit., p. 204 and n. 26, claims these criteria imply anyone without a Western sense of time is not human. He calls these terms accordion terms without clear definition. We note also that we do not know the extent to which infants have these capabilities. At least some children do not evidence a great deal of self-control, for example. Many adults don't do too well on these criteria. So the criteria are not only Western-oriented but are oriented to a particular type of person as well. On these issues, see also Gustafson, op. cit., and McCormick, op. cit., *JAMA*, 229.

Humanness is sometimes considered in terms of personhood (Robertson, op. cit.). As noted earlier (n. 6), "delayed personhood" has been suggested as one solution to the "save or let die" dilemma. Legally, the newborn is a person before the law from birth. Robertson argues against letting defective infants die on this basis. Others add to this the concept of "innocent" person for the infant has done no wrong and is not deserving of death.

40. Note that either decision, to treat, or not treat, involves "informed consent" by the parents rather than the infant. When parents decide to try for life, few argue their power of proxy consent, though such a decision may "do harm." When the proxy consent involves the death of the infant, some argue that parents do not have this power. The infant's right to life takes precedent. Historically, of course, parents have had, taken, or exercised, life-and-death decisions over their children. The variable is the extent to which society approved or disapproved. We will return to this issue in relation to children in Chapter Six. See Shaw, op. cit., and Tooley, op. cit. for the view that the infant has no right to life.

Veatch, *Case Studies*, op. cit., p. 338, notes that courts rule against parents whose religion allows such children to die rather than be treated. When the case is a defective newborn or a comatose vegetative existence (see n. 17), court rulings are more mixed, as is the ethical perspective in general. Here QOL becomes a major mitigating factor for some. See further, Ramsey, *Ethics at the Edges of Life*, op. cit., pp. 189–194.

41. Lorber, "Selective Treatment of Myelomeningocele: To Treat or Not to Treat," *Pediatrics* (Mar. 1974), **53**:307–308, and, "Early Results of Selective Treatment of Spina Bifida Cystica," *British Medical Journal* (27 Oct. 1973), **4**:201–204. Robertson and Norman Fost note that the difficulty with specific criteria is the almost unlimited complexity of individual cases. They suggest a better process of decision making. "Passive Euthanasia of Defective Newborn Infants: Legal Considerations," *The Journal of Pediatrics*, no. 5 (May 1976), **88**:883–889. Rosalyn B. Darling, "Parents, Physicians, and Spina Bifida," *HCR*, no. 4 (Aug. 1977), **7**:10–14, shares results of a survey. In twenty-five families with handicapped children from three weeks to nineteen years old, she found parents accepting and loving their children, although most would not have wanted the child born if they had known in advance. In contrast, most of the fifteen pediatricians surveyed took a strongly negative view. She suggests these attitudes influence decisions to treat or not treat. She urges informed consent for parents—information that includes the rewards of raising such a child as well as the disadvantages. In turn, medical education might redefine success as including treatment for the chronically ill. Dr. Mildred Stahlman, however, considers informed consent a legal, moral, and ethical farce. The doctor can present the information in such a way that parents will agree, whether the doctor is right or wrong. Ross Conference discussion, op. cit., p. 66. Linda Briggs Besch says getting a signed consent form is not difficult but such a signature often means very little. Full understanding is often an illusion. Meaningful consent, however, remains the goal of professionals who believe in patient autonomy. "Informed Consent: A Patient's Right," *Nursing Outlook*, no. 1 (Jan. 1979), **27**:32–35.

42. John M. Freeman, "The Shortsighted

Treatment of Myelomeningocele: A Long-Term Case Report," *Pediatrics* (Mar. 1974), **53**:311–313. Robert Reid, "The Fate of the Untreated: Euthanasia?" *HCR*, no. 4 (Aug. 1977), **7**:16–19. "Nontreatment of Spina Bifida: an 'Inbuilt Insurance Policy,' " *HCR*, no. 2 (Apr. 1978), **8**:2–3. Quoting R. B. Zachery, this report asks if oversedation of nontreated spina bifida infants makes sure they die.

43. Hippocrates also called for the treatment/cure of disease *and* the relief of suffering. In the terminal stages of incurable illness, Marvin Kohl thinks the relief of suffering should be the choice. On this basis, he argues for beneficent euthanasia (see later). Kohl and Kurtz, op. cit., p. 236. Medical historians are not all agreed that Hippocrates authored the oath. See Amundsen, op. cit. He notes also that the Oath was not typical for its day. Medical personnel commonly assisted in abortions and euthanasia, for example. Both are proscribed in the Oath, though Hippocrates himself gave directions for an abortion.

44. In 1973, the AMA House of Delegates endorsed a similar statement. *Proceedings, A.M.A. House of Delegates* (Dec. 1973). James Rachels, "Active and Passive Euthanasia," *NEJM* (9 Jan. 1975), **292**:78–80. See also, McCormick, *HCR*, op. cit., **8**:30. He notes that "The Ethical and Religious Directives for Catholic Health Care Facilities" (United States Catholic Conference, 1971) use the same language. Paul Ramsey claims the terms *ordinary* and *extraordinary* are circular until we consider concrete meanings. " 'Euthanasia' and Dying Well Enough," *Linacre Quarterly* (1977), **44**:43.

45. Op. cit., *JAMA* **229**:172 ff. Healy, op. cit., p. 71, noted some twenty-five years ago that an incubator might be difficult to obtain and thus could be classified as an extraordinary means to preserve life. Although incubators are, of course, more common today, there are still areas of the world in which they are scarce. He notes that medicine and ethics do not always mean the same thing by *ordinary* and *extraordinary*. Protestant Paul Ramsey makes a similar point in *The Patient as Person*, op. cit., p. 120. On the one hand, it is the state of medical science or the healing art. Ethically, it is the state of the patient's condition. McCormick points out we are considering the patient's QOL rather than the availability of the machinery. *HCR* **8**:31–34, op. cit.

46. Op. cit., pp. 185–192. Lasagna notes that the obstetrician and a prominent expert in mental retardation saw the child as normal. The diagnosis was made by the family pediatrician. Lasagna underscores the difficulty in determining potential. Ten years later, these difficulties often remain (personal communication from Dr. Warren G. Thompson).

47. "Critical Decisions in The Intensive Care Nursery: Three Cases," pp. 16–30, Jonsen and Garland, op. cit.

48. Dr. Bradley E. Smith asks, "Who is responsible for the depressed baby?" He quotes *ACOG Technical Bulletin*, no. 5 (Mar. 1965), "Infant Resuscitation," as indicating resuscitation is the obstetrician's responsibility. Smith suggests that in practice, several categories of personnel may be involved. He thinks that few babies under 1,200 grams will survive if the Apgar score is one at one minute, regardless of the skill of personnel. "Resuscitation, Apgar and Outcome," pp. 54–58, Ross Conference, op. cit., pp. 54–55. "Swiss Guidelines of Care of the Dying," *HCR*, no. 3 (June 1977), **7**:30–31, rely on the competent patient's wishes, but for the incompetent or comatose, or the newborn with grave abnormalities, "the final decision belongs to the physician." The British Working Party (Newcastle Regional Hospital Board) emphasized the technical (medical) basis for decisions. Parents and others might be consulted, but decisions are the doctor's responsibility. Quoted by Robert M. Veatch, "The Technical Criteria Fallacy," *HCR*, no. 4 (Aug. 1977), **7**:15–16. Veatch calls decisions based on objectively measurable criteria such as Apgar scores or Lorber's selection for treatment/nontreatment in spina bifida a fallacy. They, in fact, medicalize value choices such as the meaning of life with various handicaps. Reid, op. cit., notes that Lorber's criteria were developed after experience with more than 1,000 cases. One suspects that subjective judgment and intuition were a part of the development of his objective criteria. This is not wrong, but it might caution one not to mechanically apply the criteria without experienced judgment. Duff and Campbell, op. cit. Ingelfinger, "Bedside Ethics for the Hopeless Case, *NEJM* (25 Oct. 1973), **289**:914. D. H.

Smith, "On Letting Some Babies Die," pp. 129–138 in *Death Inside Out*, ed. by Peter Steinfels and Robert M. Veatch (New York: Harper & Row, Publishers, 1975), pp. 131–132. Paul Ramsey concurs with Smith. *The Patient as Person*, op. cit., 136–137. Ramsey goes on to insist very strongly on the distinction between a baby that is actually dying and one that could live, as in the Down's child with duodenal atresia. He sees Lorber's work in the latter category as a selection for death. He insists that the Christian ethic is to care for the dying. The "benign neglect" of nondying defective newborns is not care, but euthanasia. He considers a possible exception or two, but these are only theoretical. Life is a gift from God and must be treated with respect without regard for human potential or quality of life. *Ethics at the Edges of Life*, op. cit., pp. 191–201, 265–n. 35, 212–227. See n. 38.

49. *Euthanasia* is from the Greek *eu* meaning *well*, and *thanatos* meaning *death*. Traditionally, it means *good death*, that is, without suffering. In the Bible, a good death was living to a ripe old age and being buried with the ancestors. In ethics, it refers to letting die or actively causing death to avoid or relieve suffering. The 1973 AMA statement, noted earlier, rejected mercy killing (Rachels, op. cit., p. 78). Withholding extraordinary means of treatment, however, might be considered indirect or passive euthanasia.

One argument against euthanasia is that it will result in hardening people against infants and the aged, that it will cheapen life. That did not happen in the Duff and Campbell situation, op. cit., p. 892. Euthanasia has been linked to Nazism. Leo Alexander, "Medical Science Under Dictatorship," *NEJM* (14 July 1949), **241**:39–47. The Nazis, however, were not killing out of mercy but as a policy of genocide. Davis and Aroskar, op. cit., p. 113. Joseph Fletcher, "Ethics and Euthanasia," *AJN* (1973), **73**:675. He quotes the story of Robert Louis Stevenson, which was noted earlier, in which Stevenson found that the Polynesians who practiced infanticide had a deeper love for their remaining children than did Europeans. Fletcher, *The Ethics of Genetic Control*, op. cit., pp. 159, 186. Dyck's *benemortasia* (*Bene*, good; *mors*, death) sounds like the Latin equivalent of the Greek euthanasia. He says it differs. His concept involves the relief of pain and suffering. Jonsen and Garland, op. cit., p. 144, also see this as including the use of analgesics, even if this hastens death. This, too, is the principle of double effect. We noted this earlier for Catholic ethicists who accept removal of a cancerous uterus even when the woman is pregnant. See John Arras and Robert Hunt, "Euthanasia," pp. 179–181, in *Ethical Issues in Modern Medicine*, ed. by Arras and Hunt (Palo Alto, Calif.: Mayfield Publishing Co., 1977).

50. Robertson, op. cit., n. 16. Rachels, op. cit., objects to the distinction between active and passive, claiming there is no moral difference between them. Engelhardt in "Aiding . . . ," op. cit., pp. 191–192, n. 22, takes a similar position, as does Joseph Fletcher, "Moral Aspects," *Ross Conference*, op. cit., pp. 70–71. Walter Wadlington, professor of Law, University of Virginia, points out that this distinction is a part of our legal system (discussion, *Ross Conference*, op. cit., p. 85). In introducing Wadlington's presentation, Tom D. Moore notes a certain irony in the thought that medical ethics is being determined by the courts (*Ross Conference*, op. cit., p. 77). The legal and ethical spheres, of course, have always overlapped and interacted. One way of understanding the law is that it institutionalizes ethical perspectives. People, of course, differ on these perspectives and they differ on the acceptibility of laws. Reid, op. cit., p. 19, notes some argue that "man has managed without euthanasia for most of his civilized existence." Historically, of course, the statement is questionable. Euthanasia has been around a long time. Some current cultures ban it but on other grounds (racism, antisemitism, treatment for the poor) might be judged less civilized than those cultures openly practicing euthanasia.

51. Robertson and Fost, op. cit., p. 886, caution that both passive and active euthanasia can be considered illegal. Charges could range from neglect, maltreatment, child abuse to malpractice and murder. Parents, nurses, and hospitals could be held liable, as well as physicians. They do not recommend prosecution but note the potential, though very few prosecutions have taken place, with even fewer convictions for active euthanasia for defective newborns. At the time they wrote, no prosecutions had been instituted against parents or medical personnel for pas-

sive euthanasia of defective newborns. See Lasagna, op. cit., p. 236.

52. In this and the following, "treatment which causes lingering death," we are on the horns of an ethical dilemma (Fletcher suggests this whole area involves dilemmas, trilemmas, quadrilemmas and mutilemmas, op. cit., *Ross Conference*, p. 70). The medical tradition is to do good and if you can't do good, at least do no harm. Here we have harm, that is, suffering, no matter what we do. It may be a matter of the lesser of two evils. Which procedure causes the least harm? That may not be easy to decide. Under ambiguous circumstances, one is tempted to go with the absolutes of "no treatment" or "treat at all costs." Others say the individual situation calls for its own consideration. On the issue of lifesaving surgery for the defective newborn, Dr. Judson Randolph suggests the surgeon who always operates and the surgeon who never operates are both "cop-outs." "Surgical Decisions—Is there a Choice?" *Ross Conference*, op. cit., p. 58. See Shaw, op. cit., p. 889. Dyck, op. cit., p. 243. As noted earlier, Kohl and others argue for beneficent euthanasia in terminal cases; that is, of the two choices to treat disease *and* relieve suffering, they choose the latter. Op. cit., p. 236.

On present-day euthanasia, Paul Ramsey cites a study showing that stillbirths of spina bifida infants dropped from 40 percent to zero when treatment became technically possible in the late 1950s. *Ethics at the Edges of Life*, op. cit., pp. 193–194, no. 12.

53. Inflation since this date would alone double this figure. The figure of $250,000 was also the estimate of lifetime care of a defective child in 1971. This amount has presumably also doubled. See Avery, op. cit., p. 11. The HMD data is from C. A. Smith, op. cit., pp. 34–35. Money is part of the allocation of scarce resources. Jonsen and Garland note here the concept of triage in military and civil disaster. Priority medical treatment goes to those who need it to survive. Those who can survive without it wait their turn, while those who will not survive, regardless of treatment, presumably don't need it. See "A Moral Policy for Life/Death Decisions in the Intensive Care Nursery," pp. 142–155 in Jonsen and Garland, op. cit., pp. 151–153, 175, n. 14. The French adoption of triage in World War I was

the first example of such a rule of selection. Hans Jonas, "The Right to Die," *HCR*, no. 4 (Aug. 1978), **8**:31–36. Ramsey, *Ethics at the Edges of Life*, op. cit., pp. 232, n. 5, 244–245, 262, objects strenuously to this analogy. In a military disaster, those in need of an ICU would be treated last or not at all. He claims that in triage medicine, those who need it least get first treatment so they can help bury or aid the rest. Kramer, op. cit., notes that the allocation of scarce resources cannot be ignored. However, he observes that a decision not to treat may result in a severely impaired survivor. This could result in costs to society much higher than the NNIC, so the concern with financial costs need not result in an automatic decision for "no treatment." In the ordinary versus extraordinary distinction noted previously, financial burden may make an ordinary means into an extraordinary one. Engelhardt, op. cit., justifies "no treatment" if there is a severe financial burden and considers this required when life will be short or painful anyway. Finances, of course, are only one aspect of the cost-benefit ratio. The burden of pain for the infant and for the family are also part of the costs. In turn, these costs are a part of the distinction between ordinary and extraordinary means. It needs to be noted that NNICU costs per patient are less than ICU or cardiac care units. Personal communication, Dr. Warren G. Thompson. See also, Dr. Richard E. Hatwick, and others, "Economics and the Impact on Society," pp. 41–44, *Ross Conference*, op. cit. Dr. John W. Graef notes that the decision not to treat a defective newborn, or at least not to treat aggressively, may turn on the financial resources of the parents. He believes society should assist the parents, if necessary. "House Staff Reactions," pp. 61–62, *Ross Conference*, op. cit.

The financial issue is perhaps not as apparent in the affluent West as in underdeveloped areas where this kind of money would mean life to many people. This problem was noted earlier in our discussion of genetics. It was raised after the California conference reported by Jonsen and Garland, op. cit., by Laura Nader, who asked why our society spends so much time and money on neonatal care without similar attitudes toward children born healthy but later deprived? See "Conference on Neonatal Intensive Care

Issues Ethical Guidelines," *HCR*, no. 6 (Dec. 1975), **5**:3, 12. A current estimate is that the 30,000 defective neonates take 20 percent of the United States health care costs. Adams and Ferrell, op. cit.

Finances, of course, are a major problem in many areas of health care, for example, "Prenatal and Intrapartum Care," Perry A. Henderson, pp. 49–50, *Ross Conference*, op. cit.

54. Op. cit., pp. xix, 1, 59. The 1972 Peel Report in England was concerned with "The Use of Fetuses and Fetal Material for Research." It says that when a viable fetus is delivered, the ethical thing is to sustain its life. It is both immoral and illegal to carry out experiments on it that are inconsistent with its life. Peter Steinfels suggests it would be a mistake to consider fetal research as only a subcategory of the abortion debate. Although fetuses do not precisely fit our thinking on the ethics of human experimentation, they are human. See Steinfels' "The National Commission and Fetal Research," *HCR*, no. 3 (June 1975), **5**:11–12. Some, of course, disagree with these points. See also, Leroy Walters, "Fetal Research and the Ethical Issues," *HCR* no. 3, **5**:13–18. The National Commission for the Protection of Human Subjects of Biomedical and Behavioral Research made a series of recommendations for the control of fetal research. Generally, it was thought acceptable when there was minimal or no risk to the fetus. See Stephen Toulmin, "Exploring the Moderate Consensus," in "The Commission Report: Deliberations and Conclusions," "Commission Recommendations," *HCR*, no. 3 (June 1975), **5**:31–46. "Protection of Human Subjects: Fetuses, Pregnant Women, and In Vitro Fertilization," *Federal Register*, no. 154 (8 Aug. 1975), **40**:33526–33552. See also, Jan Wojcik, *Muted Consent* (West Lafayette, Ind.: Purdue University Press, 1978), pp. 20–25. André E. Hellegers notes that the Commission recommended that the life of the nonviable fetus should not be maintained outside the uterus for research purposes. The Department of Health, Education and Welfare suggested this could be done "to develop new methods for enabling fetuses to survive to the point of viability." "Fetal Research," *EB* **2**:489–493. "Protection of Human Subjects: Proposed Amendments Concerning Fetuses, Pregnant Women, and In Vitro Fertilization," *Federal Register*, no. 9 (13 Jan. 1977), **42**:2792–2793.

55. Joseph Fletcher, "Pragmatists & Doctrinaires," *HCR*, no. 3 (June 1975), **5**:36–37.

56. *The Ethics of Fetal Research*, op. cit., pp. 89–99. *Ethics at the Edges of Life*, op. cit., pp. 208–212. Here Ramsey objects to using defective newborns for research. It has been noted that medical research may influence decisions about their care. Such decisions might go beyond the individual patient's own interest and thus raise this same question. See Jonsen and Garland, op. cit., pp. 146, 153.

57. Hemphill and Freeman, op. cit., p. 721. On consent here, see Shaw, op. cit. Richard A. McCormick claims there is little moral problem when experimental procedures represent the most hopeful therapy. "Fetal Research, Morality, and Public Policy," *HCR*, no 3 (June 1975), **5**:26–31. Others suggest that good intentions are not sufficient grounds for deciding experimentation is acceptable.

58. Op. cit., p. 892. Jonas, op. cit., considers the right to die, with a primary focus on the competent consenting adult. He includes also the comatose who is incapable of informed consent but for whom others might give such consent. This adult situation is often compared to the neonate who obviously is incapable of informed consent.

59. Op. cit., p. 26.

60. Op. cit., p. 721. Similarly, oxygen therapy several decades ago was noted as increasing the incidence of blindness. Such iatrogenic (treatment-caused) illness is said by some to be a rationale for withholding treatment. C. A. Smith, op. cit., p. 34. Jane V. Hunt, op. cit., p. 44. Tooley and Phibbs, op. cit., p. 12.

61. Michael G. Blackburn, Jeanette R. Pleasure, and John H. Sorenson, "Research in Neonatology: Improved Ratio of Risk to Benefit Through A Scientifically Based Alteration in Research Design," *Clinical Research*, 24, No. 5 (Dec. 1976), 317–321.

62. Jonsen, "Introduction," op. cit., p. 7. Daniel L. Robinson, Jerome A. Shaffer, John W. Bowker, "Pain and Suffering," *EB*, **3**:1177–1189.

63. The alert reader will note the limited appeal to Natural Law in neonatology. If we left it all to nature, we would not have NNICU's. We would be back to a 30 percent to 70 percent infant mortality rate and few of

the problems of the type discussed here, for the newborns would simply die. Although the practice of medicine is obviously unnatural, most ethical standards prefer this to the natural.

64. Cheryl H. Harris, "Some Ethical and Legal Considerations in Neonatal Intensive Care," *Nursing Clinics of North America*, no. 3 (Sept. 1973), **8**:522.

65. See Andrew Jameton, "The Nurse: When Roles and Rules Conflict," *HCR*, no. 4 (Aug. 1977), **7**:22–23.

66. Shirley M. Steele and Vera M. Harmon, *Values Clarification in Nursing* (New York: Appleton-Century-Crofts, 1979, p. 25. We note here again the distinction between deontology (rules, duty) and the utilitarian approach to ethics.

67. Davis and Aroskar, op. cit., pp. 175–177.

68. Jonsen and Garland, op. cit., p. 16.

69. Harris, op. cit., p. 526. Personal communication, Kathryn Rosasco, RN, member of ethical task force, Babies Hospital, Columbia-Presbyterian Medical Center, New York City.

70. Dagmar Cechanek, "Nursing Reactions," pp. 59–60, in *Ross Conference*, op. cit. Personal communication, Ms. Kathryn Rosasco, RN, 1979. Mila Aroskar and Robert M. Veatch, "Ethics Teaching in Nursing Schools," *HCR*, no. 4 (Aug. 1977), **7**:23–26. Margaret O'Brien Steinfels, "Ethics, Education and Nursing Practice," *HCR*, no. 4 (Aug. 1977), **7**:20–21.

71. Op. cit., p. 894.

72. See n. 48. See Steinfels, op. cit., p. 21.

73. Cechanek, op. cit., p. 60.

74. See Ramona T. Mercer, "Crisis: A Baby Is Born With a Defect," *Nursing*, no. 11 (Nov. 1977), **7**:45–47, for a discussion of nursing attitudes toward newborns with defects and their potential influence on care giving. Barbara L. Tate, *The Nurse's Dilemma: Ethical Considerations in Nursing Practice* (Geneva: International Council of Nurses, 1977), pp. 2–5. Cathy C. Floyd, "A Defective Child Is Born: A Study of Mothers of Newborns with Spina Bifida and Hydrocephalus," *Journal of Obstetric, Gynecological, and Neonatal Nursing*, no. 4 (July/Aug. 1977), **6**:56–62.

75. Colleen McElroy, op. cit., p. 27. See M. Josephine Flaherty in Mila Aroskar, Flaherty, and James M. Smith, "The Nurse and Orders Not to Resuscitate," *HCR*, no. 4 (Aug. 1977), **71**:27–28. Gustafson, op. cit.

76. Jonsen and Garland, op. cit., p. 16. Michael J. Garland, "Care of the Newborn: The Decision Not to Treat," *Perinatology/Neonatology*, no. 2 (Sept./Oct. 1977), **2**:14–21, 43.

77. Cechanek, op. cit., p. 60. For the view that one *is* responsible for decisions, see n. 48. For the collegial view, see also James M. Smith, op. cit., p. 28.

78. J. W. Graef, "House Staff Reactions," in *Ross Conference*, op. cit., p. 61.

79. See Mercer, p. cit., p. 45. Note discussion on p. 47 of nurses seeking support and assistance from colleagues regarding individual reactions to caring for gravely ill newborns.

80. Jonsen and Garland, op. cit., p. 16.

81. Ibid., p. 23.

82. Leah L. Curtin, "The Nurse as Advocate: A Philosophical Foundation for Nursing," *Advances in Nursing Science*, no. 3 (Apr. 1979), **1**:1–10.

83. Joyce E. Beebe and Henry O. Thompson, "A Paradigm of Ethics for the Maternal Child Nurse," *MCN*, no. 3 (May/June 1979), **4**:141–142, 144, 147, 184.

Chapter 6

Childhood and Ethics

INTRODUCTION

The United Nations General Assembly declared the year 1979 as the "International Year of the Child." IYC was to highlight the needs of the world's children. Far too many, especially in developing countries, have inadequate health services, are undernourished, miss the basics of education, and are deprived of the elementary amenities of life. The UN Declaration of the Rights of the Child includes such things as the right to affection, love, and understanding, nutrition and medical care, free education, play and recreation, a name and nationality, special care if handicapped, to be the first to receive relief in time of disaster, to be useful members of society developing individual abilities, and to be brought up in peace and brotherhood. These rights are theirs without regard to race, color, sex, religion, national or social origin.[1]

There are moral and ethical elements in virtually every word of these concerns. One of the most obvious is the distribution of scarce resources, which we will look at in more detail in Chapter Seven. Here we hold it up, as we have done with previous concerns, with the reminder that many pieces of the bioethic picture appear in various parts of the life cycle.

Some of the items in the UN Declaration might be listed as values or beliefs, rather than moral or ethical principles. One might see the right to play as a peculiarly Western concern. Although children all over the world and in every culture do, in fact, play, lifting it up as an international human right seems trivial to some whereas others consider it vital. The Western world, on the other hand, does not have the best record in history for affection, love, and understanding of its children. For such ethicists as Joseph Fletcher, love is *the* crucial ingredient in ethics.[2] One could see this underlying concern in all the IYC and Rights of the Child statements. Or one might look at it all as a matter of respect for persons and sooner or later get back to the value one places on life, as in our earlier discussion of abortion and neonatology, with the subsequent issues of quality of life as compared to quantity of life.

Concerns

Out of all these values and beliefs, moral and ethical codes, and underlying concerns, we have selected three areas of discussion for this chapter. We will look at research and children, child abuse, and adolescent sexuality. These overlap several of the Rights of the Child. They are major points of contact with children for health personnel, points of conflict and conflicting opinion, points with long roots in the history of medical ethics, and points in the life cycle where modern medicine has new impact.

CHILDREN AND RESEARCH

We have touched on research in earlier chapters. We noted that many medical procedures may carry an experimental element.[3] These may be a matter of trial and error. If one thing does not work, try something else. The experiment may or may not be a matter of research records and protocol. When something is tried for the benefit of the child, it could be classified as therapeutic. When it is not for the benefit or immediate benefit of the child, it might be called nontherapeutic. Some work with children is a mix of the two. The National Commission for the Protection of Human Subjects of Biomedical and Behavioral Research prefer to speak of the prospect of direct benefit for the individual.[4]

Informed Consent

One of the basic issues in health care or medical research with children is the focus on informed consent.[5] We have noted this earlier with the obvious acknowledgment that neonates, fetuses, and the unconceived do not have informed consent. There are those who argue that they *do* have rights. It is doubtful that anyone would argue that they are able to give any kind of consent, informed or otherwise. Still, in the annals of ethics, stranger arguments have been heard. So in all probability, there is someone somewhere who would object that the unconceived and others *ought* to have informed consent.

Although it is tempting to play with the pro and con of such a view, we resist the temptation in order to move on to the serious, and deadly, corollary. If neonates and others do not have informed consent, someone has it for them. At first glance, and for the first few years, it is obvious that someone has consent for children. In the unfortunate case of the mentally incompetent, that situation may go on for years. Thus, it is common to include children and the incompetent in one category of the issue of informed consent. Incompetent may be extended to include the aged, the unconscious, and the mentally ill, as well as the retarded. In sum, our concern here is with those who are not in a position by age, mental condition, or legal status to be able to understand sufficiently to give their own consent to treatment, therapeutic or nontherapeutic.

This is a legal concern as well as a moral/ethical one.[6] Much guidance has come in recent years through law and decisions in the courts. This text will consider in Chapter Nine patients of all kinds, as well as the rights of health personnel, interested parties, and society at large. Here we want to focus on persons who might not be able to give informed consent for medical procedures.

Who Consents?

As in previous situations, the range here is from the generally accepted to the generally nonaccepted. Most people would agree that the neonate, the one-year-old, the two-year-old, the three-year-old are not able to give consent. At what age *is* a child able to give consent? Legally, in times past, children have been the property of their parents or guardians. They could be dealt with pretty much as the controlling adults chose. Herod the Great, king of Israel or Palestine when Jesus of Nazareth was born, was what today we might call paranoid. He feared for his throne. He killed several of his sons whom he suspected of plotting against him. The Roman Emperor, Augustus, is quoted as saying it would be safer to be Herod's dog than Herod's son. Herod's actions were not approved. But they were tolerated. The Roman empire gave the father complete power over his children.

This power was modifed, of course, by parental love for children. In the Judeo-Christian tradition, this came to have the force of law in the mutual relationship of parent and child. Saul or Paul, a Jewish follower of Jesus, instructed Christians with this mutuality (Ephesians 6:1; Colossians 3:20–21), based on the commandment to "Honor thy father and mother" (Exodus 20:12).

In practice, parental power remained nearly supreme to the age of majority, traditionally twenty-one, more recently lowered in various places to eighteen and nineteen with consent in sexual matters at lower ages. In many states, teen-agers can receive medical treatment for such problems as drug dependency or venereal disease. They may have both advice and materials for contraception and may get abortions without parental consent. In law, there is a general attitude that older teens and, more generally yet, mature children are capable of giving informed consent, or withholding it.[7]

At one point, the National Commission considered the age of seven as a time for requiring assent for medical procedures. We see here a move away from the legal language of consent. Instead of seeking proxy consent from parents or guardians, the move is toward "permission." James J. McCartney sees here an acknowledgment of the developing autonomy of children on a sliding scale from nonautonomy to full autonomy. The proxy power of parents and guardians thus slides also, in the opposite direction, from complete (or rather nearly complete) power to none, or at least very little.[8]

Therapeutic Research

Within this framework of autonomy and proxy, we can note that medical procedures of research for the benefit of the individual are generally acceptable. Even in therapeutic procedures, however, there is not complete agreement. The least problem, ethically speaking, appears when parents and children (if old enough) and medical personnel are in agreement on treatment. This was also noted in neonatology. There, also, we saw the problems mount when parents refused treatment. In life-threatening situations, the courts have frequently sided with the medical world, that is, when religious beliefs of the parents were against blood transfusions. The often quoted phrase is that parents can make martyrs of themselves but not of their children. When the situation is not life-threatening, the courts tend to go with the parents. There have been exceptions, however, as when a child with a facial deformity was given the operation over parental objection for the sake of the child's psychological and social well-being. In another case, medical personnel were overruled when parent and child agreed in not having the surgery to correct a hare lip.[9]

Nontherapeutic Research

Nontherapeutic research on children is much more problematic. Some ethicists, such as Paul Ramsey, are against it.[10] The Commission allows it subject to a number of restrictions, such as minimal risk, appropriate benefits, permission of parents or guardians, and so on. Some would argue that children have a duty to the larger society. Persons in a proxy position can consider what the children would want to do or ought to do as responsible members of society. Even here, the argument has emphasized that the risk must be minimal.[11]

A frequently cited case of abuse of children in research is that of Willowbrook State Hospital. Several thousand patients in this New York state hospital were part of an experiment in the use of gamma globulin for infectious hepatitis. Those who find the experiment acceptable point out that it was done with parental or guardian consent and that it was of potential benefit to the experimental children as well as to others. Those who argue against it claim the parental consent was, at least, possibly under duress and that the experiment could have been carried out with adults or that the hepatitis could have been cleared from the institution by known, although more expensive, means.[12]

The case illustrates something of the difficulties involved in this area of health care. It was an experiment. It was designed to acquire new knowledge and test an hypothesis.

It had proxy consent. The experimenters thought the children would benefit, as well as bringing benefits to others in the institution. They thought the children would get infectious hepatitis anyway, so deliberately infecting them under controlled conditions with extra care and treatment would help them. Critics either call it nontherapeutic research or claim that the risks outweighed the benefits.

Summary

Research with children remains a problematic area in bioethics. In one sense, all treatment can be seen as research or experimentation. When it is for the benefit of the individual, it tends to be more acceptable, providing the benefits are greater than the risks. Nontherapeutic procedures remain the most problematic. Informed consent, at least by proxy of parents and guardians, and preferably by the child where possible, is more and more seen as essential but, even then, procedures may be questionable.

CHILD ABUSE

Like informed consent and concern with experimentation and research, child abuse is a relatively new kind of concern. The history of childhood has been called a nightmare. It has been suggested that childhood was not discovered until the thirteenth century and that a very large percentage of the children before the eighteenth century were what today we would call abused or battered children.

In 1826, New York State still allowed gross abuse. Pennsylvania began intervening in 1838. Kempe and Helfer note that in 1875, the Society for the Prevention of Cruelty to Animals was used to get a little girl named Mary Ellen unchained from a bed. Thus began the Society for the Prevention of Cruelty to Children (SPCC) in New York City.[13]

The term *battered child* was introduced by C. Henry Kempe in 1961 at a symposium of the American Academy of Pediatrics. In 1962, the Children's Bureau convened a meeting on a model law. Today, all states have laws on child abuse. These laws require health personnel to report suspected cases of child abuse. Thus, like research, it is a legal matter as well as a moral/ethical one.[14]

Scope of Problem

The tendency has been to think in terms of physical abuse and battering. More than ten years ago, it was reported that seven hundred children are killed every year in the United States by their parents or parent figures. Today, estimates range from 1,000 to 50,000 deaths per year. Estimates of abused children run as high as 2.5 million.[15]

In 1976, Kempe began using the broader term of *child abuse* or *abused child*. In addition to the physical abuse, there is verbal abuse, sexual abuse, mental and emotional abuse, maltreatment, and neglect. The latter might be the deprivation of food, clothing, shelter, medical attention, or complete abandonment.[16]

No socioeconomic class, educational level, occupation, language group, race, ethnic group, or marital status is free of the problem of child abuse. Having said that, one can go on to say it is more prevalent in large families, poor ones (20 percent of the children of America live in poverty), alcoholic ones (there are about 30 million children of alcoholics in the United States), and in families in which the parents as children were abused, neglected, misunderstood, unloved, unhappy. Parents who are socially isolated adults are also among the more frequent child abusers.[17]

Characteristics of the Abused Child

It has been common to look at adult abusers as having problems. More recently, some children have been seen as particularly prone to being abused. Low birth weight children are more likely to be abused than others; so are handicapped children. A child's appearance, irritability, responsiveness to adults and discipline, and activity level are among characteristics that may invite abuse. There is an element of interaction here, a vicious circle. The more a child shows characteristics that invite abuse, the more it will be abused, and the more the child is abused, the more it takes on those characteristics. It is important to note, however, that the child may not exhibit any characteristics of this type. The adult caretaker may see the child in this way. The adult may be upset by someone or something else (a spouse, another child, too many children, personal problems, a crisis), and take it out on the child.[18]

Intervention

The origins of the problem point to work with parents, including therapy, as a long-range solution and prevention approach. Some parents report an inability to control themselves and to deal with their problems. Groups such as Parents Anonymous have appeared throughout the country. These self-help groups function in a somewhat similar pattern to that of the more well-known Alcoholics Anonymous. Parents help and support one another to overcome their abusive actions. Other therapeutic efforts have involved marital counseling, reparenting of parents, the teaching of more effective parenting techniques, and direct aid with the problems (psychological, financial, family planning).[19]

The abused child is not infrequently part of a larger picture of abuse. Many of the same elements as in the child abuse syndrome appear in the abused wife syndrome. An abused teen-aged wife is also an abused child. The battered wife syndrome is a growing concern in this country. In both situations, the victim is often blamed: "She asked for it." This view is common where rape is concerned as well. Abusive families tend to have multiple problems, requiring the coordination of health personnel, law enforcement, social workers, schools, and churches for relief or solution.[20]

Moral and Ethical Perspective

History: The moral and ethical perspective on battered children may at first glance be obvious or intuitive. Historically, however, children were sometimes thought to be in the grip of the devil. They were believed to be conceived in sin. Children and the mentally ill have thus shared the dubious distinction of being demon-possessed. In turn, concepts of deity have at times been that of a harsh parent who punished his children severely for any infraction of the rules. That included killing, sometimes by what today we would call epidemics, and, of course, war. Parents were like gods to their children—owning them, punishing them, and at times killing them. Martin Luther said, "I would rather have a dead son than a disobedient one."[21]

The theological justification, of course, may have been simply an after the fact attempt to explain what was going on, as in the case of slavery and war. Benjamin Disraeli (1804–1881), the English statesman, lived in a day when London police thought no more of finding a dead child on the streets than a dead dog.[22] From that day to this, there has been a major shift in religion away from the "sinners in the hands of an angry God"[23] to the idea of God as a God of love. This alone might account for the major shift in the attitude toward children. More likely, there has been an interaction between religion and culture. The early movements to get children out of factories and mines were no doubt a major factor. Humanitarian and economic interests combined to save the children for the healthier atmosphere of the schools while freeing up the jobs for adults supporting families. At the same time there was an increased need for education to meet the burgeoning technology that has been our constant companion in these pages.[24]

Concept of Person: Somewhat more recently, the Nuremburg Code (1946) on human experimentation grew out of the Nazi war crimes trials, specifically that of Karl Brandt. One way of looking at this Code is to see it as a growing respect for persons in the face of the horrors of the Nazi concentration camps. The Code does not mention children, but gradually its strictures have been extended to include children. In turn, we could see this as an extension of the concept of *person* to include children, a concept we have discussed earlier in abortion and neonatology. Until modern times, children were seen as extensions of their parents, a concept which psychology suggests is still with us, as in mother-infant bonding.[25]

Thus, we could say that although at first glance the concern for child abuse seems obvious and intuitive, it is an intuitiveness of short duration. For the masses of humanity, it is a phenomenon of recent generations. The evidence that abusive parents were themselves abused as children suggests that the modern phenomenon of concern for children has not caught up with all generations as yet. The battered wife syndrome would appear to be at least another generation behind the concern for children. This factor of being recent may help our understanding in dealing with the problem. This understanding can go on in parallel even as we also understand the shift in the moral and ethical standards of the modern world to a greater concern for the physical and emotional well-being of people, the respect for persons and individual dignity, rights of privacy and self-determination, and the concern for increased quality of life as well as quantity of life that is now reflected in our ethical codes.[26]

ADOLESCENT SEXUALITY

There is a story about President Calvin Coolidge going to church one time when his wife was unable to attend. When he returned, she asked about the sermon. "Silent Cal" said that it was fine. "What was it about?" "Sin." "Well, what did the minister have to say about it?" "He's agin it."

History: At first glance, one might expect the traditional view toward adolescent sexuality to be simply "agin it." A study of history, however, presents a picture that is neither simple nor simply "agin it." Life expectancy was more limited in earlier ages. Families were concerned that the family line be preserved. Female children were often considered a liability, and the sooner they were married, the better. The result was a combination of early betrothals and marriages. At one point, the Christian church tried to forbid marriages before the age of twelve, and betrothals before age seven, which might be at birth or as early as the age of three. It was not unusual for a first birth to be to a mother, and perhaps a father too, who were in the mid-teens. Nor was it unusual for a woman to have seven to ten children by the age of twenty-five.[27]

Nonmarital adolescent sexual activity in times past apparently was real enough. The extent of it is more difficult to determine.[28] Not all are agreed even today on how much there is, in a time when studies abound and statistics clutter the air.[29] Illegitimate births are one indicator.[30] The history of infanticide, abortion, and contraception commonly assumes that much of this activity involved illicit, premarital or extramarital sexual intercourse. The facts are more difficult to determine.[31]

Adolescent sexuality is, of course, a part of the larger picture of human sexuality. In ancient times and in primitive cultures, bodily discharges and other natural phenomena ranging from lightning to locusts, were not understood. The natural was often seen as supernatural, sometimes demonic. Thus, fertility and barrenness were seen as the gift or the curse of the deity in the Bible and elsewhere. This is still part of the thinking of some people today (see the earlier discussion of contraception).[32]

Dilemmas

The major change has been that although many people, including adolescents, are ignorant of sexuality and sexual functioning, there is less tendency to ascribe it to the supernatural and simply remain ignorant. Some, however, have seen even this ignorance as having its roots in the ancient taboos. Many parents find it difficult to talk with their children about sex. In the absence of factual sex education, the common educator of today's youth is the peer group, and secondarily, the mass media. These are frequently the source of much misinformation. The latter also shows a peculiar quirk of the ancient taboos. Sex, especially scatological sex, is common in the media. What is missing is contraceptive information (banned by law) and healthy attitudes toward sex. Although our technical knowledge of sexuality and reproduction has increased over recent decades, teen-agers and older persons, too, are often still living in primitive ignorance.[33]

Thus, we live in a contradictory situation in which we are almost constantly bombarded with sexual stimuli even as the older strictures on sexuality continue. Adolescents face additional confusion because of other developments as well. There is some evidence to suggest that originally human society was matriarchal in character. The development of war led to the accumulation of "booty" and property. An economic theory of social development suggests that the warrior who wanted to leave his property to his heir also wanted to make sure it was *his* heir. As primitive knowledge of reproduction developed, this economic concern led to a higher valuation of virginity. A virgin female child was more marriageable than a nonvirgin. The economic asset concept was reinforced by religious taboos, or perhaps they were simply interacting and reinforcing each other. Today, the religious perspective is still with us, but the bulk of the population is not actively committed to religious observance. The economic asset theory has largely disappeared, but the economics of adolescence has added a new twist.[34]

Until recent decades, children could be either a burden (food, clothing, and housing) or an asset. Children as young as five were put to work on the farm, in the mines, in factories, and mills. A hundred years ago, the abuse, neglect, and death of many of these children led to a reform movement and the child labor laws. Somewhat parallel to this, the developing technological society in which we live led to the increasing need for education. Thus, the adolescent of today is under pressure to stay in school and not compete in the job market. Economics now encourages and even requires later marriage, as does the population explosion. But in the meanwhile, sexual development continues and, in fact, appears to be earlier now than a few decades ago. Increased nutrition and health have led to earlier maturation. Concurrently, for sexually active teen-agers there is thus a higher chance of pregnancy, a lessened tendency to spontaneous miscarriage, and an increased tendency to carry the fetus to term.[35]

Current Concerns

Much of the current concern with adolescent sexuality is with pregnancy. Morally and ethically, the focus has been on unwed motherhood and the obvious evidence of the often unacceptable premarital or extramarital sexual intercourse. The latter has involved up to half the teen-age population. Interestingly, the half who do not have intercourse get less attention, so much so that on occasion counselors are asked if it's all right *not* to have intercourse. The common statement, "everybody's doing it," refers to one half but not the other.[36] Medically, the concern is both within and without marriage. Teen-age mothers have a higher mortality rate and teen pregnancy has a higher rate of miscarriages, defective fetuses, premature births, and infant mortality. Syphilis is 60 percent higher and gonorrhea is 300 percent higher in teen-age women than in those in their twenties.[37] Economically, there is a growing concern for unwed mothers, who frequently end up on welfare with their children. In turn, their economic future is less than optimal because of interrupted education.[38] The ethical and moral concerns in this may be a question of the allocation of scarce resources (money that might go for other things), the continuation of a poverty cycle from generation to generation, the right to consent and confidentiality for adolescent health care, the quality of life for both mothers (parents) and children, and the quantity of life in the face of higher mortality statistics, as well as the traditional moral concerns with sexual intercourse outside of marriage.[39]

Women's Movement: Other currents of thought also affect the teen-ager of today. The women's liberation movement has helped focus attention on an ongoing process. Women as property was in part an outgrowth of warfare in which females were often part of the "loot." This is no longer acceptable to many people, although, as noted earlier, the legal rights of women are changing only gradually. The growing rights of women include the right of sexuality, both within and outside of marriage. The double standard, in which men "sowed their wild oats" and "boys will be boys" while women must remain chaste and pure, is less acceptable for some people today. Surveys suggest that sexual activity among males has not increased to any extent, but it has increased among women substantially. The result may be increasing numbers of pregnancies but, as noted earlier, this could be a factor of physical health rather than increased sexual activity.[40]

Sexual Revolution: Another, and perhaps *the* major current of the day, is what is frequently called the sexual revolution.[41] This is sometimes looked upon as the moral breakdown of society. It includes the breakdown of the family, pornography, the increasing number of pregnancies in teens below the age of fifteen, and extramarital pregnancies in general, as well as what is sometimes called "free sex." Others look at the positive side of the new sexual attitudes with the increasing regard for mutuality and relationship both within and outside of the marital bond. For some, at least, the new openness toward sexuality is a plus to be preferred to the hush-hush attitudes of the past.[42] Health personnel face all this in terms of sex education in the schools and clinics, in family planning clinics, in treatment for venereal disease that appears to be increasing in incidence, in abortions, in prenatal care for pregnant teens, and in postnatal care and instruction for infants and new parents.[43] We will look at the role of health personnel in more detail in a moment. First, let us look at two additional factors.

Teen-age Male

The teen-age male is often overlooked. This may be because of the old double standard. It may be because women get pregnant, rather then men. At least one study suggests that if the teen-age father gets too much attention, there is an increased likelihood of marriage and a second pregnancy.[44] The same has been said for teen-age girls, for some of whom attention has been sorely lacking until they became pregnant. There is some evidence that the pregnant teen who has the attention of her male partner is better able to deal with the pregnancy physically and emotionally. Many teen-age pregnancies are conceived within marriage, or end in marriage (either prenatally or postnatally), so the adolescent father is or can be of major significance even though the studies and the literature have largely overlooked him. At times, the push for contraceptive information and materials for the adolescent girl may have encouraged the idea that she is responsible for birth control, whereas the male is left irresponsible or led to believe that he has no responsibility.[45]

Changing Roles

A second factor to consider is the changing roles of men and women in Western society. The traditional role of the man who goes out to work and the woman who works in the home is still with us. But many women work outside the home both before and after marriage. In some cases, the women are the major support of the family. So sexual roles are changing. Young people now face a greater choice in roles, with more men involved in housework and caring for the children than in some earlier periods. And it is not only the heterosexual roles that are in flux. There is a greater degree of acceptance of homosexuality today, or at least it is more out in the open. Whether there is an increase in homosexuality as such may be more debatable. The single life, single parenthood, and childless marriages are more common or at least more openly discussed than in an earlier day.[46]

Summary

Traditionally, religion and society have accepted sex in marriage and were "agin it" outside marriage. The practice of premarital and extramarital intercourse has been in contrast to official teachings, as we noted earlier for contraception, abortion, and infanticide. In our present sexual revolution these practices are either increasing or are more open. Sexual ethics, morals, mores, values, and customs appear to be undergoing major change even as the traditional morality continues.[47]

THE ISSUES

Informed consent is a major issue in work with children. To treat children humanely is another. The ethical and moral overtones of sexuality have long historical roots. Weaving in and around these major issues are such traditional concepts as human beings as an end in themselves, rather than a means to an end (Kant). The dependent, as the poor or helpless in general, are often seen as having a moral claim on the powerful. This principle goes back at least as far as the Hebrew prophets. Children range from totally dependent to near independence. One might see a parental or societal responsibility to help them become independently functioning adults. Related to this is the old idea that for every right, there is a responsibility. If people have a right to bring children into the world, they have a responsibility to care for them. If they cannot care for them, they do not have the right to have them.

Cost/benefit ratio is involved in all this. Many people have children for the benefits they derive, such as care in the parents' old age. This has been a major bar to contraception in the developing countries. In Western nations, the idea that children should be wanted and loved for their own sakes has come to prominence in more recent years, with parents looking to social security and pension plans for care in their old age.

Research was noted to have a major cost/benefit component. If the research benefits the child, it is more acceptable. With no benefit to the child, it is more questionable. Even with benefit, the cost in pain, discomfort, and money might outweigh the benefits and make research unacceptable.

The modern world has come to look more carefully on emotional as well as physical well-being of children. To this is added an increased concern for the dignity of all persons and the extension of personhood to more people, including children and women. Rights of privacy and self-determination as well as an increased concern for the quality of life have been added to the right to life itself.

Sex has been a part of moral codes from most ancient times. Partly, this may have been an economic concern, with women treated as property, and a concern for inheritance to one's own issue. It was often seen as a divine command in the tradition of the deontological approach to ethics. Sexual intercourse has long or often been forbidden outside of marriage in Western tradition. Sociologically, this has included a concern for offspring and the integrity of the family. In more recent times, the focus has often been on unwanted or unplanned and often out-of-wedlock pregnancies. Sexual mores appear to be undergoing extensive change as we move toward the twenty-first century.

NURSES AND THE CARE OF CHILDREN AND ADOLESCENTS

The extent of nursing involvement in the care of children and adolescents is wide-ranging, covering the spectrum from principal care giver in health promotion programs (well-baby clinics, young adult contraceptive services) to observer-advocate in some research situations. In between, nurses are often the first health professionals who meet the sick child in the emergency room or hospital setting and set into motion the system that will care for their needs. Nurses also tend to have the most responsibility for care of children and spend the most continuous time in contact with them.

Working with and caring for children and adolescents is an exciting challenge for most nurses as they seek to support normal growth and development from infancy to adulthood and also recognize that the child may have special health and sickness needs that can interfere with this needed growth, at least temporarily. Providing health and illness care for children and adolescents also presents some unique ethical issues for nurses and other health personnel to consider.

Nurses and Research with Children

As discussed earlier, one of the major issues involved in research with children revolves around the idea of informed consent and who gives consent when a minor is to be involved in a research study. The role of the nurse in relation to the child and research may be that of principal investigator of a given study, participant in carrying out someone else's study, principal caregiver of a child involved in a research study, or member of an institutional review board responsible for the protection of any human subject proposed for use in a research project. In all of these roles, nurses must know the legal status of research on minors in their state,[48] and be aware of the ethical concerns that might arise. This is one area in which the mix of ethical and legal aspects of nursing practice is quite evident. How the nurse carries out both the legal and ethical responsibilities of his/her role will probably depend to some extent on how he/she views research in general, and research on infants and children in particular.

Nurses are encouraged as professionals to initiate and support research for the advancement of knowledge, particularly knowledge related to the effects of nursing practice on the health and illness states of clients. Nurses are also often called upon by physician colleagues to carry out some aspects of their research, such as administering experimental treatments or drugs, witnessing informed consent, recording patients' reactions to a given experimental treatment, or collecting laboratory samples of blood or urine.

Advocacy

Most nurses who support the client's right to make decisions about health and illness care and involvement in research studies based on informed consent have little difficulty working with competent adults involved in research studies. When children/minors are proposed for participation in a research study, however, some nurses do not view the child's right of involvement as clearly. Nurses in such situations (particularly with the infant and very young child) often assume the role of advocate and become personally involved in the decision-making process. The trust relationship she has built up with the child can be used to influence the child's decision one way or another. Whether this should be done is an ethical issue. The nurse's personal involvement may range from active protests if the nurse decides that the study is not "in the best interests" of the child (see Chapter Five on neonatology) to insisting that she be present while consent is being obtained so she is certain that the study has been explained clearly and that both parents and child realize they have a choice. Nurses' tacit approval of research on children without questioning may be just as objectionable to ethical practice as deliberately influencing parents to decide for or against participation. It would appear that the nurse cannot carry out her responsibility to protect the patient if she ignores the fact that someone is carrying out research on the children for whom she is caring.

Age of Consent

Nurses and other health professionals are concerned about the age at which a child's permission, in addition to the permission of parents, should be obtained. The general rule of thumb is that a child of seven years or older should give informed consent in addition to that of the parents.[49] Some nurses also use the yardstick of "intrusive" versus "nonintrusive" research as a factor in insisting on informed consent of the child, insisting on such consent in cases where the experiment requires some type of painful procedure. The ANA *Code for Nurses*, Statement Seven, speaks to the nurse's responsibility to protect the "life, health, and privacy of human subjects (in research) from unanticipated as well as anticipated risks . . . and rights must be especially safeguarded if they are unable to protect themselves . . . because they are in a dependent relationship to the investigator."[50] One might quickly note that although the overall intent of the statement appears clear, it lends itself to individual interpretation. That is, some nurses may accept parental consent on behalf of a child, but others may insist on informing and requesting the child's permission.

Research Guidelines

In keeping with ANA *Human Rights Guidelines for Nurses in Clinical and Other Research*,[51] we offer the following suggested approach to nurses for carrying out their responsibility to children who are proposed for research study.

1. Know the study protocol: is the research consistent with professional duties toward clients and can you support its aims/goals?
2. Know whether Institutional Review Board (IRB) approval has been obtained: insist on it.
3. Observe the explanation of the study to ensure informed consent:
   a. Do parents/child understand the study and what it entails?
   b. Do parents/child understand that they can withdraw their consent at any time

without influencing the care they receive?

   c. Are the parents/child free of pressure to participate (captivity or fear of not having child taken care of)?

It should be noted here that nurses who cannot support a given research study because of a conflict with moral beliefs have the right not to participate in the study. However, the nurse does not have the right to impose her beliefs on the child or parents unless the child is, in fact, in danger from the study protocols. When possible, it is best if the nurse can remove herself from the study setting when her own personal beliefs cannot support a valid research aim.

NURSES AND THE ABUSED CHILD

Working with abusing families can be one of the most difficult roles that nurses accept. One's feeling of reaching out to protect the abused child often runs headlong into one's feelings of anger, disgust, and, sometimes, fear of the abusing parent(s). The danger of trying to rescue the child from the abuse of others often leaves the nurse in a less than effective helping position. Scharer notes that when the nurse attempts to rescue the child from its abusers, the anger and hostility held toward the abusers can lead one to give extraordinary attention to the child. This attention often includes a failure to set appropriate limits on the child's behavior and, finally, to rejection of the child when he fails to respond with the behavior the nurse expects in return for her attention.[52] Thus, the cycle of abuse continues as the child is now rejected by the health professional as well as by the parents. Nurses can benefit from examining and understanding their own reactions to abuse of children and adults and making a conscious decision as to whether they can remain effective care givers in situations of abuse. If not, the nurse might be more effective as a professional caregiver if she does not work with the abusing families.

Nurses are in a unique position to detect potential abusers of children as well as the actual abusers. It is often the nurse who has sufficient contact with the pregnant and newly delivered woman to observe her reaction to her pregnancy and newborn infant. Public health nurses have the opportunity to observe parent-child interaction in the home setting during their regular visits to a family, and they can be on the lookout for clues that things are not going well for the child and/or parents. Other settings where nurses have the opportunity and responsibility to detect actual abuse are emergency rooms where children are brought for treatment of their injuries, or in schools where nurses may be asked to examine a child who appears ill or bruised.

Primary Intervention

Primary intervention in the child abuse cycle implies prevention of abuse with intervention before an actual episode of abuse. The National Center for the Prevention and Treatment of Child Abuse and Neglect suggests the following conditions need to be present before abuse actually takes place, and the nurse can keep these in mind when working with families. These conditions include 1) parents who have the potential for abuse (history of being abused, lack of support for each other), 2) the existence of a "special child" (different sex than wanted, resemblance to disliked family member), and 3) existence of a crisis or series of crises (poverty, unemployment, death).[53]

Primary intervention is possible with the nurse and nurse-midwife caring for the pregnant woman and parturients and listening for cues that the infant will not be able to satisfy the mother's (parents') expectations—unwanted, wrong sex, ugly, cries too much.[54] Emergency room nurses can often pick up child behaviors that seem to be irritating to parents, especially when a child is brought repeatedly for treatment of vague symptoms, such as a stomachache, with no apparent physical basis. The nurse may pick up that the parent is asking for help in dealing with the child, and she can lend a listening, sympathetic ear before the parent actually strikes out at the child. Reinforcing positive parenting behaviors (bringing the child for care) and listening sympathetically may be the beginning of help for a distraught parent who is fearful of striking out at the child. The nurse who has dealt with her own feelings about hitting children and reactions to those who may wish to can be more comfortable and possibly more helpful to such a parent in this situation.

Referral

The nurse would also do well to know when referral to other professionals and sources of help is needed to help the family in question. It is suggested that the nurse try to clarify what she can and cannot do for a given family in these circumstances and to know when to refer to another colleague if her own values and attitudes prevent her from establishing a therapeutic relationship.

Secondary Intervention

Secondary intervention in the abuse cycle occurs after some form of abuse has actually occurred, whether physical, emotional, or verbal. Nurses are frequently the ones to obtain the initial history of the illness or injury of a child brought for treatment.[55] School nurses also have a responsibility to question children about cigarette burns or injuries such as visible strap marks on the back, recognizing that fear of future abuse from the parent may keep the child from responding. These types of injuries should alert the school nurse to potential abuse, however, and the need for further follow-up with the parents.[56] Detection of physical abuse is easiest and generally results when the nurse realizes that the parent's description of how the child was injured does not seem to correlate with the actual injuries. Falls, burns, and broken bones are the most common types of injuries from physical abuse.

Reporting: If the nurse suspects that some form of abuse has taken place, she faces a difficult moral decision. Does she/he proceed to validate the suspicion of abuse by further questioning and risk the antagonism and possible assault of the parent? Does she/he share suspicions with the physician and let him decide what to do? Or does she/he accept what the parent says happened and treat the child's injuries, sending the child back into the home with no benefit of protection? Nurses who have not been in such situations caring for abused children often state that the path of decision making is clear-cut. You must protect the child and determine whether the suspected abuse is actual. On the other hand, nurses who daily work with abusing families know that no decision is clear-cut.

Sophisticated Intervention

A sophisticated level of nursing intervention is required if a caring, helpful, advocacy relationship is to be cultivated instead of an adversarial one that includes fingerpointing, snoopervision, and accusatory actions intent on removing the child from the parents, no matter what.[57] This sophisticated intervention may include a delay in reporting suspicions until they are confirmed through repeated contacts with the family and a slow search for the truth within the framework of a trusting relationship. One aim of intervention is to support and assist the parents to recognize their need for and ability to seek counseling and help. If the decision is made to delay reporting, the nurse may need to accept the fact that abuse may continue if the child stays in the family unit, until the parents are willing to accept help in changing their behavior patterns.

Legal Mandate

One of the major problems for nurses who work with children and suspect some form of abuse is the legal mandate for reporting and documenting one's suspicions of abuse. One theory about why nurses hesitate to document and report such evidence is that they are taught to be less than diagnostic when describing a patient's condition, so careful not to use words that might hint at having made a diagnosis lest they be accused of practicing medicine. Reporting abuse requires proof, documented, written descriptions of injuries, and so on. Another reason nurses may hesitate to report suspected or actual abuse is their discomfort in taking such responsibility for intervention (though the ANA

Code and modern nursing practice insists on responsibility taking), as well as the ease of deferring in such difficult decisions to the physicians (see Chapter Five).

In such instances of responding to both a legal and professional mandate for advocacy, nurses must examine their own value system and decide who/what carries highest priority for action in a given situation—personal feelings, protection of a defenseless child, desire to help the entire family cope with their problems, fear of reprisal from the parents or legal system, or something else.[58] Josten[59] suggests that accepting one's legal mandate as a family advocacy activity may help the nurse to respond to this mandate.

Professional Relationship: Josten[60] points out that the nurses who are working with an abusing family would do well to work through their own feelings toward the abused and the abuser(s). In order to proceed with a supportive relationship, one needs to accept the fact that the entire family needs and is worthy of help. She supports other authors and practitioners in suggesting that even though anger toward the abuser is common, a nurse who wishes to "punish" the abuser probably should not be working with the family. The caring professional relationship so necessary in working with abusing families is based on honesty and an accurate view of what the nurse can and cannot do for or with the family. Dependability, genuine helpfulness, and role modeling positive parenting behaviors leaves little room in this relationship for the need to punish the "offenders." We would hasten to add that sharing one's appropriate feelings toward specific behaviors of children and parents does have its place in the caring relationship, including offering one's reasons for these feelings.

Nursing Roles

The roles of the nurse working with abusing families include advocacy, teaching, counseling, and coordination of resources available to help the family change its behaviors and ways of relating to each other in a positive direction. One of the problems in coordinating resources, especially those in the community, revolves around the inade-

quacy of some and the lack of knowledge of others. In 1966, the Committee on Infant and Preschool Child of the American Academy of Pediatrics pointed out the need for immediate, accurate reporting of abuse plus adequate follow-up services in the community if child abuse statistics were to be reduced.[61] In a follow-up report in 1972, the community resource coordination was still nonexistent, or nearly so.[62] It is little wonder that nurses working with abusing families often make decisions about reporting or not based on their knowledge of the adequacy or track record of a given agency. If you believed that abused children should be treated in the context of the family, and the major community agency responsible for that section of the city always removed children to foster homes with minimal or no follow-up care for parents, might you hesitate in referring families to this agency? It is important for the nurse to *know* the community resources available to abusing families and their previous record of helping these families constructively.[63]

Information or Invasion?

The final problem to be discussed here involves the issue of how to probe for information that can refute or substantiate abuse without invading another's privacy unnecessarily. Some suggestions on approach can be offered although it is recognized that each nurse will have to decide for herself how to proceed in keeping with her understanding of the interface of privacy, protection, and legal reporting when child abuse is suspected or evident. One good approach to discussing parental reactions to children is to observe the child's behavior that appears to be upsetting to the parents, and then to ask them for verification. Questions such as "how do you feel when Johnny does that?" may be a helpful opener. Some nurses find it helpful to recognize their feelings of "there but for the grace of God go I" when faced with disturbing child behavior and the urge to "let them have it." This recognition of one's own frailty may encourage greater sympathy and understanding of why some parents abuse their children and provide the bases for a truly understanding, helpful relationship.

Documentation of actual abuse situations generally requires repeated, yet slow, probing of what happened, tempered with the reality that the story does not seem to fit the injury the child has. Asking for specifics while sharing concern that this injury can be prevented in the future may help the parent to face the reality of his/her actions. On the other hand, the parents may become hostile, accuse the nurse of not being willing to care for the child, and then take the child elsewhere for treatment.

Summary

Working with abusing families carries the risk of forcing parents to choose between care for the child or protection of their behavior patterns to the detriment of the child. It also exposes the nurse to repeated episodes of testing and questioning of motives for care, with minimal or no rewards evident when the family refuses care. A nurse who seeks/values immediate reward from one's job would do well to avoid this aspect of nursing practice. How the nurse deals with these types of situations is often reflective of her personal value system and the extent of commitment to the professional role and responsibilities. Seeking out and forming peer support groups helps nurses deal with their negative attitudes or reactions to caring for abusing families and helps them to maintain long-term contact and caring with difficult families.

NURSES AND ADOLESCENT SEXUALITY

As in other areas of health care, nurses who work with adolescents can benefit from first exploring and understanding their own values related to adolescent behaviors in general, and adolescent sexuality in particular. It is then more likely that nurses who provide health care for adolescents will be truly committed to providing the services needed by this segment of the population and less prone to punishing them for their sexual behaviors, or, worse, ignoring the adolescent's request for care.

Legal Aspects

Provision of health care services for adolescents has legal as well as ethical dimensions for nurses. The legal dimension revolves around the age of majority and under what circumstances an adolescent (minor) can request and receive medical or health-related care without parental consent. The legal aspects of care will be dealt with in more detail in the chapter on rights. Suffice it to say here that the nurse providing care must know the laws of the state regarding provision of care to minors with or without consent of parents in order to avoid incurring unnecessary liability for her treatment actions.[64]

Ethical Aspects

The ethical dimensions of providing health or medical services to adolescents were summarized earlier. The issue of sex education, including provision of contraceptive information, is very real for some nurses who work in schools or family planning settings. One might assume that nurses who work in these settings are basically supportive of the right of all people to choose to contracept or not. This is not, in fact, true because nurses tend to represent a variety of attitudes toward situational choices; that is, it's permissible for the married teen but not the unmarried teen; it's all right for the eighteen-year-old but not for the fourteen-year-old, and so on.

Sex Education: A recent survey of school nurses in an eastern state exposed widely divergent attitudes and practices regarding the teaching of subjects related to sex education or adolescent sexual behavior.[65] This is not one of the states that prohibits sex education in the schools. Yet, here is a group of professionals who seem to ignore responsibility for providing sound information on contraception and conception, let alone sexuality in general. The Osofskys point out that sex education is a right of every person.[66] If this is true, to what extent are school nurses responsible for meeting this need of adolescents? The Osofskys argue that sex education allows for prevention of undesired sexual exposure and unwanted pregnancy, but only if information on how to prevent pregnancy is also offered. Sex education also implies helping adolescents explore their attitudes about sex, including the right not to be sexually active plus values on sexuality, and helping them to talk comfortably about sexual behavior.[67] Nurses are often in an excellent position to provide this kind of sex education and information in a nonthreatening manner.

Contraception: Some nurses feel strongly that providing information on contraceptive methods only enhances the desire of adolescents to engage in sexual intercourse. Sol Gordon, among many, takes a more pragmatic approach in stating that many teenagers are engaging in sexual activities already and this cannot be prevented by *not* telling them about birth control measures.[68] What can be prevented may be an unwanted pregnancy. Whether a nurse decides pro or con the teaching or prescription of contraception for teen-agers may reflect the nurse's personal values about unwanted children as well as adolescent sexual behaviors.

Care Needs: Working with adolescents, whether they are sick, seeking contraception or abortion, or pregnant, can be trying for any health professional. Knowledge and understanding of adolescent growth and development can help the nurse understand and work with teen-agers more constructively. Identity formation is central to the adolescent's growth, and peer support, body image, and magical thinking (I can't get pregnant) pervade the adolescent's behavior. Adolescents often seek out adults other than their parents to discuss their thinking and behaviors, and, if given the opportunity, their most intimate feelings. Health professionals often can be these "other adults" and may play a significant role in the adolescents' maturation. School nurses in particular can be supportive and informative on aspects of healthy adolescent sexuality when the teen-agers appear for excuses from physical education classes with a myriad of reasons for not "exposing" their bodies to others.[69] Steinman suggests that health professionals who cannot tolerate anything other than following routines and strict appointment keeping be-

havior should not be working with the adolescent.[70] She goes on to note the importance of health professionals dealing with their own feelings regarding sexual activity among adolescents so that conflicting values are not projected onto the adolescent, causing rejection of the services being offered.[71] Adolescent health services are best received when provided in a nonjudgmental, objective, matter-of-fact manner. Chanis and colleagues add that having a separate waiting area for pregnant teens is one way to remove them from the judgmental atmosphere of the general clinic and thus to encourage ongoing participation in pregnancy care.[72]

Pregnant Teen: The needs of the pregnant teen-ager are many. They have been written about in many books and journals, and have been the subject of many professional conferences in recent years. The nurse and nurse-midwife who provide pregnancy care for teens need to be cognizant of the many social, emotional, educational, as well as physical needs of a teen-ager who is pregnant. The nurses' values of education and properties for "good mothering" need to be explored so that they do not inhibit their abilities to respond to the teen-ager's special needs at this time.

Caring for pregnant teen-agers seems best accomplished in collaboration with many members of the health team—nurse, nutritionist, teacher, nurse-midwife, social worker, and physician. Needless to say, a supportive, caring relationship that is built on mutual trust and acceptance is important to the success of pregnancy care (encouraging the teen-ager to return for each visit), as well as the fostering of positive parenting behaviors when the teen has decided to keep and raise her infant. This type of relationship is possible when the health professionals are comfortable working with adolescents and are willing to provide the needed care.

Attitudes: The teen-ager in labor can pose a variety of moral dilemmas for the professionals taking care of her. Extremes of behavior from screaming, biting, and kicking to a desire for intimate physical contact with the nurse (surrogate mother) can give rise to many responses from the caregivers. Nurses who are comfortable with their role as support person during labor and who can respond to the teen-agers' needs just as with any other laboring woman probably provide the best care.[73] Yet it is difficult for many to tolerate physical and verbal assaults from patients over extended periods of time even when one can understand that these arise from fear, pain, and other emotions. Nurses who seem to have the most difficulty working with teen-agers in labor are those who may not think it right for this person to be having sex, yet alone a baby, and may be tempted to "punish" the child for past behavior by now

leaving her alone during labor and ignoring her requests for pain medication.

Again, we stress the need for nurses to examine their own feelings, attitudes, and values regarding the practice situations they are working in so that patients receive needed care in a positive, helpful manner. If one's values are in direct conflict with those of a patient, the chances that good care will be provided are lessened. Nurses have the responsibility to know their own limits of tolerance of client behaviors and to seek colleague relief of duties if the care situation demands more than they can give at that moment.

CASE STUDIES

Case #15

Infants and Research

D. J., a pediatric nurse-practitioner, was approached by Dr. J. and asked to participate in a special research study involving infants from two to twelve months of age. The study would involve taking six capillary tubes of blood from the infant at specified time intervals, scheduled during the normal visits for well-child care. The physician shared the research protocol with the nurse, and the approval from the Institutional Review Board. In return for participating in the study, these infants would receive free child care at a special research center. D. J. agreed to participate in the study after observing the informed consent process with the parents and being assured that the parents knew they could withdraw their infant from the study at any time and still continue to receive care in the center.

Questions for consideration in addition to applying the *Guidelines:*

1. Would you have agreed to participate in this study? On what conditions?
2. Would knowing why the blood studies were needed be helpful to you in making such a decision?
3. What is your response to the idea of parents giving consent for such an invasive procedure as heel or fingersticks on their young infants? Does any research merit such a physical invasion or causation of pain, though momentary?
4. Did D. J. respond in an ethically sound manner to Dr. J.'s request?

Case #16

A Child's Consent

You are a staff nurse in a pediatric section of a regional medical center. You have been caring for Jonathan, a twelve-year-old child who has leukemia. The doctors are interested in trying out a new drug as therapy for leukemia and need permission to use it on Jonathan. The study is discussed with the parents as permission is sought, and the parents respond that Jonathan will have to be asked first before they can agree to allow the drug to be used. The doctor agrees and proceeds to talk with Jonathan about the new drug. After the doctor leaves, Jonathan looks to you and asks you what you think he should do. He adds that he knows he is dying and is not sure he wants any more "needles."

In addition to applying the *Guidelines,* please consider the following questions for study:

1. How would you respond to Jonathan's request?
2. What further information about the nature of the drug and expected results would you need to know in order to understand the nature of the research?
3. How might you respond if Jonathan were your son?

Case #17

Child Neglect

D. A. is a pediatric nurse clinician working in the outpatient department of a hospital. One day she greets Mrs. P. and her children and begins to ask some questions about the children. The nurse weighs the newborn and discovers that she is in the less than 5 percent range of normal and appears not to be growing. When the mother is questioned about what the infant is eating, she responds, "She drinks four or five bottles of formula a day." When asked how she was preparing the formula, the mother did not seem to remember. At this point, the nurse observed the two-year-old grunting and pointing, but not talking. She asked the mother if the child talked at home, and the mother said no—he was "kind of slow, just like my other two children." The nurse decided that a home visit was in order to check on the home environment and just how Mrs. P. was feeding the newborn. Mrs. P. agreed to the visit, and the Public Health Nurse agency was notified.

In addition to applying the *Guidelines,* consider the following questions during study:

1. Was the nurse correct in calling on the PHN agency to verify the home situation, or could this be considered an "invasion of privacy"?
2. What would you have done in this situation if you were the nurse in the clinic?
3. What kind of feelings do you experience when you care for a family in which child neglect seems evident? How do these feelings influence your approach to the parents/mother?
4. What is the role of the public health nurse in this type of situation?

Case #18

Child Abuse

H. P. is a nurse working in the emergency room. One evening a woman appears with her three-month-old infant, who appears very ill and pale. Upon examination, the infant is found to have many bruises over the body, especially the back, and a broken arm. The mother is questioned about what happened to the infant, and she responds that the infant "fell out of her crib," The nurse's knowledge of the behavior patterns of three-month-old infants signals to her that the story does not seem to fit together. The nurse decides to proceed with questioning and states, "It doesn't seem possible for a three-month-old infant to fall out of a crib, especially since you said there were siderails all around. Do you think maybe something else happened?" The woman is nearly in tears, and responds, "I wasn't home when it happened, but that's what my old man said. What's going to happen to my baby? Will she be all right?" The nurse senses that the mother is really concerned about the infant, but that she is not telling what really happened. The nurse decides to confer with the physician about her suspicion of child abuse, and let the physician decide what should be done next.

In addition to applying the *Guidelines,* consider the following questions in your study:

1. What would you have done at this point if you had been the nurse interviewing this mother?
2. What further information would you need from the mother, and how might you go about obtaining it?
3. What are the nurse's responsibilities in this situation, and why do you think she deferred to the physician for a decision on action?
4. Was the nurse fulfilling her duty to the child? the parent? the physician?

Case #19

Adolescent Pregnancy

A. B., thirteen years old, appeared for pregnancy care at the nurse-midwifery Teen Clinic. She was twenty weeks pregnant and gave a history of being exposed to "measles" a week ago, with a "light rash" appearing on her back two days ago. A rubella titer indicated no prior immunity. A follow-up titer one week later was slightly elevated, though not definitive of disease. The physician urged the nurse-midwife to gain consent for an immediate abortion because this fetus could be damaged by rubella. She added that A.B. was just too young to have a baby anyway. A. B. refused to consent to the abortion and continued with the pregnancy.

In addition to the *Guidelines,* please consider the following questions:

1. To what extent do you think the physician's plan for abortion was based on medical/scientific rationale, and to what extent was it based on her personal views of adolescent sexual behavior?
2. If you were the nurse counselor, how might you present the options concerning this pregnancy to A. B. so that your own beliefs about thirteen-year-olds who are pregnant do not influence your manner of counseling? Do you think this is possible?
3. Does the nurse have the right/responsibility to always follow the physician's plan? On what grounds might the nurse choose to follow another plan?

Adolescent Sexuality

B. D. is a family planning nurse-practitioner working a large, urban setting. One evening during the young adult session, a thirteen-year-old girl appears, requesting a prescription for pills. When asked what kind of sexual activity patterns she currently has (how often she has sex), the girl responds, "Oh, I haven't had it yet, but I may sometime in the next month or six months." B. D. begins to discuss the advisability of using the pill when it is not really needed, and suggested that the young girl consider some other alternative. The girl responds that she wants the pill, and if B. D. won't give it to her, she'll get it somewhere else. Besides, she adds, she doesn't intend to use it until she's ready to have sex. B. D. gives in, and gives the teen-ager three packs of pills.

Consider the following questions, applying the *Guidelines:*

1. Would you have given this teen-ager the pills as requested? State your rationale.
2. What are your feelings/beliefs about prescribing contraception for teen-agers who have not begun to have sexual relations, but are planning to?
3. Would you prescribe oral contraceptives for any thirteen-year-old?

NOTES AND REFERENCES

1. Brochure No. 1110, International Year of the Child, 1979. UN General Assembly Resolution 1386 (XIV), 20 Nov. 1959, *Official Records of the General Assembly*, Supplement 16, 1960. Daniel P. Hallahan and James M. Kauffman. *Exceptional Children* (Englewood Cliffs, N.J.: Prentice-Hall, Inc., 1978), "Rights of the Handicapped," pp. 28–19. All this is in striking contrast to the heartlessness and cruelty with which children have been treated for centuries. Florence Lieberman, "Special Children," pp. 171–176, in *Bioethics and Human Rights*, ed. by Elsie L. and Bertram Bandman (Boston: Little, Brown and Company, 1978). A. E. Wilkerson, ed., *The Rights of Children* (Philadelphia: Temple University Press, 1973). Lloyd deMause, ed., *The History of Childhood* (New York: The Psychohistory Press, 1974). Philippe Aries, *Centuries of Childhood* (New York: Alfred A. Knopf, Inc., 1962). Samuel X. Radbill, "A History of Child Abuse and Infanticide," pp. 2–17, in *The Battered Child*, 2nd ed., ed. by Ray E. Helfer and C. Henry Kempe (Chicago: The University of Chicago Press, 1974). Paul Adams and others, *Children's Rights* (New York: Praeger Publishers, Inc., 1971). We shall look at "rights" in more detail later in the text. Here we might note the grounding of children's rights in the larger concern of human rights. Our founding fathers said God has created all people equal and has endowed them with certain inalienable rights. Bernard J. Coughlin, "The Rights of Children," pp. 7–19, in Wilkerson, op. cit., describes these as natural rights. Humans hold these "naturally." They are not given by anyone else, individual or organization. Others point to the curiosity that it has taken so long to discover this "natural" endowment, a discovery that we have yet to apply to all people equally. The Constitution originally applied only to adult male property owners. Obviously, not everyone agrees on who has rights or what they are. Lindsay G. Arthur gives us food for thought when he asks if children should be treated equally. He answers with a no. They shouldn't have equal liberties, but less. They shouldn't have equal protection, but more. How much less or more depends on the individual child's maturity. "Should Children Be as Equal as People?" pp. 118–137, in Wilkerson, op. cit. The "mature

minor" is now a legal concept. It applies especially to the teen years. Judith B. and Daniel Offer, "Adolescents," *Encyclopedia of Bioethics* 1:39–44. The Encyclopedia is cited hereafter as *EB*.

2. *Situation Ethics* (Philadelphia: The Westminster Press, 1966).

3. Some would go so far as to say all medicine is experimental and that medicine has always experimented. Robert M. Veatch, *Case Studies in Medical Ethics* (Cambridge, Mass.: Harvard University Press, 1977), p. 266. The history of experiments "on humans is as old as medicine itself." Gert H. Brieger, "Human Experimentation: History," *EB* 2:684–692. George J. Annas quotes a doctor as claiming the title of physician confers the right to experiment and merely presenting oneself for treatment means presenting oneself for experimentation. *The Rights of Hospital Patients* (New York: Avon Books, 1975), pp. 103, 199. Annas and others disagree. Generally, it is against the law though the legal history is mixed. Jay Katz, *Experimentation with Human Beings* (New York: Russell Sage Foundation, 1972). Annas goes on (p. 100) to limit the meaning of "experiment" to treatment that departs from standard practice for the purpose of getting new knowledge or testing an hypothesis.

4. "The Commission's Recommendations for Research on Children," *The Hastings Center Report*, no. 5 (Oct. 1978), 8:28–29. The Report is abbreviated hereafter as *HCR*. See also Jean D. Lockhart, "Pediatric Drug Testing Today: Obstacles to Research," *HCR*, no. 3 (June 1977), 7:8–10. No research may harm or deprive children. This violates the "do no harm" ethic, just as some research may do more harm than good.

5. James J. McCartney, "Research on Children: National Commission Says 'yes, If . . . ,'" *HCR*, no. 5 (Oct. 1978), 8:26–31. Katz, op. cit., pp. 955–1011. Karen Labacqz and Robert J. Levine, "Informed Consent in Human Research: Ethical and Legal Aspects," *EB* 2:754–761, cite several bases for informed consent. Philosophically, it is respect for persons. Religiously, it is concern for the sanctity of life and the idea of covenant (faithfulness). Legally, the concept is based on battery and negligence doctrines. Hans Jonas looks at it from the perspective of social contract. "Philosophical Reflections on

Experimenting with Human Subjects," *Daedalus* (Spring 1969), 98:219–245. Reprinted, pp. 317–339, in *Ethical Issues in Modern Medicine*, ed. by Robert Hunt and John Arras (Palo Alto, Calif.: Mayfield Publishing Co., 1977). Annas, op. cit., p. 104, notes that the Nuremberg judges trying the Nazis said Nazi experiments without informed consent violated Natural Law. See also, William J. Curran and Henry K. Beecher, "Experimentation in Children," *The Journal of the American Medical Association* (6 Oct. 1969), 210:77–83. Anne J. Davis and Mila A. Aroskar, *Ethical Dilemmas and Nursing Practice* (New York: Appleton-Century-Crofts, 1978), pp. 76–79. Jan Wojcik, *Muted Consent* (West Lafayette, Ind.: Purdue University, 1978), pp. 17–19. Veatch, op. cit., p. 290, claims the notion of consent is relatively new in history. He suggests it is based on the "principles of individualism and autonomy which form the basis of Anglo-American political philosophy. Coughlin, op. cit., p. 7, sees the special right of children to protection as residing in their dependency. This is implied also in the American Nurses' Association code, *Human Rights Guidelines for Nurses in Clinical and Other Research*, Publication no. D–46 (Kansas City, Mo.: The Association, 1975). Florence S. Downs, "Whose Responsibility? Whose Rights?," *Nursing Research*, no. 3 (May–June 1979), 28:131. The Offers, op. cit., pp. 42–43, find informed consent crucial for research with adolescents. It is not only an ethical principle but helps accuracy as well. Linda Briggs Besch, "Informed Consent: A Patient's Right," *Nursing Outlook*, no. 1 (Jan. 1979), 27:32–35.

6. Annas, op. cit. Susan Webb notes that fifty years ago children were the exclusive property of parents by common law. In 1967, the Gault decision established the legal rights of children, "The Rights of Parents and Children in Biomedical and Social Context," pp. 177–182, in Wilkerson, op. cit., p. 20. Janet F. Stansby, "In Re Gault: Children are People," pp. 285–302, in Wilkerson. Marguerite Mancini, "Nursing, Minors, and the Law," *AJN*, no. 1 (Jan. 1978), 8:124, 126.

7. Annas, op. cit., pp. 137–138. State laws vary and need to be checked for each item. Adele D. Hofmann, "The Right to Consent and Confidentiality in Adolescent Health Care: An Evolutionary Dilemma," pp. 183–188, in Bandman and Bandman, op. cit.

American Academy of Pediatrics, Committee on Youth, "The Implications of Minor's Consent Legislation for Adolescent Health Care: A Commentary," *Pediatrics*, no. 4 (Oct. 1974), **54**:481–485. Alexander M. Capron, "Right to Refuse Medical Care," *EB* 4:1498–1507. Paul Ramsey, *Ethics at the Edges of Life* (New Haven: Yale University Press, 1978), pp. 160–171, 268–300. Offers, op. cit., pp. 39–40.

Norman C. Fost notes the very definition of "child" is elusive, as is the age of consent. The boundary between fetus and infant is a shifting one, and that between childhood and adulthood is still harder to define. "Children and Biomedicine," *EB* **1**:150–156.

8. McCartney, op. cit., p. 27. Annas, op. cit., p. 140.

9. Annas, op. cit., pp. 86–87, 106, and n. 29, 138–139. The martyr statement is from the U.S. Supreme Court in *Prince* v. *Massachusetts*. The case involved a nine-year-old girl selling religious literature. Katz, op. cit., pp. 975–976. See also, William Ruddick, "Parents, Children, and Medical Decisions," pp. 165–171, in Bandman and Bandman, op. cit.

10. *The Patient as Person* (New Haven: Yale University Press, 1970). "The Enforcement of Morals: Nontherapeutic Research on "Children," *HCR*, no. 4 (Aug. 1976), **6**:21–30. A part of his reasoning is the idea that human beings are an end in themselves. They are not to be used as means to an end. The classical statement of this doctrine is by Immanuel Kant. *Foundations of the Metaphysics of Morals*, trans. by L. W. Beck (Indianapolis: The Bobbs-Merrill Co., Inc., 1969, original 1785), p. 52. See in the same volume, Pepita Haezrahi, "The concept of man as end-in-himself," pp. 292–318. Veatch, op. cit., pp. 266–267, notes that strict adherence to the Hippocratic Oath would prohibit nontherapeutic research because it concerns benefit for the patient.

11. Richard A. McCormick, "Proxy Consent in the Experimentation Situation," *Perspectives in Biology and Medicine*, no. 1 (Autumn 1974), **18**:2–20. Reprinted, pp. 456–465, in *Contemporary Issues in Bioethics*, ed. by Tom L. Beauchamp and LeRoy Walters (Encino, Calif.: Dickenson Publishing Co., 1978). McCormick, "Experimentation in Children: Sharing in Sociality," *HCR*, no. 6 (Dec. 1978), **6**:41–46. This view has been called "novel."

That is not to say that it is wrong. Like many decisions, it would be subject to abuse; that is, it might be difficult to separate "my" view from what my children might want. George H. Kieffer, *Bioethics: A Textbook of Issues* (Reading, Mass.: Addison-Wesley Publishing Co., Inc., 1979), p. 252. Paul Ramsey, op. cit., *HCR*, no. 4 (Aug. 1976), **6**:28. William G. Bartholome suggests the children might benefit in moral development from participation in such research. "Parents, Children, and the Moral Benefits of Research," *HCR*, no. 6 (Dec. 1976), **6**:44–45. LeRoy Walters, "Fetal Research and the Ethical Issues," *HCR*, no. 3 (June 1975), **5**:13–18.

One part of the argument is the deontological (duty or rule) ethic. For Ramsey, parents have a duty to protect their children. For McCormick, children and parents have duties to society.

12. McCartney, op. cit., pp. 26, 30. Ramsey, *The Patient . . .* , op. cit., pp. 47–54. The National Commission objected to the overuse of any one category of children, thus banning studies such as Willowbrook. Kieffer, op. cit., p. 253. Robert Ward and others, "Infectious Hepatitis," *The New England Journal of Medicine*, no. 9 (27 Feb. 1958), **258**:409–416. Reprinted, pp. 291–296, in Hunt and Arras, op. cit. Katz, op. cit., pp. 1007–1010. Veatch, op. cit., pp. 274–277.

13. See n. 1. Fost, op. cit., p. 151. C. Henry Kempe and Ray E. Helfer, *Helping the Battered Child and His Family* (Philadelphia: J. B. Lippincott Company, 1972), p. ix. Wilkerson, op. cit., p. 312; de Mause, op. cit., pp. 3, 40. The picture is not absolute. Richard R. Lyman, Jr., cites numerous efforts throughout the centuries to stop infanticide and alleviate some of the worst abuses. The efforts were ineffective for the most part. "Barbarism and Religion: Late Roman and Early Medieval Childhood," pp. 75–100, deMause, op. cit. It can also be pointed out that some things we now call abuse were considered normal in earlier times. "Earlier times" here ranges from the present to a generation ago and back to the dawn of time. See Radbill, op. cit. Deborah Adamowicz, ed., *Child Abuse and Neglect*, vol. 1 (Washington: DHEW Publication No. (CHD) 75–30073, 1976). Anne Allen and Arthur Morton, *This is Your Child* (New York: National Society for the Prevention of Curelty to Children, 1967), p. 16.

14. C. Henry Kempe and others, "The Battered-Child Syndrome," *The Journal of the American Medical Association* 181 (1962), 17–24. Kempe, "New Vistas in the Prevention of Child,Abuse," pp. 76–80, in *Child Advocacy and Pediatrics*, ed. by Eli H. Newberger (Columbus: Ross Laboratories, 1978). In this report, Jane Knitzer notes the birth of the term *child advocacy* in 1969. "Concepts of Advocacy," pp. 13–17. The legal rights of children were established in 1967 (n. 6). In 1974, Congress passed the Child Abuse Prevention and Treatment Act, which established the National Center on Child Abuse and Neglect (NCCAN). Adamowicz, op. cit., pp. iv, 4. The First International Conference on Child Abuse and Neglect was held in Geneva, Switzerland in 1976. The second was in London in 1978. The International Society for the Prevention of Child Abuse and Neglect started in 1977. See *Evaluation of Child and Neglect Demonstration Projects, 1974–1977*, vols. 1 and 2 (Hyattsville, Md.: National Center for Health Services Research, Public Health Service, U.S. DEHEW, 1978). An earlier concern was expressed by the League of Nations Geneva Declaration on the Rights of the Child, in 1924. See Wilkerson, op. cit., p. 3. See further the American Academy of Pediatrics Committee on Infant and Preschool Child, "Maltreatment of Children: The Battered Child Syndrome," *Pediatrics*, no. 1 (July 1972), **50**:160–162.

That a symposium was held in 1961, of course, indicates an earlier concern. Robert E. Shepherd Jr., suggests the current wave of interest seems to stem from the X-ray studies of John Caffey in 1946, Frederic N. Silverman in 1953, and P. V. Wooley, Jr., in 1955. The White House Conferences on Children started in 1909. This led to the establishment of the Children's Bureau in 1912. By 1930, the Conferences produced a "Children's Charter," which guaranteed every child love and affection plus protection from abuse and neglect. But it took more than thirty years to produce laws to back up the charter. Reluctance to interfere with the right of parents to discipline their children is cited as explanation for the delays. Invasion of privacy remains a primary concern in enforcement of the laws. A whole history of earlier laws goes all the way back to Hammurabi of Babylon, c. 1750 B.C. These, however, were mostly concerned with

infanticide (see earlier discussion). Shepherd, "The Abused Child and the Law," pp. 174–189, in Wilkerson, op. cit., and Wilkerson, p. 307. Radbill, op. cit., pp. 16–17. *Child Health in America* (Rockville, Md.: DHEW Publication no. (HSA) 76–5015, 1976), p. 25.

15. Katz op. cit., p. 999. Vincent J. Fontana, *Somewhere a Child Is Crying* (New York: Macmillan Publishing Co., Inc., 1973), p. 38. Fontana and Douglas J. Besharov, *The Maltreated Child*, 4th ed. (Springfield, Ill.: Charles C. Thomas, Publisher, 1979), p. 12, estimate one million cases. Adamowicz, op. cit., pp. 9–10, 12–13. *New Light on an Old Problem* (Washington: DHEW Publication no. (OHDS) 79–31108, 1978). In our previous references to child abuse, we have been talking largely about physical abuse. Infanticide fits here. As noted earlier, some look upon withholding medical treatment as a form of abuse, especially when this results in the death of the child. This might more accurately be called neglect (see following) or benign neglect. The concern may be extended to dying and the whole problem of keeping people of any age alive by machines. As noted earlier, others would suggest that letting a dying person die may be an act of mercy.

We note here too the legal concept of battery, which is any unauthorized touching, whether it harms or not. Some cite this concept as a reason for not doing research on children or incompetent persons. In research, as here in child abuse, part of the issue turns on what constitutes "unauthorized touching." At one time, teachers could physically discipline children. That's largely past. Parents and parent surrogates can still physically discipline. How far does their authority extend? At what point does discipline become abuse? Gross cases are clear. The dividing line may not be.

16. Kempe, "New Vistas . . . ," op. cit., p. 78. Jacob L. Issacs, "The Role of the Lawyer in Child Abuse Cases," pp. 225–241, in Kempe and Helfer, op. cit. Issacs notes that for legal purposes, "child abuse" means "battered child." "Neglect" is used for deprivation cases. See also, Hallahan and Kauffman, op. cit., p. 405. Nancy L. McKeel, "Child Abuse Can Be Prevented," *American Journal of Nursing*, no. 9 (Sept. 1978), **78**:1478–1482. The Journal is abbreviated hereafter as *AJN*. Sexual abuse is a smaller problem in the 5 per-

cent range of reported cases. Although a lower percentage, it remains a major concern. The American Nurses' Association House of Delegates adopted (1978) a statement extending child abuse and neglect to include child pornography, prostitution, and any commercial sexual exploitation of children. The resolution (No. 31) calls for investigation of child abuse in the diagnosis of venereal disease in children under twelve, and encourages stronger penalties for obscenity laws involving children under sixteen.

Deprivation—starvation, chronic disease, illiteracy—the whole range of human difficulties—affects and kills millions of children throughout the world. One might call this societal abuse to the extent that it is beyond parental control. Parents who continue to produce children they cannot or will not care for might be seen as child abusers. This assumes, of course, knowledge and resources for contraception. In Württemberg, Germany, economists once argued that no one had a right to produce children they could not support. Marriage was not allowed unless one could show proof that one could support the family. In 1830, there was one marriage per 121 inhabitants, and in 1854, one in 236. William L. Langer, "Checks on Population Growth: 1750–1860," *Scientific American*, no. 2 (Feb. 1972), **226**:92–99.

17. McKeel, op. cit., p. 1478. Hallahan and Kauffman, op. cit., pp. 405–506. Lieberman, op. cit., p. 171. Webb, op. cit., p. 179. Adamowicz, op. cit., pp. 5–6. "New Light . . . ," op. cit., pp. 14–15. Robert J. Olson, "Index of Suspicion: Screening for Child Abusers," *AJN*, no. 1 (Jan. 1976), **76**:108–110. Children's Defense Fund, "Second National Legislative Agenda for Children" (brochure), 1520 New Hampshire Ave. N.W., Washington, D.C. 20036, 1979. "Prevent Child Abuse" (brochure), National Committee for Prevention of Child Abuse, 111 E. Wacker Drive, Suite 510, Chicago, Ill. 60601, 1976. Brandt F. Steele and Carl B. Pollock, "A Psychiatric Study of Parents Who Abuse Infants and Small Children," pp. 1, 3, 147, Helfer and Kempe, op. cit.

Some studies vary from the outline given here. The Family Life Center (180 Main Street, Hackensack, N.J.) reports on 141 families for 1977–1978. Referrals included physi-

cal abuse (60 percent), emotional abuse (55 percent), neglect (23 percent), and sexual abuse (4 percent). The total is more than 100 percent because some children were referred for several reasons. There were four or fewer children in 85 percent of the families; 62 percent had an income of $10,000 or less; 55 percent were single parent families; in 26 percent of the families, a handicapped child was the object of abuse or neglect (43 percent had a handicapped child).

18. Hallahan and Kauffman, op. cit., p. 406. Steele and Pollock, op. cit., pp. 128–130. Adamowicz, op. cit., pp. 4–5. Donald H. Bouma, "Population Explosion," pp. 336–337, in *Birth Control and the Christian*, ed. by Walter O. Spitzer and Carlyle L. Saylor (Wheaton, Ill.: Tyndale House Publishers, 1969). Eleanor J. B. Corey, Carol L. Miller, and F. W. Widlak, "Factors Contributing to Child Abuse," *Nursing Research*, no. 4 (July–Aug. 1975), **24**:293–295. Harry H. Gordon, "Perspectives on Neonatology–1975," pp. 1–10, in *Neonatology*, ed. by Gordon H. Avery; Philadelphia: J. B. Lippincott, 1975. Arnold Sameroff, "Psychological Needs of the Mother in Early Mother-Infant Interactions," pp. 1023–1045, in Avery, op. cit. One explanation for the low birth weight child that becomes abused is the lack of mother-infant bonding. See Marshal H. Klaus and John H. Kennell, *Maternal-Infant Bonding* (St. Louis: The C. V. Mosby Company, 1976), pp. 2–3. Harold P. Martin and Martha A. Rodenheffer, "The Psychological Impact of Abuse on Children," *Journal of Pediatric Psychology*, no. 2 (Spring 1976), **1**:12–16.

19. McKeel, op. cit., pp. 1478–1479. Kathleen M. Scharer, "Rescue Fantasies: Professional Impediments in Working with Abused Families," *AJN*, no. 9 (Sept. 1978), **78**:1483–1484. Hallahan and Kauffman, op. cit., p. 406. Lavohn Josten, "Out-of-Hospital Care for a Pervasive Family Problem—Child Abuse," *Maternal Child Nursing*, no. 2 (March/April 1978), **3**:111–116. Parents Anonymous (PA), 22330 Hawthorne Blvd., Suite 208, Torrance, CA 90505. PA has more than 450 chapters in more than 300 cities. The group works with both abusing parents and parents who permit abuse. The national organization publishes a newsletter, "PA Frontiers" (a tax-deductible donation is requested). NCCAN has 10 regional Child Abuse

Resource Centers. A regional director can be contacted through NCCAN, Box 1182, Washington, D.C. 20013. The National Center for the Prevention and Treatment of Child Abuse and Neglect was established in 1973 at the University of Colorado Medical Center. It was an outgrowth of the Child Protection Team (1958) in the Department of Pediatrics, under the direction of pediatrician C. Henry Kempe and Psychiatrist Brandt F. Steele. The Center uses the team approach in education, consultation, technical assistance, demonstration programs for treatment, and research. Information is available without charge to interested parties. The address is 1205 Oneida Street, Denver, Colorado 80220. See n. 17 for the NCPCA and the CDF.

20. Josten, op. cit., p. 112. Melva Jo Hendrix, Gretchen E. LaGodna, and Cynthia A. Bohen, "The Battered Wife," *AJN*, no. 4 (Apr. 1978), **78**:650–653. Kay Lieberknect, "Helping the Battered wife," ibid., pp. 654–656. Kathleen O'Ferrall Friedman, "The Image of Battered Women," *American Journal of Public Health*, no. 8 (Aug. 1977), **67**:722–723. Barbara Parker and Dale N. Schumacher, "The Battered Wife Syndrome and Violence in the Nuclear Family of Origin: A Controlled Pilot Study," ibid., pp. 760–761. William Ryan, *Blaming The Victim* (New York: Vintage Books, 1976). Woods, op. cit., pp. 262–264. Malkah T. Notman and Carol C. Nadelson, "Women as Patients and Experimental Subjects," *EB* **4**:1704–1713.

21. Elizabeth Elmer and others, "Studies of Child Abuse and Infant Accidents," pp. 214–242, in *Vulnerable Infants*, ed. by Jane L. Schwartz and Lawrence H. Schwartz (New York: McGraw-Hill Book Company, 1977). Radbill, op. cit., p. 3. deMause, op. cit., pp. 10–11, 30, n. 148. Ewald M. Plass, *What Luther Says: An Anthology*, vols. 1 and 2 (St. Louis: Concordia Publishing House, 1959), p. 145. In the Bible, Deuteronomy 21:18–21 decreed stoning to death for a disobedient son. Later Jewish exegetes understood this as an educational commandment to encourage obedience rather than an execution to be carried out literally. A similar process is applied to the New Testament commandments of Jesus to cut off one's hand and pluck out one's eye if either of these caused sin. (Matthew 5:29–30).

22. Fost, op. cit., p. 151. The quote is from a coroner in Middlesex in 1862. Langer, op. cit., p. 97.

23. This was the title of a sermon by Jonathan Edwards (1703–1758).

24. Radbill, op. cit., pp. 11–12.

25. "Nuremberg Code," *EB* **4**:1764–1765. Children as an extension of their parents might be seen as the principle behind the idea of ownership. The extension of "personhood" to slaves has had a partial parallel. The U.S. Constitution grants them a partial personhood. The Emancipation Proclamaion and the post-Civil War amendments freed the slaves and made them legal persons. In practice, of course, this is a process still underway for the descendents of slaves, as well as for immigrants and minorities of all kinds, including children and wives. See Wilkerson, op. cit., p. viii. Historically, Robert F. Drinan notes that until c. 1900, only the husband could contract, make debts, or have legal responsibilities. "The Rights of Children in Modern American Family Law," pp. 37–46 in Wilkerson, op. cit., p. 37. See n. 6, "in re Gault."

26. Ronald S. Gass, "Codes of the Health-Care Professions," *EB* **4**:1725–1730. "Appendix: Codes and Statements Related to Medical Ethics," *EB* **4**:1731–1815. Quality of life compared to quantity of life has been noted earlier. We return to it in our consideration of death. Here, we underline its importance again. Obviously, the death of a child eliminates its quantity of life. An abused child has a lower quality of life. Sheer existence is no longer enough for many today as it was a generation ago. The quality of our existence is a growing concern. See also, Joseph Goldstein, Anna Freud, and Albert J. Solnit, *Beyond the Best Interests of the Child* (New York: The Free Press, 1973).

27. Mary M. McLaughlin, "Survivors and Surrogates: Children and Parents from the Ninth to the Thirteenth Centuries," pp. 101–181, in deMause, op. cit., p. 126 and n. 143. Elizabeth W. Marvick, "Nature Versus Nurture: Patterns and Trends in Seventeenth Century French Child-Rearing," pp. 259–301, in deMause, op. cit., p. 281 and n. 142. Langer, op. cit., p. 93. Teenage parenthood remains the situation in many cultures even today. See Phyllis T. Piotrow, "Mothers Too

Soon," pp. 3–5; Sattareh Farman-Farmaian, "Early Marriage and Pregnancy in Traditional Islamic Society," pp. 6–9; and Nani Soewondo, "Marriage Law Reform in Indonesia," in *The Draper World Population Fund Report*, no. 1 (Autumn 1975). Ramona T. Mercer, ed., *Perspectives on Adolescent Health Care* (Philadelphia: J. B. Lippincott Company, 1979), p. 246. In the United States, 32 percent of the teens aged fourteen to nineteen were married in 1960. By 1976, this had dropped to 22 percent. Frederick S. Jaffe and Joy G. Dryfoos, "Fertility Control Services for Adolescents: Access and Utilization," *Family Planning Perspectives*, no. 4 (July/Aug. 1976) **8:**167–175. This journal is abreviated hereafter as *FPP*. Of the world's 60 million women who gave birth in 1975, 13 million were parents before they were adults. See *11 Million Teenagers* (New York: The Alan Guttmacher Institute, 1976), p. 5. When Thomas Malthus foresaw the population explosion, he recommended raising the age of marriage as a way of slowing reproduction. Red China is currently attempting this. Leo A. Orleans, "New Patterns in China's Family Planning," pp. 10–12, *The Draper Report*, op. cit.

28. Lois J. Welches, "Adolescent Sexuality," pp. 29–41, in Mercer, op. cit. Phillips Cutright, "Illegitimacy: Myths, Causes and Cures," *FPP*, no. 1 (1971), **3:**25–49, and "The Teenage Sexual Revolution and the Myth of an Abstinent Past," *FPP*, no. 1 (1972), **4:**24–31. Nancy F. Woods, *Human Sexuality in Health and Illness*, 2nd ed. (St. Louis: The C. V. Mosby Company, 1979), p. 216. Karen R. Stewart, *Adolescent Sexuality and Teenage Pregnancy: A Selected, Annotated Bibliography with Summary Forewards* (Chapel Hill, N. C.: State Services Office, Carolina Population Center, 1976). *11 Million Teenagers*, op. cit., p. 10, notes that of the 1.1 million teen pregnancies each year, two thirds are conceived out of wedlock.

29. John F. Kantner and Melvin Zelnik report that about 27 percent of the never married fifteen- to nineteen-year-old teens in the 1971 survey claimed they had experienced sexual intercourse. By 1976, this had reached 35 percent. The rates rose from 14 percent at age fifteen to 46 percent at age nineteen. By 1976, the range was 15 percent to 55 percent. "Sex and Reproduction Among U.S. Teenage

Women," pp. 13–15, *The Draper Report*, op. cit. "Sexual Experience of Young Unmarried Women in the United States," *FPP*, no. 4 (1972), **4:**9–18. "Sexual and Contraceptive Experiences of Young Unmarried Women in the U.S., 1976 and 1971," *FPP*, no. 2 (1977), **9:**55–73. Mercer, op. cit., pp. 245–246, reports for 1975, 20.3 million American teens. In 1957, there were 13.1 million. In 1957, they had 557,172 births, and in 1975, they had 594,880. In 1957, the ten- to fourteen-year-olds produced 6,960 children, and in 1975, they had 12,645. *11 Million Teenagers*, op. cit., pp. 7, 10, 17, notes that 10 percent of American teens aged fifteen to nineteen get pregnant each year. Of these, 6 percent give birth. Of the one million pregnancies, 28 percent were conceived after marriage, 10 percent were conceived before marriage, 21 percent were out of wedlock births, 27 percent ended in abortion, and 14 percent in miscarriages. There are 4.3 million sexually active fifteen- to nineteen-year-old women, of whom 1.1 million are married. The title of this booklet refers to 11 million (7 million men and 4 million women) teens fifteen to nineteen, who are sexually active. An estimated 1.6 million of the 8 million thirteen- to fourteen-year-old teens are sexually active. Helen V. Burst, "Adolescent Pregnancies and Problems," *Journal of Nurse-Midwifery*, no. 2 (Mar/Apr. 1979), **24:**19–24. For the ethics of surveys, see Donald R. Nilson and Margaret O'Brien Steinfels, "Parental Consent and a Teenage Sex Survey," *HCR*, no. 3 (June 1977), **7:**13–15. This may be a case of adolescent self-determination, compared to parental responsibility for their children.

30. Kantner and Zelnik, *The Draper Report*, op. cit., p. 13, note that in 1972, 19 percent of births in the United States were to women under the age of twenty. In 1974, there were 30,000 pregnancies among women under fifteen years of age. Out of 12,600 live births, 10,600 were to unwed mothers. Jaffe and Dryfoos, op. cit., p. 174. According to *11 Million Teenagers*, op. cit., pp. 10, 13, 14, out of wedlock births among eighteen- to nineteen-year-olds increased by one third, and by three fourths among fourteen- to seventeen-year-olds, and half of all out of wedlock births are to teens.

31. Woods, op. cit., p. 225. For the present,

we can note in the Jaffe and Dryfoos study, cited previously, that out of the 30,000 pregnancies in under fifteen-year-olds in the United States, there were 13,500 abortions and 4,000 miscarriages. For 1974, single teens accounted for one fourth of all abortions. One third of all abortions were on women under twenty in 1973. "Teen-age Pregnancy: A Major Problem for Minors," Zero Population Growth, Washington, D.C. Woods, op. cit., p. 219. Diana Taylor, "Contraceptive Counseling and Care," pp. 109–143, in Mercer, op. cit. J. Parker, F. Nelson, and M. Svigir, "Legal Abortions: a half decade of experience," FPP, no. 6 (1975), 7:248–255. Alan F. Guttmacher, *Pregnancy, Birth and Family Planning: a Guide for Expectant Parents in the 1970s* (New York: Viking Press, 1973), pp. 300–301. *11 Million Teenagers*, op. cit., pp. 40–51.

32. Genesis 11:30, 25:21; Exodus 23:26. Farman-Farmaian, op. cit., p. 7. Lee Ranck, "Use It Better Than James," *Engage/Social Action* (e/sa) no. 39 (Apr. 1978), 10–16. Daniel Callahan in *11 Million Teenagers*, op. cit., p. 58.

33. Noncontraceptors report ignorance of birth control, belief they could not get pregnant "the first time" or "at that time of the month" or because they are not old enough or not in love, preference for spontaneity in having coitus, belief in oneself as "a good girl" by denying sexual activity even when it is frequent or she's pregnant, fear that birth control methods are dangerous, and the inaccessibility of contraceptive materials, or a belief that they are inaccessible. Taylor, op. cit., p. 109. Ranck, op. cit. Walter R. Aryan, Jr., *Adolescent Medicine in Primary Care* (New York: John Wiley & Sons, Inc., 1978), p. 265. Jerome R. Evans, Georgiana Selstad, and Wayne H. Welcher, "Teenagers: Fertility Control Behavior and Attitudes Before and After Abortion, Childbearing Or Negative Pregnancy Test," FPP, no. 4 (July/Aug. 1976), 8:129–200. *11 Million Teenagers*, op. cit., pp. 30, 34–37. "The Fear Barrier to Teenage Birth Control," *Psychology Today*, no. 4 (Sept. 1979), 13:109. On media, Gene Vadies of Planned Parenthood reports the National Association of Broadcasters saw nothing wrong with a nude woman selling new cars, but the NAB has a rigid ban on advertising contraceptives. "Children Bearing Children," *Engage/Social Action* (e/sa) no. 39 (Apr. 1978),

23–27. Gertrude Powell, "Sex Education: Whose Responsibility?" 39:32–39. Farida Shah, Zelnik, and Kantner, "Unprotected Intercourse Among Unwed Teenagers," FPP, no. 1 (1975), 7:39–44. Cutright, "Illegitimacy . . . ," op. cit., claims religion, ignorance, sex education, early maturation, nutrition, availability of abortion and/or contraception are not correlated with illegitimacy rates. Early and late marriage patterns are, as is Gross National Product. Illegitimacy has risen with GNP. It is not clear if this is fortuitous or if there are decisions that one can now afford to have children. When a culture switches from a late marriage pattern to an early one, illegitimacies increase. Again, the reason is not clear. Perhaps if marriage is a clear option, people are more careless on the theory that if she gets pregnant, they can get married.

34. Woods, op. cit., pp. 23, 219. Farman-Farmaian, op. cit., p. 6. Cutright, "Illegitimacy . . . ," op. cit.

35. The onset of menstruation is estimated at 13.5 years in 1940 and 12.5 years in the late 1960s. Between 10 percent and 20 percent menstruate by age 11. The 1940 illegitimacy rate may have been lower by as much as 3.4 per thousand in fifteen- to nineteen-year-olds because of a higher rate of miscarriages. It may have been another 1.6 per thousand lower because of a lower fertility rate. This could lead to the conclusion that there is no adolescent sexual revolution. Woods, op. cit., p. 216. Mercer, op. cit., p. 246. Cutright, op. cit. (both articles). Leona Zacharias, Richard J. Wurtman, and Martin Schatzoff, "Sexual Maturation in Contemporary American Girls," *American Journal of Obstetrics and Gynecology*, no. 5 (1970), 108:833–846. Alan S. Parkes, "Biological Aspects of Teenage Pregnancy," p. 20, *The Draper Report*, op. cit. Radbill, op. cit., pp. 11–13. David Solomon, "Shaftesbury, The Children's Friend," *New Tomorrow*, no. 18 (Jan. 1979), pp. 8–11. Orleans, op. cit. Burst, op., cit., p. 20.

36. Taylor, op. cit., p. 109. Woods, op. cit., pp. 100–101. Statistics vary. Taylor says 42 percent of teens are sexually active. Only 25 percent think it is all right. The contradiction may not be any more than that of older generations. Zelnik and Kantner, op. cit. (all references). Frank F. Furstenberg, Jr., "The Social

Consequences of Teenage Parenthood," *FPP*, no. 4 (July/Aug. 1976), **8**:148–164. Jaffee and Dryfoos, op. cit.

We noted the schizophrenia in some of the moralizing about abortion. The alternative of contraception is often objected to as well. In the meanwhile, as also noted earlier, the media and much of American culture promotes sexual stimulation and the exploitation of sex. In 1978, President Carter approved funds for pregnant teens but did nothing to help them from becoming pregnant in the first place. Laws are either silent in not providing for sex education or in providing education without information on family planning. The teen-agers get the message: it's okay to have sex as long as you don't use birth control. Cutright calls this the pseudomoral barrier to contraception. See "Illegitimacy . . . ," op. cit., pp. 43–44. Vadies, op. cit., pp. 26–27. Margaret Mead notes a variant of this. Our society preaches premarital chastity but rewards premarital pregnancy. "The Cultural Shaping of the Ethical Situation," pp. 4–23, in *Who Shall Live?*, ed. by Kenneth Vaux (Philadelphia: Fortress Press, 1970), p. 21. Woods, op. cit., p. 50. Harriet F. Pilpel, "Legal Rights of Minors," pp. 30–31, in *The Draper Report*, op. cit. She notes that many groups support contraceptive services for teens. These include the AMA, ACOG, AAP, APHA, and The American Bar Association. A number of religious groups now approve also in spite of some antisexual traditions. These include Unitarian-Universalists, United Presbyterians, and United Methodists among others. See Powell, op. cit., pp. 37–39, as well as our earlier chapters. Sex education is also approved by more and more groups. These include the U.S. Catholic Conference, the Synagogue Council of America, Sixth White House Conference on Children and Youth, NEA, NCC, NCPT, NAMH, ACOG, AAHPER, and AAP. See Sex Information and Education Council of the USA (SIECUS, 1855 Broadway, New York, N.Y. 10023); Social Principles of the United Methodist Church (1976), Board of Church and Society, 100 Maryland Ave., N.E., Washington, D.C. 20002; Policy Statements of the APHA (18 Oct. 1978), 7837: "Prevention of Unwanted Teenage Pregnancy," *American Journal of Public Health*, no. 3 (Mar. 1979), **69**:309–310.

37. Mercer, op. cit., pp. 247–250. Ruth R. Puffer and Carlos V. Serrano, "Teenage Pregnancies: High Risks for Infants," pp. 16–18, in *The Draper Report*, op. cit. *11 Million Teenagers*, op. cit., pp. 22–23. Vadies, op. cit., pp. 23–24. Stewart, op. cit., pp. 24–31. She notes that except for infant mortality for mothers under fifteen, the evidence is not this clearcut. Race and socioeconomic status are also major influences. American Academy of Pediatrics, Committee on Youth, "Venereal Disease and the Pediatrician," *Pediatrics*, no. 3 (Sept. 1972), reprint. "Leaders Alert Bulletin 30," The National Foundation/March of Dimes (Feb. 1979). Burst, op. cit., p. 21.

38. Furstenberg, op. cit., pp. 148–151, 155–164. "Digest," pp. 176–177, and T. James Trussell, "Economic Consequences of Teenage Childbearing," *FPP*, no. 4 (July/Aug. 1976) **8**:184–190. Mercer, op. cit., pp. 253–256. Leaders Alert, op. cit. *11 Million Teenagers*, op. cit., pp. 24–27. Stewart. op. cit., pp. 32–35, suggests that the data on this subject need to be updated.

39. *11 Million Teenagers*, op. cit., pp. 15, 28. Of 385,000 births to married adolescents, 326,500 were conceived prior to marriage. "Forced" marriages are generally less stable. Three out of five pregnant teen brides are divorced within five years. This is a sociological concern as well as a concern for traditional morality. Callahan suggests the ethical question is, what obligations do we have toward teenagers who might get pregnant, toward those who are, and toward those who have given birth? He adds other concerns such as the moral climate of the country and the allocation of scarce resources. *11 Million Teenagers*, op. cit., p. 57. Stanford Research Institute reports that teen pregnancies cost the United States taxpayers $8.3 billion a year. Without legal abortions, it would be another $1.5 billion. Costs include cash support, food stamps, medical and social services. "Teenage Pregnancies," *The Christian Century*, no. 21 (6–13 June 1979), **96**:633. Hoffman, op. cit. The law is moving in the direction of teen rights to medical care, including abortions, contraception, and venereal disease treatment. Pilpel, op. cit. See also Eve W. Paul, Harriet F. Pilpel, and Nancy F. Wechsler, "Pregnancy, Teen-agers and the Law, 1976," *FPP*, no. 1 (1976), **8**:16–21.

40. Woods, op. cit., p. 26.

41. See n. 35. Welches, op. cit., p. 29.
42. Ranck, op. cit. R. Franklin Gillis, "Values and Sexuality," e/sa, no. 39 (Apr. 1978), 17–22. "Social Principles of the United Methodist Church," op. cit.
43. Mercer, op. cit., pp. 274–383.
44. Lorraine V. Klerman, "Adolescent Pregnancy: The Need for New Policies and New Programs," *The Journal of School Health*, no. 5 (1975), **45**:263–267.
45. Woods, op. cit., pp. 225–226. Mercer, op. cit., pp. 267–269. Reuben Pannor and Byron W. Evans, "The Unmarried Father Revisited," *Journal of School Health*, no. 5 (1975), **45**:286–299. *11 Million Teenagers*, op. cit., p. 9, notes that information about teenage male sexual activity is practically nonexistent. Most of the material refers to the 4 million sexually active women aged fifteen to nineteen and to the 1.1 million who get pregnant each year. Stewart, op. cit., pp. 1, 7, 42–43. She suggests the unwed adolescent father is almost a forgotten person. APHA Policy Statements, op. cit., p. 309.
46. Woods, op. cit., 16–20, 55–59.
47. Woods, op. cit., pp. 28–29. Gillis, op. cit.
48. American Academy of Pediatrics, Committee on Youth, "A Model Act Providing for Consent for Minors for Health Services," *Pediatrics*, no. 2 (Feb. 1973), **51**:293.
49. Rowine H. Brown, "Consent," *Pediatrics*, no. 3 (Mar. 1976), **57**:414.
50. "American Nurses' Association Code for Nurses with Interpretive Statements (1976)," *EB* **4**:1796.
51. Op. cit.
52. Scharer, op. cit., p. 1483.
53. McKeel, op. cit., p. 1479.
54. Joan Hopkins, "The Nurse and the Abused Child," *Nursing Clinics of North America*, no. 4 (Dec. 1970), **5**:3, reprint. McKeel, op. cit., p. 1479.
55. Lynne L. Gorline and Mary M. Ray, "Examining and Caring for the Child Who Has Been Sexually Assaulted," *MCN*, no. 2 (Mar./Apr. 1979), **4**:110–114.
56. Hopkins, op. cit., p. 5.
57. Ibid., p. 1. Personal communication, Dorothy Allbriten, May 1979.
58. Others suggest that the nurse should not report child abuse. It is the physician's responsibility and "only the diagnostic ability of a physician is a sensitive enough instrument to sort out discrepancies between a child's physical state and the caretaker's explanation of the event." Monrad C. Paulsen, "The Law and Abused Children," pp. 175–200, in Helfer and Kempe, op. cit., p. 182.
59. Josten, op. cit., p. 112.
60. Josten, ibid., p. 111.
61. Op. cit., *Pediatrics*, **37**:379.
62. Op. cit., *Pediatrics*, **50**:160.
63. Ibid., pp. 160–161; Hendrix, op. cit., p. 652. A suggested approach for nurses to find out what community resources are available for abusing families is as follows:
1. Call or visit the local health department and request information on which agency(ies) is by law designated to follow up on suspected and actual abuse cases, and which private agencies participate in providing services to abusing families (children).
2. Call or write the county or city clerk of records for a copy of the law relating to child abuse in your state.
3. Call or visit the local Bureau of Child Welfare, if available, and gather information on how they process child abuse reports, what and how they provide services to the abusing families.
4. Check with public health nursing colleagues for word of mouth information on voluntary and official agencies working with abusing families, what services each provides, and what is their track record for helping abused children and families.
5. See footnotes 17 and 19 for additional sources of information.
64. Mancini, op. cit., p. 126. See also Taylor, op. cit., p. 141.
65. Virginia Gorosh, *Orientations of New Jersey School Nurses Toward Adolescent Sexual Behavior and Contraceptive Needs*, unpublished doctoral dissertation, Columbia University School of Public Health, October 1979.
66. H. J. Osofsky and J. D. Osofsky, "Let's Be Sensible About Sex Education," *AJN*, no. 3 (March 1971), **71**:532.
67. Woods, op. cit., pp. 100–101.
68. Sol Gordon, "What Adolescents Want to Know," *AJN*, no. 3 (March 1971), **71**:535.
69. Welches, op. cit., p. 39.
70. M. E. Steinman, "Reaching and Help-

ing the Adolescent Who Becomes Pregnant," *MCN*, no. 1 (Jan./Feb. 1979), **4**:18.

71. Compare with Woods, op. cit., p. 228, who notes the need for congruence of attitudes, knowledge, and behavior so that the health professionals can present a consistent approach to persons under their care who are most vulnerable to the positive and negative responses of staff persons. See also, Welches, op. cit., p. 40.

72. Margaret Chanis, Nancy O'Donahue, and Alicia Stanford, "Adolescent Pregnancy," *Journal of Nurse-Midwifery*, no. 3 (May/June 1979), **24**:18.

73. Mercer, op. cit., pp. 302–345.

Chapter 7

Bioethics and Adults

INTRODUCTION

The astute reader will recognize that we have been dealing with adults all along. It is not the unconceived who make ethical decisions. Nor is it the fetus and the neonates. It is adults who make decisions about genetics and contraception and abortion and defective infants. The same is often true for the use of children in research, and battered children are battered by adults. In childhood, however, we are into a more problematic area. As noted in Chapter Six, the line of demarcation has become vague on both ends of the child scale. At some point along the way, whether age seven or fourteen or some other magic number, or simply the awareness of the gradual maturation of the human being, the young person may get in a word or participate in the decisions or actually make them. But the point is, we have been concerned with adults and bioethics throughout this book.

DISTRIBUTIVE JUSTICE

Thus we do not come to an entirely new area of decision making in this section. Rather, we focus here on a particular concern: the allocation of scarce resources. This concern spreads across the life cycle. Genetic counseling, contraception, abortion, NNICU's, and help for battered children and battering parents are not available everywhere without exception.[1] But advancing years tend to develop or exaggerate defects in the human body. So at least some things catch up with us beyond the teen years. Various parts of the system start breaking down; cancer begins to take a heavier toll. In a nation that overeats and underexercises, health becomes a greater concern. The right to health, influenced by the availability or delivery of health care, which involves the allocation of resources, is an issue we can appropriately consider at this point.[2] The basic ethical issue is distributive justice.[3]

History: Historically, the problem has always been with us. The matter has traditionally been resolved in a fairly simple, straightforward way. Those who had the money and/or the power got; those without went without. The rich got richer and the poor got poorer. That is to say, available resources were available to those who could pay, or who had the power to take without paying. But the knowledge of health care, antiseptic technique, sanitation in general, nutrition, medical technology, prenatal and postnatal care was not all that advanced. So health, or perhaps unhealth, was the great leveler. The plague might take a heavier toll in the rat-infested slums, but it did not stop there. It was no respecter of persons. Microbes feasted on rich and poor alike without discrimination.

What has changed is our knowledge of sanitation, nutrition, and medical procedures.[4] Such knowledge is more available to the educated, and the attainment of that knowledge is more available to those with the ability to pay.[5] But that has limits, except for the truly wealthy, as some techniques outdistance the financial resources of some knowledgeable but materially limited folk.

SCARCE RESOURCES

Funding is not now a problem for hemodialysis, the classic example in modern writings on scarce resources. Since 1973, thanks to Public Law 92–603, the federal government has been financing the procedure. It turns out that funding is not the only problem. The comment on geographical availability remains. Simply having the money there does not guarantee adequate numbers of trained personnel. There has been a move to home dialysis, supported by some but not others. The procedure may put undue strain on a family even as it relieves the patient of extended time in treatment centers. It is cheaper, and not even the federal government has unlimited funds. Those concerned with funds also point out the ethics of unequal funding, for governments do not fund treatment of all other health problems, including some with high costs.[6]

Kidney Transplant: Terminal renal failure can sometimes be dealt with by hemodialysis.[7] Alternately, a kidney transplant may be a possibility.[8] Because the body tends to reject foreign tissue, kidneys from cadavers and unrelated donors have a higher ratio of rejection.[9] Thus, a subtle coercion may descend on family members to donate a kidney, a coercion that violates the principle of free consent. The donated kidney may still be rejected, leaving the recipient as bad off as before and the donor minus one kidney.[10]

The kidney of an identical twin is least likely to be rejected, with other family members next in line. Tests can sometimes determine in advance the family members with the most incompatible tissue, thus narrowing the selection process. This can increase the psychological pressure just noted. There have been several cases in which the best donor (on medical indications) was a minor or mental incompetent. Some of these cases have reached the courts. Children as young as seven have been allowed, with parent/guardian permission and the child's own agreement, to donate a kidney to a needy sibling. Decisions here and in mental or legal incompetency cases have often turned on a cost-benefit ratio. When the recipient was a sibling who could care for the incompetent after the death of the parents, or the recipient was the potential donor's chief contact with the real world, the tendency has been to agree to the procedure.[11] A recent hypothetical case was reported in which a man was tired of dialysis. His wife offered to get pregnant, have an abortion at six months, and remove the kidneys from the fetus for her husband. Even here, of course, there could be no guarantee that the father's body would not reject the transplant.[12]

Ethically, the last situation would be rejected by those who see the fetus as a person or worthy of protection because of its dependency. One ethicist, approached on this issue, admitted that for him personhood is not an issue until birth, and possibly, viability in the womb. He could find no ethical stance against the procedure. Aesthetically, he was appalled. The idea somehow seemed bizarre, wrong, and even insane. But when pressed for a reason, the ethicist could find none other than his feelings. Either his conscious standard was inconsistent with his emotional standard, or it might be seen as a case of "natural law" in the sense of someone being naturally (intuitionism) appalled at something that seems wrong.

For those recognizing the personhood of the fetus, the issue of informed consent compares with that for incompetents. There is, of course, no way that the fetus could give informed consent. It is doubtful that a retarded person could be fully informed, though that would depend on the degree of the retardation. The child of seven might or might not be capable of informed consent. Presumably, the fetus would die (if it were aborted prior to viability and/or kidneys were removed). The risk of death is there for the child and the incompetent, although one can live with only one functioning kidney. The degree of risk that the donor might in turn succumb to kidney malfunction is unknown.[13]

Value of Human Life: The sale of kidneys, or at least the willingness to buy, raises a question about the value of human organs and of human life in general. This refers to all transplants, of course, including the famous heart transplants and the lesser known liver transplants.[14] The permission not to go to extraordinary lengths to preserve life is one perspective. The earlier discussion noted cost as one factor in deciding what is extraordinary. The ordinary-extraordinary means distinction is held by numbers of people and groups. It has been upheld by Catholic leaders in terminal cases, as noted earlier. At least one Roman Catholic thinker has said that transplants are un-Christian and immoral because they deny what Christians traditionally believe about this life and the afterlife. Transplants such as corneas that improve the quality of life are all right because the people will continue to live anyway. Those that extend life can be seen as immoral on the basis that God controls the beginning of life (no contraception or abortion) and the end of life as well.[15]

It is, of course, an interesting argument that could be used against all medicine, not to mention the sanitation, nutrition, and miracle drugs that are generally seen as lowering the Western mortality rates. The acceptance of an improved quality of life, however, is a crucial aspect of dialysis and transplants. Some object to being "hooked to a machine" or having their lives dependent on a machine. They might be excused from what for them is an extraordinary means. Others do not seem to have such great antipathy. They feel better for the dialysis and see it as a gift of life.[16]

Catholic theologians have debated more thoroughly than others the merits of live donor transplants (*inter vivos*). For example, do we have a right to do what we please with our bodies?[17] The principle of totality says organs must not be diverted from their primary use in relation to the body. Some have seen this as a ban on transplants, whereas others find it acceptable because the intent is for the organ to continue its primary function in the recipient. There have also been attempts to justify organ donation on the basis of responsibility to community or humanity, and as an altruist expression of the Judeo-Christian commandment to love thy neighbor (Leviticus 19:18; Mark 12:31). This has tended to turn, however, on the cost-benefit factor. Thus, the transplantation has been restricted to paired organs. It is not permissible to risk death by such donation, and the recipient's benefit must be proportionate to the donor's loss.[18]

The cost-benefit factor has a large application as well. There are questions about the justification of spending huge sums to keep kidney patients or heart transplant patients alive. Those monies might go for other less serious but more productive treatments for more people. Those who argue the utilitarian position of the greatest good for the greatest number could justify letting the kidney and heart patients die while all that money was used for other needy persons.[19] The need extends, as noted earlier, to the ill-fed, ill-clothed, ill-housed, ill-educated millions of the world. The heart transplant cost of $36,000 (1975) could buy a lot of milk for a lot of children.[20] We also noted this issue in NNICU costs as compared to the neglect of millions of born-well but now deprived children.

How to Allocate?

One solution to the allocation of scarce resources has been a lottery. Scarce resources can be divided by drawing straws or numbers out of a hat. That at least makes for some equality for those in the geographical area. Another solution has been the "first come, first served" idea, which also has some limited equality, assuming all those in need in a geographical area do in fact know about the service. Some suggest allocation on the basis of need. Although health needs are unlimited, there are or may appear to be priorities.[21] Another solution has been consideration of social worth, either potential (prospective—future contribution to society) or past (retrospective—in gratitude for services rendered). One aspect of this is the concept of gift. We give; we receive; we repay. The repayment may be a matter of passing on to others that which we received. Thus, gratitude is seen as a legitimate moral/ethical standard or principle.[22]

Scarce medical resources compared to scarcity of resources in general (food, clothing, shelter) has sometimes been dealt with by what is called lifeboat ethics. The imagery is a lifeboat that can only hold so many. Others are swimming from the shipwreck. They want to climb in the lifeboat. If they do, the boat will sink. Some would say the boat occupants have a right to shoot or beat off the newcomers. Others say let them in and take the chance the boat will sink. Still others say, sink the boat and let no one in in the first place.[23] The latter two have the appeal of some kind of equality although both violate commonsense. The first appeals to self-interest and would presumably have more appeal to those in the boat than those struggling in the water. Those who already have medical resources may find that they aren't too worried about those who don't. They may even justify having these resources because they've earned it or deserve it.[24]

Concept of Social Worth: Generally, ethicists do not like to make moral/ethical decisions based on who has the money or the power or who has been a good person.[25] The concept of social worth may become crucial in dealing with an alcoholic liver that could be replaced by a transplant, except that the available organ for transplanting is also desired by a nonalcoholic patient. The lung cancer victim who has been smoking all his/her life may now require rare treatment that might more justifiably go to a nonsmoker. The aged person in the intensive care unit might be displaced by a younger one who has potential contributions to make to society. On money and power we noted earlier the concern of some that the Hyde Amendment denied abortions to the poor and thus was discriminatory. Do the wealthy and the powerful have the right to treatment that is not available to the poor? The reality of life is that this is what happens, but the concepts of justice embodied in the Bible, the American Declaration of Independence, the various medical codes, and other statements of human rights suggest that such a division of resources is wrong.[26]

Unnecessary Treatment: There's another division of resources, which at first glance appears more an abundance than a scarcity. Several studies have shown that some procedures such as surgery may be provided when they are not strictly necessary. Gall bladder specialists manage to find a higher percentage of gall bladder attacks that require operations in their area than appear in other areas without gall bladder experts. Other specialities find their concerns in a higher ratio where they are. The allocation of scarce resources is a concern here on several counts. It may be that people in other areas who need a particular treatment are not getting it, or are getting the wrong treatment. It is generally agreed as well that unnecessary treatment, especially hospitalization, drives up costs, including insurance rates. Thus, monies are going for iatrogenic problems that might better go for nutrition and sanitation or restoration of the ecology.[27]

ETHICS AND WOMEN

Finally, we come to an ethical concern in adults that covers half the human race. We have been concerned with women on several earlier points. In Chapter Six, we touched on the problem of battered wives as compared with battered children. Occasionally one hears of a battered husband. That too is a wrong by traditional standards of respect for persons. Whether people have a right to love and affection is debated, but it is often seen as a desirable feature in human relationships, a desire rooted in the biblical tradition to "love thy neighbor" as well as the right to live in safety.

In our culture, the battered wife is the much more common occurrence. As with the battered child, the abused wife is often blamed for the situation. "She asked for it" is a not uncommon statement. The rape victim also has too often reported the crime only to be treated as the criminal rather than the victim.

We noted earlier, too, the fact that it is women who get pregnant. Traditionally, it has been men, often celibate men, who have made the rules on conception and birth control. Would the rules have been any different if it had not been so? We do not know. As more women enter the ranks of ethicists and moral theologians, it will be interesting to see what happens.

A side issue has been the responsibility that men have been willing to take or not take for either the prevention of pregnancy or the child that results from their sexual activity. The double standard has at times prevailed. Men sowed their wild oats and women got pregnant, but men demanded virgin brides for marriage. This double standard has been breaking down, according to some studies. It has moved primarily in the direction not of less nonmarital intercourse for men but of greater freedom in sexual activity for women. One force behind this movement has been the technical advances in contraception and abortion. Another has been the women's health movement or liberation movement.[28]

We noted earlier the allocation of scarce resources problem in the availability of contraceptives and abortion. This has been partly geographical, partly economic, partly a withholding by religious groups and individuals. On a different level, infertility tests are costly. Such things as the transplantation of an ovary, test-tube babies, and artificial insemination are all expensive. The suggestion here is that overcoming infertility may be a luxury limited to those who can afford it. Or, one could say these are a misuse of funds that could be used to feed the children we already have. Among related feminine issues we can note the questionable procedures that have sometimes been used in the development and testing of contraceptives and the excessive use of X-rays for infertility tests. The lack of research on menopause, uterine fibroids, and other concerns in women's health has hindered treatment. Excessive numbers of hysterectomies, mastectomies, and other surgeries have been noted.[29]

Women as Patients

In the medical field, many doctors are men. Women patients not uncommonly find themselves in a double bind.[30] The patient seeking help is already in an inferior position. It's a dependency relationship. In the terms of Fritz Perls' Gestalt therapy, the patient is the Under Dog and the doctor is the Top Dog. In terms of Eric Berne's transactional analysis, the doctor has often been Parent (either Critical or Nurturing) and the patient has been Child. It's the old classification of the powerful and the powerless, the rich versus the poor, the established versus the disestablished.

This relationship is, of course, not a necessary one. We have had personal experiences with doctors who treated the patient as an equal. Yet, the person in need of health care may be, often is, usually is, already "down," in need, perhaps depressed, in some sense a supplicant, a "Not OK Child." Health care personnel can reinforce such negative feelings by taking the superior role (Top Dog, Parent), and this happens, in fact, all too often, judging by the literature and personal experience.[31]

The Patients' Rights movement is one response to the allocation of the scarce resource known as equality in relationships.[32] This is discussed fully in Chapter Nine. Here we note the women's movement has a medical and health care component. Culturally, men have been in the position of power and women have been expected to take the subservient role. Faced with male doctors, women are programmed by our society to be good patients, that is, passive, undemanding, cooperative, ignorant, and unable to learn. The good patient and the traditional description of femininity are roughly equal, for both men *and* women health care personnel.

The increasing concern for *informed* consent, respect for persons, the dignity of the individual, the right to self-determination, justice and equality all point to a stronger position for women patients. As noted earlier, the concept of personhood has been grudgingly extended to Blacks and children and now women. Discrimination, battered children, and the expectation that women be good patients are all still with us and will be for the foreseeable future. Liberation movements are steadily pushing to overcome and change past attitudes.

There is a corollary that might be kept in mind. We might call it the ethics of responsibility. The right to informed consent implies that the patient is willing to be informed, willing to learn. On numerous fronts, the women's movement has moved to self-help and to educate through such studies as *Our Bodies, Ourselves.*[33] The educated consumer is truly informed and can more accurately cooperate with the health care team, that is, not just passively be undemanding but genuinely cooperative.[34]

In the larger sense, biothics for women remains to be written. But it will be, if for no other reason than that so many medical issues, from in vitro fertilization to cancer of the breast are specific to women.[35]

Women As Health Care Providers

An ethical concern of some interest, too, is the role of women in the health care professions.[36] Women have been systematically, or by implication, excluded from a number of health care roles. The focus historically has been on the role of physician. From time immemorial there have been female as well as male doctors. The rise of medical schools facilitated the exclusion of women from the occupation. Schools specifically for women were set up. The Flexner report of 1910 eliminated many so-called substandard schools. Numbers of these just happened to be schools for women. It has been suggested that here again we have a parallel with the Black experience. Blacks have on occasion found themselves excluded by standards set up by whites. Ostensibly, of course, the standards were objective.

The situation may have eased somewhat today, under the impact of nondiscrimination laws and the proposed Equal Rights Amendment (ERA) to the Constitution. Yet there remain reports that show major fields such as obstetrics lack significant numbers of women. On the international scene, current history reflects Western history. When the physician's role has been downgraded, the percentage of women has increased. When the physician's role has been upgraded, the percentage of women has gone down. The inclusion or exclusion of women from major fields or roles seems to reflect the evaluation of women in the general society.

This can be noted too within fields that in recent decades or centuries have been primarily female enclaves. Nurses at one time were often criminals and prostitutes, with long hours and low pay. Florence Nightingale (1820–1910) led a nursing reform movement that included a school in 1860, following her monumental efforts during the Crimean War (1854–1857). Her work met opposition from physicians who thought of nurses more as "hewers of wood and drawers of water." The "handmaid of the physician" image of nurses is still with us, although nurses and nursing organizations have sought and are seeking increased responsibilities.[37] A growing ideal that is being realized in at least some settings is the health care team, with nurses and other female members functioning on a collegial basis with the men on the team.

Equality of treatment in the allocation of educational monies and places, the acceptance of persons without prejudice and bias, the whole thrust of the human rights movement, the concept of people as an end in themselves rather than a means to an end, the dignity and worth of the individual and such basic biblical concepts as men and women created in the image of God, the acceptance of women as persons are concepts supporting equality for women and men in the health professions.

THE ISSUES

As noted at the beginning, allocation of scarce resources is the central focus of this chapter. The basic principle here is the just distribution of resources. The concept of just distribution implies some kind of concern for equality or equity, some doctrine of fairness that implies various people have some kind of claim, some right, to just distribution. Although in the practical world, the rich often get richer while the poor have children, it is doubtful if anyone but the rich are satisfied with such a state of affairs. Religion, government, sociology, philosophy, and several other branches of human endeavor raise questions. The Judeo-Christian tradition calls for care of the poor and the helpless. It's a call that may at last be reaching the ears of those powerful enough to do something about it. Bismarck found out a hundred years ago that nation building required healthy people. Today, government has a stake in health, a stake that has appeared in the United States in the form of burgeoning programs.

The care of renal failure was a focus of this chapter. Research money has poured into cancer labs and other efforts to cure and care. Many hospitals have been built with the scarce resource of money. At least some of them are trying to serve those who are ill. Jesus of Nazareth said those who are well need no physician. We are coming to recognize, however, that preventive maintenance can help keep people well, so although those who are well may not need a physician, they do need preventive care.

In all of this, ethics and morality raise the issue of just distribution of scarce resources. People, whether men, women, or children, are seen by some, if not most, ethical systems as an end in themselves, worthy of being treated as persons. In centuries past, personhood has been conferred, mostly on adult males. Today, we are seeing more and more the demand that Blacks, women, children, and others be accepted as persons. The American Indian, the poor, the immigrant, the non-English speaking, the foreigner are stepping forward to be counted as persons. *Person* is being equated with *human*. These persons need health care. They are saying they have a right to it or at least equal access to it as a human right. Time will tell if such a right becomes a reality.

In this concern for the allocation of scarce resources, women are a particular concern. In many cultures, they have been the underdog, getting a short allocation. Yet, they have much to do with the welfare of children and future generations. They are themselves a scarce resource, improperly utilized in terms of their brains and skills, frequently shut out and even battered by the Top Dogs. Equal access is a long way from reality, but it may be the wave of the future.

NURSES CARING FOR ADULTS

There are many situations when nurses provide services for adult clients within the health and illness care systems. These include the care of women during childbearing and men and women choosing some form of contraception, as noted in earlier chapters. It would be impossible to discuss all nursing contacts with adults, so we have been deliberately selective in order to illustrate some common ethical issues in working with adults. Our focus is on the role of nurses working with patients involved in the allocation of scarce medical resources and situations of sexual discrimination for patients and staff, particularly those who are female. The issue of truth telling will also be discussed as it relates to working with adult clients.

Nurses and the Allocation of Scarce Medical Resources

There are two roles for discussion here regarding nurses and the allocation of scarce medical resources. The first is that of nurses who are involved in making decisions about how to allocate scarce resources, and the second role is that of nurses who are providing direct care for those clients who are recipients of the scarce resources. Some of the ethical dilemmas to be addressed are unique to this area of nursing and many are common to all areas of nursing practice but are discussed here.

The Decision Maker

One encounters little or no argument that health and illness needs/wants are endless and that the resources to provide for these are finite. As long as there is a limit to the resources that can be offered by any health program, a decision must be made about the appropriate use of these resources—what is offered and to whom? Some of the ethical components of these decisions have been discussed earlier. Nurses as professionals and as members of a community have many opportunities to become involved in this decision-making process and may find it helpful to understand the kind of ethical issues and/or conflicts that can arise when allocating scarce medical/health resources.

One of the more obvious opportunities for nurses to participate in decisions on how to allocate health monies, personnel, and treatment comes as an integral part of the role of nurse administrator. Whether working in a community agency or large, acute care hospital, nurse administrators participate in deciding what health/illness programs will be offered, which need to be discontinued, and what population of clients will be served by the available resources. Some writers suggest that these kinds of decisions can be made on the basic of economics,[38] that is, cost-benefit; yet others suggest the tremendous difficulties of placing a dollar value on human life, and, especially, health.[39] All might agree that the decisions on allocation of scarce/finite resources are best made not on the basis of the personality and conviction of individual health team members.[40] Yet, many have not spent time and energy learning other ways of making such weighty decisions.

Approaches: There are many variables to consider when nurses are called upon to participate in allocating scarce resources. Aroskar[41] suggests that such considerations in the focus of care as health promotion, community resources available, and personal life-styles exhibited by the population to be served help to define what nursing services are needed and who should get them.

Nurses may also elect an individualistic or aggregate approach to ethical decision making about problems of distributive justice. The individualistic approach focuses on providing care to individuals and families in an episodic, demand-response pattern, characteristic of acute care settings and most community nursing agencies. The aggregate approach considers the health needs of population groups at risk, such as pregnant teen-agers or adults with hypertension.[42] The

definition of health needs of individuals and groups and how these needs are met in a given community will reflect the values of the decision makers as well as the community as a whole to the extent that the larger community has participated in defining needs and priorities for resource allocation.

Example: A specific example of nurses as decision makers can be found in most clinical research units where procedures such as organ transplants are done. Nurses are important members of the team in preparing and caring for patients undergoing transplant procedures, and are respected for their judgment in helping to decide which clients are appropriate recipients.[43] Often a team approach is used to determine the suitability of an individual donor and recipient, as many factors need to be evaluated.[44] Medical suitability is prerequisite, but emotional stability and willingness to work with the health team and treatment regimen are also vital. All have value components because professional judgment is required at each step in the evaluation process. Nurses often have the most direct contact with the prospective clients and can evaluate their expectations of the transplant, willingness to follow a treatment regimen, and important psychosocial variables acting in the client's life at the moment that may determine how the client and family will respond to the transplant procedure and its sequelae.

One of the important benefits of nurses actively participating in decisions on who gets what resources is the sense of responsibility gained and of having one's judgment respected. Clients benefit also when such difficult decisions are shared by all team members and consumers, diminishing the chances of one individual's value bias determining the fate of other people. We also suggest that having the entire staff participate in decisions on who should receive scarce resources (transplants, ICU care) helps to ensure equality of allocation as well as appropriateness. Tinker and others[45] note that nurses who are required to provide intensive care for patients who cannot possibly benefit while others who can benefit are denied such services gradually become very discouraged and apathethic in their care giving, or simply quit. One way to avoid this untenable situation is to include nurses in the decision-making process.

Difficulties: Nurses who respond to the challenge as decision makers in the allocation of scarce resources would do well to recognize some of the difficulties of this role. In the real world, everyone cannot have everything he/she wants or needs. Tradeoffs are the rule. Such tradeoffs are necessary when allocating scarce resources; some people will gain and some will lose, even their life. Questions that are involved in decision making are, can we continue to allocate scarce and costly resources such as heart transplants to persons who may not live longer than a few weeks and, at the same time, make feeble efforts to prevent malnutrition in the well-born children in our rural and inner city clums? Are we capable of allocating resources fairly, with just distribution?[46] What or who gives us the power to make such decisions over life and death? Wouldn't it be simpler if nurses refused to participate in such decisions so that they would not have to face such agony? These questions reflect some of the reality of allocating health and illness resources, and we encourage nurses' efforts and willingness to participate in such decisions.

The Care Givers

Nurses who work with dialysis and transplant patients and in intensive care units are a special breed of professional care giver. A sensitive, caring, highly skilled person, willing to work with the challenge of life and death daily, characterizes many. Levine notes that nurses are often the principal care givers of dialysis patients. Some authors speak of the high levels of stress encountered, with resultant high turnover of staff working in such specialized units,[47] but this is not true of all nurses in all units.

The Investment: Some nurses, who seem to thrive in the midst of caring for patients who are recipients of scarce medical resources, exhibit a sense of professional and personal maturity—a keen sense of self-awareness. They invest a lot of themselves in the care of their patients, often treating them as "family." These nurses are willing to laugh when their patients laugh, and cry when they cry. They describe their major role as helping others to find greater meaning in life and a sense of increased self-dignity. The nurses' rewards include a greater sense of satisfaction and feelings of self-worth.[48]

When nurses establish long-term relationships with patients who are on dialysis or the recipients of organ transplants, many ethical problems arise and need to be considered. One of these arises from the great emotional investment that nurses put into their relationship with these patients. The results of this investment may be illustrated by De-Nour's and Czaczkes' study of the reactions of the medical team to chronic dialysis patients.[49] Nurses were found to be possessive and overprotective towards the patients, and exhibited signs of withdrawal from the patient if the patient refused treatment or seemed not to be responding well. One might question whether nurses can provide needed supportive care if they refuse to let other team members know of progress and constantly "do for" the patient rather than encourage independence in care.

In situations where patients are receiving dialysis or an organ transplant, nurses would do well to balance their supportive care-giving with the goal of promoting increased independence and greater patient control over his treatment and his life.[50] Working as a "family" carries all the risks of families in the normal sense, ranging from supportive to destructive relationships. A nurturing surrogate-mother-nurse role can be helpful to the fearful patient-child. But as treatment progresses and fear of failure is reduced, the patient needs to progress to adult responsibility—caring for himself. Nurses who can progress to adult-adult relationships with patients in such situations are probably most beneficial in their care giving, even if this progression is difficult to accomplish with people who have chronic, debilitating, progressive disease conditions. Yet, we must ask if we are practicing in a truly ethical manner if we foster dependence unnecessarily in dialysis or transplant patients.

The Questions: Nurses who care for patients receiving organ transplants will probably have examined their own views and values relative to the use of human organs in such fashion. It is tempting to suggest that those who cannot support organ transplant procedures would choose to work in other areas of nursing. Probably closer to reality is the situation where nurses can accept transplants in some situations and for some patients, but not in others. What is the nurse to do with the anger engendered by a transplant recipient who destroys the organ by not following the specified regimen, especially when the nurse predicted this might happen? This would seem to be justifiable anger in view of the scarcity of organs available for transplant and the intense preparation of the patient that preceded the transplant procedure. Or how does the nurse respond to the dialysis patient who decides to discontinue treatment, choosing death over lifetime dependence on a machine? The nurse's value of sanctity or quality of life, including attitudes toward a machine-dependent life, will often dictate how he/she will respond to the patient in such a situation. The Interpretive Statements of the Code for Nurses suggests the responsibility of supporting the client's right to self-determination,[51] but how is this done if a nurse does not believe in suicide for whatever reason?

One means of dealing with these emotion-laden reactions is the use of weekly team conferences. Here staff are free to share their feelings and attitudes and are supported as they search for answers to their internal dilemmas. Alternatives for action and responses toward patients can also be shared and discussed. A supportive administrative environment where all staff can share their innermost feelings without fear of reprisal can go far in reducing high turnover rates[52] in such units, as well as helping all team members work toward a more ethical mode of practicing their professions.

Summary

These are just a few of the dilemmas posed for nurses working with patients who are recipients of scarce medical resources. Others include how one reacts when the resources are given to an "undeserving" person, when the resources are not allocated as an individ-

ual thinks best, or when it is time to stop the use of resources for a given patient so that another may benefit. Chapter Eight will include further discussion of that situation, and the case studies in this chapter will offer some of these problems for further analysis and thought.

SEXUAL DISCRIMINATION

Women as Patients

Women as patients have been the recipients of many acts of discrimination at the hands of health and medical workers. Earlier we discussed the characteristics of the "good" patient as being equated with traditional feminine behaviors—obedient, dependent, easily influenced, and emotional.[53] That doctors and nurses expect this type of behavior from patients, especially female patients, is untenable but too often true. We suggest that it is not in the best interests of any patient (hence unethical) to promote dependent, indiscriminatingly compliant responses to caregivers. Nurses may wish to consider the potential detrimental effects of their "maternal caring" that can promote an extension of illness instead of promoting wellness in their clients.[54]

Nurses often witness other acts of sexual discrimination toward women who are patients in the health care system. Nurses' unwillingness to speak out on behalf of women and their rights to informed self-determination often lends tacit approval of such procedures as unnecessary mastectomies and/or hysterectomies. The fact that the majority of nurses are women on whom these unnecessary procedures may someday be performed does not appear to give some nurses the strength to overcome their "allegiance" to the doctor-nurse relationship in favor of the nurse-patient relationship based on truth telling, trust, and informed decision making.

Caring: Another example of a potential impact nurses can have on diminishing discriminatory acts against women involves situations of abuse—wife battering and rape, for example. Often abused women are treated as the offenders and not the victims of abuse by health team members in emergency rooms.

Nurses concerned about this unfair treatment of women, in keeping with the Code for Nurses statement on responsibility to care for patients regardless of the nature of the health problem,[55] have organized crisis centers and manned telephones to counsel such victims. Some nurses have also recognized the need for a supportive, female caregiver as the first contact with a rape victim, and have elected to work with such patients. Nurses generally develop advanced skills in listening and counseling during their educational process, and they can be very supportive of women who are battered or raped. These nurses, however, need to be aware of their own feelings and fears of being abused before they can offer counseling in a comfortable, nonjudgmental manner. Otherwise, one can ward off her own anxiety and feelings of helplessness by denying the patient's story and blaming her for the abuse.[56]

Educating: Possibly one of the most important roles of the nurse as a professional is that of educator. Nurses' willingness to teach others about their bodies and how to care for them is central to fulfilling their responsibility to encourage self-determination in others based on sound information. Sound information about health and illness and care is best given by the health team. Without this health education process, no patient will ever be able to exercise his/her right to self-determination, and the "mystique of the profession" will be perpetuated to the detriment of consumers. Nurses often have led the health team in teaching others to care for themselves, possibly because of their educational focus on the promotion of health rather than the medical model of curing disease. This need for health education is particularly evident for women who are often placed in an inferior position in the medical establishment by virtue of their sexual identity. Nurses can promote women's rights to self-determination by offering information about health, illness, and medical and nursing care that allows the client to decide what care is indicated and whether the care being given is appropriate to the needs defined. The principle of equality suggests sound health education for all clients. This implies equal treatment of women and men, with no discrimination against males in the system simply because that discrimination has been practiced against females. Rabbi Hillel's form of the Golden Rule is "Do not do unto others that which is hateful to thyself."

Women As Care Givers

Much has been written about the status of women as caregivers in health and illness systems. Our particular interest here is the fact that the majority of nurses are women, as contrasted with the majority of physicians who are men. The ethical dimensions of this professional reality are related to the extent to which nurses assume or are allowed to assume responsibility for management of patient care, decision making, and adherence to the Code for Nurses rather than to the unwritten allegiance to the subservient "handmaiden of the physician" role.

Suffice it to say that as nurses are more and more willing to place optimal care of the patient at the center of their practice and accept responsibility for ensuring that all health team members practice in an ethical manner, the recipients of care will benefit. Wouldn't it be a delightful situation if nurses no longer needed to practice "deceptive decision making?" These are the type of decisions that are made when the experienced nurse decides what is best for the patient (generally based on sound knowledge and judgment) but cannot convince the physician of the soundness of her decision. She then proceeds to find a physician who will listen to her, or simply goes ahead with the plan against the physician's orders. This is a dangerous game to be played when patients' lives are at stake, and one would hope that the combination of nurses openly expressing their willingness to be active decision makers and mutual respect for all members of the team, no matter what profession or sex, will lead to better patient care for all people.

Female nurses have much opposition to overcome in establishing themselves as colleagues in the health care system, as do male nurses, though for other reasons. And much of this opposition comes from other nurses, who, for whatever reasons, thrive on being low person on the totem pole.[57] The nurse-practitioner movement has legitimized decision making on the part of nurses, as have nurses who have been willing to openly participate in difficult ethical decisions (allocation of scarce resources, for example). The struggle continues, however, as evidenced in a recent Michigan court decision, which stated that nurses were not permitted to exercise judgment in the diagnosis or treatment of symptoms. Her duty was to report them to the physician.[58]

Many nursing roles are ambiguous and often overlap traditional medical practice, but unless nurses are willing to use their intelligence and knowledge to make decisions on health care and treatment, how can they practice in an ethical manner? Nurses must take the time to educate colleagues, physicians, and clients to their new roles and responsibilities. We suggest that all people will benefit from the nurse's exercise of responsible decision making.

CASE STUDIES

The following cases are presented for your analysis and discussion. We suggest that you apply the *Guidelines for Identifying and Analyzing Ethical Dilemmas in Nursing Practice* as well as consider the questions posed at the end of each situation.

=Case #21

Dialysis

B. T. is the nurse assigned to work in the dialysis unit of a local hospital. T. N., a twenty-nine-year-old man, arrives for his biweekly treatment and, as they both are preparing to begin the dialysis, T. N. remarks that he really is tired of this whole process and is trying to decide whether to continue dialysis. He adds, "I'm beginning to think I would rather die than have to depend on this machine forever. You know I am going to die soon, anyway. Why prolong the inevitable?" B. T. responds "What you are saying is really distressing to hear. We have spent all this time caring for you and making sure you get the right treatments, and you're just going to give up? You're too young to think about dying. Think about it."

Questions
1. Was the nurse being ethical in her response to the patient? Share the rationale for your decision.
2. What value do you think the nurse places on using dialysis to prolong or maintain life?
3. What other values are represented in the nurse's statements?
4. What values is T. N. sharing with the nurse?
5. How would you have responded to the statement made by T. N.?
6. How do you think B. T. would have responded if the patient were fifty-eight years old?

=Case #22

Transplant

D. R. is a thirty-five-year-old man who received a kidney transplant at his request two months ago. The postoperative course was uneventful, and D. R. was discharged home with full instructions about diet and rest. He missed two return appointments before arriving this morning in acute distress. When questioned by the nurse as to where he had been and why he did not return before now, D. R. responded that he was so glad to not have to be on dialysis and tied to a machine that he took off on a vacation. His current condition was evaluated, and it appeared that the kidney was destroyed by the eating and drinking binge D. R. engaged in while on his "vacation" from treatment. The nurse finds herself very angry at this behavior, and tells D. R. that she is not sure she can continue caring for him if he is not going to take care of himself.

Questions

1. Do you think the nurse responded to this situation in an ethical manner?
2. How would you have responded, knowing that the transplant was deliberately destroyed by D. R.'s behavior?
3. Are there any care giving situations where it is appropriate to threaten the patient with loss of care?

Case #23

Women As Patients

A. S. has worked as the charge nurse on a large gynecological unit of a hospital for the past four years. During the course of obtaining the admission history on D. U., a thirty-five-year-old married woman, she notes that the patient is admitted for a hysterectomy. When asked the reasons for this surgery, D. U. responds that she didn't want any more children and wanted the uterus taken out. She added that her mother had died from uterine cancer, and she decided "this was a good way not to have to worry about cancer.

A. S. discussed this case with the patient's physician to determine if there was some pathological condition necessitating hysterectomy. The physician confirmed that he was removing the uterus at the request of the patient. He added, "Why not? She doesn't need it any more and she'll be less anxious about cancer if the uterus is removed." A. S. expressed concern that the patient did not understand the risks of such a decision, and wondered if the surgery was really necessary.

Questions

1. Did A. S. have a legitimate concern for unnecessary surgery?
2. Comment on her course of action and results of same.
3. What value conflicts are evident?
4. What would you have done in this situation? State your reasons.
5. Define the values operant in your choice of actions.
6. Do you think a physician would agree to remove the testes if a man requested it for fear of cancer and at the conclusion of his procreation activities? Discuss the values operating in this situation.

Sexual Identity and Care Giving

K. W. is a nurse in the maternity unit of a large municipal hospital. As he begins morning rounds on postpartum, he enters the room of S. H., a twenty-three-year-old para 1001 who delivered her first child six hours ago. As K. W. explains what he proposes to do during the postpartum examination, S. H. says, "You're not going to examine me. I want a nurse." K. W. explains that he is the nurse assigned to the unit today and it is important that all new mothers are examined to make sure everything is progressing normally. S. H. says, "You will not examine me! Get out of here!" K. W. is the only nurse assigned to this unit, and he leaves the room wondering how he can continue to provide good care for S. H. when she refuses to let him examine her uterus and perineum.

Questions
1. What kind of ethical issues are raised in this situation?
2. What options for care are available to S. H.?
3. What would you do if you were the male nurse in this situation?
4. What are your personal attitudes/feelings about male nurses examining female patients, and female nurses examining male patients?

Distributive Justice

J. B. is the director of a community health nursing agency in a small midwestern county. Today she is attending a meeting of the county Board of Supervisors to discuss the budget for health programs for the next fiscal year. J. B. has come prepared to support her request for initiating a primary care clinic for adults, to be staffed by nurse-practitioners. Her supporting data includes an increase in the adult population in the community with a concomitant decrease in the number of family physicians. The social worker from the health department has also come prepared to substantiate his request for provision of counseling services for drug addicts. The Board of Supervisors reminds each participant that there is a ceiling on funds available for new programs, and new programs can only be initiated if one is willing to give up some portion of the existing health programs. J. B. responds that there are many more adults in need of health supervision than there are drug addicts in need of care, and that the healthy adults deserve more attention and money to keep them healthy.

Questions for Discussion
1. What values are evident in the discussion, and whose are they?
2. What ethical issue(s) are present in this case?
3. What further information would you like to have before making a decision on how limited funds should be allocated?

NOTES AND REFERENCES

1. Albert R. Jonsen, "Health Care: Right to Health-Care Services," *Encyclopedia of Bioethics* **2:**623–630. The Encyclopedia is cited hereafter as *EB*. Health care personnel are themselves a scarce resource in many areas. This is obvious for undeveloped countries but is also true in developed areas. Sweden has been trying for more than thirty years but has never been able to produce enough medical personnel. Daniel Juda, "An Interview with Bror Rexed: Planning for Scarcity in Sweden," *The Hastings Center Report*, no. 3 (June 1977), **7:**5–7. The Report is cited hereafter as *HCR*. In the United States, there are understaffed geographical areas as well as areas of need. Mila A. Aroskar points out that the vast majority of nurses practice in hospitals and nursing homes, but the majority of patients are elsewhere in private homes, schools, work, clinics, doctors' offices, and so on. "Ethical Dilemmas and Community Health Nursing," *The Linacre Quarterly*, no. 4 (Nov. 1977), **44:**340–346, and, "Ethical Issues in Community Health Nursing," *Nursing Clinics of North America*, no. 1 (Mar. 1979), **14:**35–44. Edmund D. Pellegrino, "Medical Morality and Medical Economics," *HCR*, no. 4 (Aug. 1978), **8:**8–11.

2. Proponents of a right to health see it as a natural right. Others say it is nonsense to talk of such a thing. Health is a gift of God or nature. Frank DeGraeve, "Health and Disease: Religious Concepts," *EB* **2:**585–590. Others speak of the obligation we have to our own health. Ruth Macklin, "Moral Concerns and Appeals to Rights and Duties," *HCR*, no. 5 (Oct. 1976), **6:**31–38. Samuel Gorovitz, "Health as an Obligation," *EB* **2:**606–610. Bernard Häring, *Medical Ethics* (Notre Dame: Fides Publishers, 1973), pp. 66–73. This is an issue also in medical care when the patient has "brought it on himself."

The "right to health care" is approved in the "Interpretive Statements" of the ANA *Code for Nurses*, 1976. See *EB* **4:**1699. This is a moral, general, or conditional right, according to some. It arises from personal autonomy, prior to special relationships such as that of nurse-patient or doctor-patient, but it is conditional on availability. Jonsen, op. cit., p. 629. Robert M. Veatch, *Case Studies in Medical Ethics* (Cambridge, Mass.: Harvard University Press, 1977), pp. 89–90. Charles Fried says the right to health care does not mean the best care or equality. We can't afford the best and our system is full of inequalities such as food and housing. "An Analysis of 'Equality' and 'Rights' in Medical Care," pp. 452–464, in *Ethical Issues in Modern Medicine*, ed. by Robert Hunt and John Arras (Palo Alto, Calif.: Mayfield Publishing Co., 1977). Garvan F. Kuskey says there is no right to health care. People in need can seek help, but need does not create a right. "Health Care, Human Rights, and Government Intervention," pp. 465–471, in Hunt and Arras, op. cit. On the other hand, Jesus of Nazareth interprets the biblical command to "love thy neighbor" in the story of the Good Samaritan. The Samaritan responded to someone in need. It may not be a "right," but our "Good Samaritan" laws recognize the need. Leon Kass, "Regarding the End of Medicine and the Pursuit of Health," pp. 99–108, 371–378, in *Contemporary Issues in Bioethics*, ed. by Tom L. Beauchamp and LeRoy Walters (Encino, Calif.: Dickenson Publishing Co., Inc., 1978). Edward V. Sparer, "The Legal Right to Health Care: Public Policy and Equal Access," *HCR*, no. 5 (Oct. 1976), **6:**39–47.

"Right" has various meanings. Veatch, op. cit., pp. 100–101, suggests that in ethics, it is a morally justified claim on others doing for us, rather than a duty, which is something we do. As such, it is on the level of a rule or moral, as compared to the more abstract principles of ethics as we have noted earlier. Another way to put it is that a right to health care means health care providers are obligated to give care.

One thing people seem to agree on is that health does not equal health care. Paul Starr, "The Politics of Therapeutic Nihilism," *HCR*, no. 5 (Oct. 1976), **6:**24–30. Ivan Illich, *Medical Nemesis* (New York: Pantheon Books, Inc., 1976). Carol Levine, "Ethics, Justice, and International Health," *HCR*, No. 2 (Apr. 1977), **7:**5–7. Anne J. Davis and Mila A. Aroskar, *Ethical Dilemmas and Nursing Practice* (New York: Appleton-Century-Crofts, 1978), pp. 184, 193. There is, of course, an interaction and both involve the allocation of scarce resources.

3. Beauchamp and Walters, op. cit., p.

347. One way to look at this is the idea of equal *access* to health care. Some call such equal access absolutely essential, but others see it as nonsense, even an artificial creation that ignores individual choice of life-styles. Carol Levine, "Ethics and Health Care Containment," *HCR*, no. 1 (Feb. 1979), **9**:10–13. Pellegrino, op. cit., p. 8. Starr, op. cit. Illich, op. cit. Nancy Milio, "Ethics and the Economics of Community Health Services: The Case of Screening," *The Linacre Quarterly*, no. 4 (Oct. 1977), **44**:347–360.

4. Some medical procedures are quite new. Renal dialysis has been around only since the early 1940s. Kidney transplants have been with us since 1951 and heart transplants since 1967. Other concerns here are older. The cleanliness of midwives lessened the incidence of puerperal sepsis, compared to doctors a few centuries ago. Nutrition is still debated in some quarters. Natural food proponents point to growing evidence of harm from additives. The basic principles of just distribution, equitable treatment, health care delivery, and the allocation of scarce resources have been around for some time. Veatch, op. cit., pp. 221–222. Starr, op. cit., p. 26. Renée C. Fox and Judith P. Swazey, "Kidney Dialysis and Transplantation," *EB* **2**:811–816. Carol C. Nadelson and Malkah T. Notman, "Women and Biomedicine: Women as Health Professionals," *EB* **4**:1713–1720. Louise Juliani and Bonita Reamer, "Kidney Transplant: Your Role in Aftercare," *Nursing*, no. 7 (1977), **77**:46–53.

5. Some studies suggest health is more closely related to living standards, education, and income, than to health care. Evelyn M. Kitagawa and Philip M. Hauser, *Differential Mortality: A Study in Socioeconomic Epidemiology* (Cambridge, Mass.: Harvard University Press, 1973). Starr, op. cit., pp. 27–28. Illich, op. cit. We've noted this type of thing before, for example, with birth control. The state of Kerala in India raised the living standard and the birthrate went down. This is notable in the United States. Among all religious and nonreligious groups, as socioeconomic level rises, the birthrate goes down.

6. Fox and Swazey, op. cit., p. 812, note that these procedures continue to have experimental overtones with the ethical requirements of research. Hunt and Arras, op. cit., p.

403. Paul Ramsey, *The Patient as Person* (New Haven: Yale University Press, 1970), pp. 211–212, 240–241. Levine, "Ethics and Health . . ," op. cit., p. 12. Benjamin Freedman, "The Case for Medical Care, Inefficient or Not," *HCR*, no. 2 (Apr. 1977), **7**:31–39, and, "Efficient Allocation: Mystique and Myth," *Health Values: Achieving High-Level Wellness*, no. 1 (Jan./Feb. 1978), **2**:7–15. Carol Levine, "Home Dialysis and the Medicare Gap," *HCR*, no. 6 (Dec. 1976), **6**:5–6, and, "Dialysis or Transplant: Values and Choices," *HCR*, no. 2 (Apr. 1978), **8**:8–10. In 1979, the End Stage Renal Disease (ESRD) program cost the federal government $1 billion in medical bills and unknown amounts in disability and other costs. Dialysis cost per patient was about $28,000. Since passage of the ESRD program in 1972, patient population has shifted from younger, working people to older persons, some with terminal cancer and heart disease, and some senile patients delivered three times a week to the dialysis centers from their nursing homes. Gina Bari Kolata; "Dialysis After Nearly a Decade," *Science*, no. 4443 (2 May 1980), **208**:473–474, 476.

7. Estimates range from one to ten treatable out of fifty cases. Each year, about 50,000 people die from kidney failure. Over 23,000 people were on dialysis in 1976. By 1980, it was 48,000. Veatch, op. cit., p. 236. Davis and Aroskar, op. cit., p. 192. Kolata, op. cit., p. 473.

8. In March, 1977, it was reported that about 100 people now hold the title of kidney transplant coordinator. Lowered speed limits have meant fewer accidents and fewer available kidneys, making this project more difficult. More than 10,000 people want kidneys and the number is growing. "Shortage of Kidneys Creates New Occupation: Transplant Coordinator," *HCR*, no. 2 (Apr. 1977), **7**:2. Juliani and Reamer, op. cit., p. 46. In April 1978, it was reported that only 3,000 transplants are done a year, for lack of cadaver kidneys. Only 5 percent of the patients can get a matching kidney from a willing family donor. Levine, "Dialysis," op. cit., p. 10.

9. Richard A. McCormick, "Organ Transplantation: Ethical Principles," *EB* **3**:1169–1173. The use of cadaver organs violates ancient taboos against mutilating dead bodies. Part of the background here is the idea that in the resurrection of the dead, we

will be brought back to life. If we are going to be resurrected, most of us would prefer to be in one piece. The primitive concept has now been largely spiritualized. More ancient taboos turn on fear of the dead, fear that the spirits of the dead will retaliate for lack of respect for their bodies and simple respect for that which was once alive. In the biblical tradition, desecration of the body was a sacrilege (Amos 2:1). In traditional Christianity, this concern worked against autopsies and the use of cadavers for medical studies. The first public dissection in Montpelier in 1375 was declared obscene. In 200 years, dissections were part of carnival programs. But mutilation remains problematic. Mutilation of live patients is acceptable if it is to save the whole body or for replaceable aspects as in skin grafts. The basic principle is totality, discussed later, and the impairment of the primary function of the organ or tissue. Edwin F. Healy, *Medical Ethics* (Chicago: Loyola University Press, 1956), pp. 121–123, 142–143. Lloyd Bailey, "Death in Biblical Thought," *EB* 1:242–246. William May, "Attitudes Toward the Newly Dead," pp. 139–149, and, Ivan Illich, "The Political Uses of Natural Death," pp. 25–42, in *Death Inside Out*, ed. by Peter Steinfels and Robert M. Veatch (New York: Harper & Row, Publishers, 1975). In Judaism, the law against mutilation can be suspended in order to save a life ("Pikuach Nefesh"). Mutilation of a corpse has had a mixed reception. The dead body should not be violated. There has been some greater latitude for scientific study and autopsies. Today's attitudes are split pro and con. Immanuel Jakobovits, *Jewish Medical Ethics* (New York: Philosophical Library, 1959), pp. 49–52, 132–152. Fred Rosner, *Modern Medicine and Jewish Law* (New York: Yeshiva University, 1972), pp. 132–154 (autopsy), 155–176 (transplant).

In England and France (Caillavet Law, 1976), cadaver organs can be removed for therapeutic or scientific purposes without consent unless the deceased has made his refusal known during his lifetime. "The French Solution: Removing Cadaver Organs Without Family's Permission," *HCR*, no. 3 (June 1977), **7**:2–3. In the United States, consent is still required. After death, this is, of course, from the next of kin. The Uniform Gift Act (1968) is a way in which persons can plan before death to donate their organs after death. Jess Dukeminier, "Organ Donation: Legal Aspects," *EB* **3**:1157–1160. "Uniform Anatomical Gift Act," *Uniform Laws Annotated* **8**, *Estate, Probate and Related Laws* (St. Paul: West Publishing Co., 1972), pp. 15–44. Approved by the National Conference of Commissioners on Uniform State Laws and the American Bar Association in August 1968. Dukeminier notes that the Act has had little effect on the shortage of organs. Ramsey, op. cit., pp. 196–215. Advisory Commission to the Renal Transplant Registry, "The 12th Report of the Human Renal Transplant Registry," *The Journal of the American Medical Association* (1975), **233**:787–796. Cadaver graft survival is about 35 percent to 40 percent, and family graft survival is about 50 percent to 60 percent.

A special problem in using cadaver organs is the newly dead. The pronouncement of death for purposes of organ removal has been heavily debated. It overlaps into the legal realm, as well as the philosophical concepts of death.

10. Andrew L. Jameton, "Organ Donation: Ethical Issues," *EB* **3**:1153–1157. Ramsey, op. cit., p. 196. Carol Levine, "Another Choice: The Gift of Life," *HCR*, no. 2 (Apr. 1978), **8**:9. In Australia, only 2 percent of transplants are from living, related donors. In Europe, it is 15 percent. In the United States, it is 33 percent.

11. Jameton, op. cit., p. 1154. Veatch, op. cit., pp. 222–227. Ramsey, op. cit., pp. 171–172. William J. Curran, "A Problem of Consent: Kidney Transplantation in Minors," *New York Law Review* (May 59), **34**:891–989. "The French Solution . . ," op. cit., p. 3, allows adults to donate organs if consent is freely given. Minors are allowed to donate only to a sibling and then only with the approval of a three person committee of experts. If the minor can be consulted and refuses, his/her decision is to be respected.

12. Mary Anne Warren, Daniel Maguire, and Carol Levine, "Can the Fetus be an Organ Farm?," *HCR*, no. 5 (Oct. 1978), **8**:23–25. Nick Fotion, Howard Brody, R. D. Guttman, Virginia McFarland Feldman, "The Fetus as Organ Farm," *HCR*, no. 3 (June 1979), **9**:4. Maguire calls his objection the horror of the new. Levine suggests both the fetus and the mother are being used as means to an end. The proposed plan thus violates the

moral/ethical principle that human beings are ends in themselves. She suggests that creating life in order to destroy it is a perversion of both planned conception and planned abortion.

13. It does happen, of course. Three out of 287 donors in 1974 at the University of Minnesota developed the same disease. Levine, "Another Choice . . ," op. cit. See Ramsey, op. cit., pp. 173–174. "Ethics for the Use of Live Donors in Kidney Transplantation," Annotations, *American Heart Journal* (May 1968), **75:**711–714. A question of informed consent might also be raised about "Death Row" prisoners who wish to be executed in a way that allows organ donation. Apart from problems of capital punishment, reviewers were concerned that Death Row might become an organ farm. Hugo A. Bedau and Michael Zeik, "A Condemned Man's Last Wish: Organ Donation and a 'meaningful' Death," *HCR*, no. 1 (Feb. 1979), **9:**16–17.

14. Jameton, op. cit., p. 1156, notes that the marketing of kidneys has not yet been accepted. Blood is sold in this country, but in England it is all voluntary. In France, hospitals can be reimbursed for expenses, but there are no sales of organs. "The French Solution . . ," op. cit., p. 3. Dukeminier, op. cit., pp. 1158–1159. Veatch, op. cit., p. 112. Ramsey, op. cit., pp. 211–215, 272. There are seventeen organs plus a number of tissues that are of potential transplant use. Artificial spare parts is a $700 million a year business and growing rapidly. These include pacemakers, plastic hips, heart valves, and so on. "Human Spare Parts: 'The Bionic Man' Meets 'The Price is Right,' " *HCR*, no. 4 (Aug. 1978), **8:**2–3. Steven Solomon, "Human Spare Parts," *Forbes Magazine* (29 May 1978), pp. 52–54. Bruce Hilton, "The Ambiguities of Medical Ethics," *Physician's World* (Apr. 1973), pp. 18–19.

15. Sister Patricia Knopp, "Organ Transplants are Immoral," *U.S. Catholic* (Jan. 1977), **42:**12–16. Life extensions for kidneys may be as long as twenty years or less than a dozen, whereas heart transplants are quite limited in life extension. Ramsey, op. cit., pp. 230–238. Juliani and Reamer, op. cit., p. 52.

16. Fox and Swazey, op. cit., pp. 813–814. Veatch, op. cit., pp. 230–233. Levine, "Dialysis. . ," op. cit., p. 8. Shana Alexander, "They Decide Who Lives, Who Dies," *Life* (9 Nov. 1962), **53:**102–128, reprinted, Hunt and Arras, op. cit., pp. 209–424.

17. One view is that we are only stewards, not the owners of our bodies. Susan T. Nicholson, "Abortion and the Roman Catholic Church," *JRE Studies in Religious Ethics*, **2:**84. Häring, op. cit., pp. 66–73. Even if a donor has a right to donate, health care personnel may not necesarily have to participate. Paul Ramsey, *Ethics at the Edges of Life* (New Haven: Yale University Press, 1978), p. 147. Gerald J. Gruman traces the stewardship concept back to Mercantilist economic theory (1498–1714), rather than to the Bible and the idea we are stewards of our bodies, the temple of God (I Corinthians 3:16). "Death and Dying: Euthanasia and Sustaining Life I. Historical Perspectives," *EB* **1:**261–268.

18. Healy, op. cit., pp. 139–142. McCormick, op. cit., pp. 1170–1172. Note that the tradition *primum non nocere*, "do no harm," is suspended with live donors. Jameton, op. cit., p. 1154. Ramsey, *The Patient . . ,* op. cit., pp. 165–197. Nicholson, op. cit., p. 42. The death rate on dialysis is 5 percent the first year, and 10 percent for transplants. The costs to recipients may include many negative physical and psychological side effects. The ancient taboos against mutilation are also part of this concern. Levine, "Dialysis . . ," p. 8. Cost to the donor may be unemployment for several months, heavy medical expenses, social upsets, and physical debilitation for some time. Levine "Another Choice . . ," op. cit., p. 9. In "Man and Transplant," *HCR*, no. 5 (Oct. 1976), a two-year transplant patient's wife (name withheld) makes a passionate appeal for advance information and adjustment help. Medical personnel must start realizing they are dealing with live people, not products on an assembly line (compare ANA Code, Item 1 on the dignity of patients). She suggests it might be kinder to let some chronically ill patients die.

19. Jeffrey Blustein points out that policy decisions on the allocation of scarce resources kills people. It might be more gentle to say these decisions let some people die, but it amounts to the same thing. With unlimited needs, each and all decisions will be life-and-death decisions. "Allocation of Scarce Life-Saving Resources and the Right Not to Be

Killed," pp. 285–289, in *Bioethics and Human Rights*, ed. by Elsie L. Bandman and Bertram Bandman (Boston: Little, Brown and Company, 1978). Ramsey, *Ethics.* . , op. cit., pp. 148–153; *The Patient* . . , op. cit., pp. 240, 268. He sees these larger issues of medical and social priorities as almost beyond reasonable decision. On how to decide who lives and dies, much more can be said.

20. Cost may run more than $160,000 per case. This becomes more excruciating when the difference between survival with or without a transplant is only a matter of days. Harmon L. Smith, "Heart Transplantation," *EB* **2**:654–660. Ramsey, *The Patient.* . , op. cit., pp. 230–231. An artificial heart is being developed. Estimated total costs are $1 billion for the up to 50,000 candidates. Albert R. Jonsen, "The Totally Implantable Artificial Heart," pp. 425–430, in *Bioethics*, ed. by Thomas A. Shannon (New York: Paulist Press, 1976). Kidney dialysis ranges from $7,000 at home to $24,000 in a center to $30,000 in a hospital. In 1976, costs were $450 million. In 1979 they reached $1 billion a year. A transplant is from $25 to $35,000 plus $3,000 to $5,000 in maintenance a year. Veatch, op. cit., pp. 236–237. Kass, op. cit., pp. 510–511. Davis and Aroskar, op. cit., p. 192. Ramsey, *The Patient.* . , op. cit., pp. 240–243. Juliani and Reamer, op. cit., p. 52. Levine, "Dialysis. . ," op. cit., p. 10. Kalata, op. cit., p. 473. We have noted cost-benefit concerns earlier. These figures can be compared to institutionalization for mental patients, for example.

21. Jan Wojcik, *Muted Consent* (West Lafayette, Ind.: Purdue University, 1978), p. 118. Gene Outka, "Social Justice and Equal Access to Health Care," pp. 352–363, in Beauchamp and Walters, op. cit. Pellegrino, op. cit., pp. 8–10. Priorities cut many ways. Pellegrino notes that billions could be saved if we eliminated smoking, alcohol, poor diets, poor driving, and dangerous working conditions.

22. James F. Childress, 'Rationing of Medical Treatment," *EB* **4**:1414–1419. Dr. Donald G. Jones, personal communication, June 1979. Beauchamp and Walters, op. cit., p. 350. Renée C. Fox, "Organ Transplantation: Sociocultural Aspects," *EB* **4**:1160–1164. Fox and Swazey, op. cit., pp. 812–813. The retrospective concern is as old as Aristotle who spoke of "just desserts." The Bible speaks of

harvesting what we plant (Galatians 6:7), but it also talks about grace or undeserved kindness (Gal. 1:15). Richard Titmuss, *The Gift Relationship* (New York: Pantheon Books, Inc., 1970). Nicholas Rescher makes a utilitarian appeal for future services. Society has a right to a return on its investment. But he counts past services on the basis of equity. "The Allocation of Exotic Medical Lifesaving Therapy," pp. 425–443, in Hunt and Arras, op. cit. Ramsey, *The Patient.* . , op. cit., pp. 252–259, favors a lottery. He is against allocating scarce resources on the basis of social worth. The judge favored a lottery in the famous *United States* v. *Holmes* case. An overloaded lifeboat could not survive so fourteen men were thrown overboard. Holmes was convicted of manslaughter. It is not clear how he could have set up a lottery in high seas and a sinking boat.

23. George R. Lucas, Jr., and Thomas W. Ogletree, eds., *Lifeboat Ethics* (New York: Harper & Row, Publishers, 1976). Garrett Hardin, "Living on a Lifeboat," *Bioscience* (1974), **24**:561–568. Hardin, *The Limits of Altruism: An Ecologist's View of Survival* (Bloomington, Ind.: Indiana University Press, 1977). Peter Singer, "Survival and Self-Interest: Hardin's Case Against Altruism," *HCR*, no. 1 (Feb. 1978), **8**:37–39.

The "all saved or none saved" is suggested by Edmond Cahn, *The Moral Decision* (Bloomington: Indiana University Press, 1955), pp. 61–71. An English court ruled in this way in 1884. See Ramsey, *The Patient.* . ., op. cit., pp. 259–266.

24. A related concept is that of triage, which we noted earlier in neonatology. Those who are going to die anyway get nothing. Those who are going to live anyway get nothing, or they get a minimum so they can function to help the middle group, those who will live *if* they get help. Beauchamp and Walters, op. cit., p. 350. Ramsey, *The Patient.* . , op. cit., pp. 273–275.

25. The right to medical care implies that no one should lack medical care for lack of money. Jonsen, op. cit., p. 627. It would, of course, be naive to think it doesn't happen otherwise. Private patients pay and those with coverage have insurance companies that pay. Hospitals have been known to turn away people who did not have proof of payment.

Power here includes the power of lobbies, which persuade governments to provide funds, for example, for kidney problems or anemia. Davis and Aroskar, op. cit., p. 192.

26. Rescher, op. cit., p. 464. Childress, op. cit., pp. 1415, 1418. Ramsey, *The Patient . . ,* op. cit., p. 259. Jonsen, op. cit., p. 628. Veatch, op. cit., pp. 106–107, 233–234. Roy Branson, "Health Care: Theories of Justice and Health Care," *EB* **2:**630–637. "ANA Code for Nurses, 1976," *EB* **4:**1789–1799. Report of the Judicial Council: "Cost-Benefit Analysis and Decision Theory," AMA Report A (I–78) says the primary concern is the patient, rather than the theoretical economics. Again, one is tempted to note that if these sentiments were carried out in practice, poor people would be receiving as much and as good health care as anyone else. And it is not only the poor. Roger E. Coene tried to arrange a kidney transplant. The team was concerned about getting paid and was inflexible about commitments. When the day came, the team straggled to the hospital over a five-hour period, long enough for the donor kidney to deteriorate to uselessness. Coene was then billed for services he never received. "Dialysis or Transplant: one Patient's Choice," *HCR*, no. 2 (Apr. 1978), **8:**5–7.

Harry R. Moody, "Is It Right to Allocate Health Care Resources on Grounds of Age?" pp. 197–201, in Bandman and Bandman, op. cit. Davis and Aroskar, op. cit., p. 192. Age was a factor in Seattle Swedish Hospital committee decisions. Prepuberty children were not chosen for dialysis, for it interferes with development. Those over forty-five years were not chosen because of the tendency to complications. Alexander, op. cit. Those over fifty-five are still considered poor risks for either dialysis or transplant. Children are now on dialysis, which stunts physical, emotional, and social growth. Transplants are more successful for them. Levine, "Dialysis or Transplant. . ," op. cit., p. 8.

27. Personal communication, Dr. Warren G. Thompson. Illich, op. cit. Starr, op. cit., p. 26. Malcah T. Notman and Carol C. Nadelson, "Women As Patients and Experimental Subjects," *EB* **4:**1704–1713. Hysterectomies in Saskatchewan dropped 32.8 percent when the procedure required a review committee's supervision. Outka, op. cit., p. 361, indicates

twice as many per capita surgeries in the United States as in Great Britain.

28. Margaret A. Farley, "Sexual Ethics," *EB* **4:**1575–1589. Victoria V. Ozonoff and David Ozonoff, "On Helping Those Who Help Themselves," *HCR*, no. 1 (Feb. 1977), **7:**7–10. Perry London, "Sexual Behavior," *EB* **4:**1560–1569, notes that historically, the repression of sexuality has been allied with the subjugation of women. He sees education and economic independence as being as important as contraception.

There is a voluminous literature on sexuality and sexual ethics today. One thrust of the literature is to "do your own thing." Ethically speaking, the greater emphasis has been on mutuality. It is ethical egoism versus a balanced approach of responsibilities and rights. The "new" on the scene is the discovery or acknowledgment that women have sexual feelings or that their feelings should or need to be considered. See also adolescent sexuality in Chapter six.

29. Notman and Nadelson, op. cit., pp. 1705–1711. Judith L. Woodward, "Infertility Issues," *The Christian Century*, no. 3 (4 Oct. 1978), **95:**934. A hotly debated concern is home births. Some insist on hospitals for delivery for the safety of mother and child. Others note the lower costs of home births. One ethical issue is this use of economic resources and another is self-determination. George J. Annas, "Homebirth: Autonomy vs. Safety," *HCR*, no. 4 (Aug. 1978), **8:**19–20. The ANA *Code for Nurses*, 1976, in its "Interpretive Statements," includes self-determination "whenever possible," *EB* **4:**1789. The safety issue has been heavily emphasized. The improvement in infant mortality rates probably owes more to improved sanitation and nutrition than to hospital births. If that is the case, then allocation of scarce resources might loom as a larger issue than safety.

30. Notman and Nadelson, op. cit., pp. 1704–1705. Tom L. Beauchamp, "Paternalism," *EB* **3:**1194–1201. "A Drug to Ease Menstrual Cramps," *Newsweek* (9 July 1979), p. 63. Some doctors say the pain is in the brain. The problem is certainly not limited to the health field. See Karen McCarthy Brown, "Heretics and Pagans: Women in the Academic World," pp. 266–288, and, Elizabeth Janeway, "The Power Relationships: A View

from Below," pp. 289–307, in *Private and Public Ethics*, ed. by Donald G. Jones (New York: The Edwin Mellen Press, 1978), Janeway's concern is politics and government.

31. This is not a woman's issue in the strict sense. In the health care system, men may also be treated as incompetent. They may experience this at the hands of women who are in power positions in the system. It is not a "necessary relationship" with a male patient either. But again, as noted before for battered spouses, the bind for women is more commonly a "double bind."

32. George J. Annas, *The Rights of Hospital Patients* (New York: Avon Books, 1975). Annas, "Patients' Rights Movement," *EB* **3:**1201–1206. "A Patient's Bill of Rights, American Hospital Association, 1973," *EB* **4:**1782–1783.

33. Boston Women's Health Book Collective, 2nd ed. (New York: Simon & Schuster, Inc., 1976). Ozonoff and Ozonoff, op. cit., pp. 9–10. This concern might be seen as allocation of scarce resources (saving money on medical expenses and distributing it to other priorities) and/or as autonomy, as in the home birth controversy.

34. Donald G. Jones (personal communication) has noted the disparity between the lay person's expertise and the professional person's. The relationship is thus inherently unequal. This reflects the Top Dog-Under Dog, or, Parent-Child perspectives. Jones goes further, however, in claiming that the professional has a responsibility to close the gap by educating lay persons to care for their own health. This is not just a matter of preventive health care but an ethical issue of equity, or establishing equity so that patient and health care personnel can have a relationship of equality or, at least, greater equality. Jones then goes on to note that professional conduct equals ethical conduct and unprofessional conduct equals unethical conduct, i.e., professional health care personnel have an ethical responsibility to educate patients. Aroskar, op. cit., p. 344, notes a dilemma when nurses must choose between their caring and teaching functions and seeing a certain number of patients, as required by their institution or agency.

35. Nonspecifics are also of concern. At one point in the history of kidney dialysis, 66 percent of the patients were men, excluding Veterans Administration hospitals. There is no evidence that twice as many men have renal failure as women. Ramsey, *The Patient . . .*, op. cit., pp. 250–251. Childress, op. cit., p. 1418.

36. The following paragraphs draw on the excellent overview by Nadelson and Notman, op. cit., pp. 1713–1720. See also, Barbara Ehrenreich and Deidre English, *Wtiches, Midwives, and Nurses: A History of Women Healers*, 2nd ed. (Old Westbury, N.Y.: Feminist Press, 1973). The failure to fully utilize the services of women in health care has been called a misuse of, or failure to allocate scarce resources.

37. The law is still somewhat ambiguous, but there appears to be a trend toward holding nurses liable for malpractice, where earlier, nurses were excluded from exercising independent judgment. In addition to Nadelson and Notman, op. cit., see the ANA *Code for Nurses*, op. cit. Teresa Stanley, "Nursing," *EB* **3:**1138–1146. Davis and Aroskar, op. cit., pp. 197–199.

38. Freedman, op. cit., p. 11. Jack Tinker, "General Intensive Therapy," *Nursing Times* **74:**266–268.

39. Aroskar, op. cit., p. 42–43. V. A. Bishop, "A Nurse's View of Ethical Problems in Intensive Care and Clinical Research," *British Journal of Anesthesiology* **50:**515–518. Luther Christman, "Moral Dilemmas for Practitioners in a Changing Society," *Nursing Digest*, no. 1 (Summer 1978), **6:**47–49.

40. Bishop, op. cit., p. 516.

41. Aroskar, op. cit., p. 36.

42. Ibid., pp. 36–37.

43. Levine, "Dialysis . . .," op. cit., p. 10.

44. Personal communication, Ms. Rita Ryan, Nursing Supervisor, Transplant and Dialysis Unit, Columbia-Presbyterian Medical Center, New York City. A. K. DeNour and J. W. Czaczkes, "Emotional Problems and Reactions of the Medical Team in a Chronic Hemodialysis Unit," *The Lancet* (1968), **2:**987–991. Juliani and Reamer, op. cit., p. 52.

45. Tinker, op. cit., p. 268. Bishop, op. cit., p. 41.

46. Christman, op. cit., p. 48.

47. DeNour and Czaczkes, op. cit., p. 987.

48. Ryan, op. cit.

49. Op. cit., p. 987f.

50. Juliani and Reamer, op. cit., p. 52.

51. *ANA Code for Nurses with Interpretive Statements* (Kansas City, Mo.: The ANA, 1976), p. 4. Compare Freedman, op. cit., p. 14. H. Abram and others, "Suicidal Behavior with Chronic Dialysis Patients," *American Journal of Psychiatry*, no. 9 (Mar. 1971), **127**:1199–1204.

52. Ryan, op. cit. DeNour and Czaczkes, op. cit., p. 990.

53. Notman and Nadelson, op. cit., p. 1704.

54. Christman, op. cit., p. 48. Rita Payton, "Information Control and Autonomy," *Nursing Clinics of North America*, no. 1 (Mar. 1979), **14**:23–33. Notman and Nadelson, op. cit., p. 1704.

55. *Code for Nurses*, op. cit., p. 5.

56. Notman and Nadelson, op. cit., 1709.

57. Francis Lewis, "The Nurse as Lackey: A Sociological Perspective," *Supervisor Nurse* (Apr. 1976), pp. 24–27.

58. Notman and Nadelson, op. cit., pp. 1718–1719.

Chapter 8

Ethics and the Later Years

INTRODUCTION

Older people are treated in a variety of ways in various cultures. Some wandering hunter and gathering or nomadic tribes have been known to leave the aged behind on an ice floe or along the desert trail. That may have been routine or only when the food supply was short. At times, it may have been at least partly a matter of choice when the old person knew she/he was no longer a productive member of society, a society that lived a marginal existence. Other cultures have honored their older members. They have been the political leaders and the teachers, the "wise ones" honored for their wisdom, the gurus of the seekers and the religious.[1]

As we have seen all along, attitudes and ethics are interwoven. A society that does not honor women and children may not treat them with respect for their human dignity, or respect their self-determination and autonomy, or include them in a just distribution of scarce resources or even resources held in abundance. So it is with older citizens. If we see people as a means to an end, and let us say the perspective is that of seeing people as a means to production, then the older person who can no longer produce is likely to be cast aside. Alternatively, of course, gratitude for past services or the reward of the "just desserts" may bring respect.

The deontological rule approach to ethics might say that the aged are human beings whose lives are to be respected.[2] Life is to be respected regardless of age or productivity.

The utilitarian approach might be that the greatest good for the greatest number is being served by leaving the old ones behind on the trail so that the life of the tribe is preserved. Then again, a utilitarian approach, the practical, pragmatic approach so dear to American hearts, might also see the greatest good coming from respect for the aged. People are smart enough to see that if the old are respected, they, too, can work hard and when they are old, they will retire with respect. But if the aged are simply cast aside, why work hard now, only to be dumped when you can no longer produce?

The American scene is mixed, as the perceptive reader will have realized by now. Our "ice floes" and desert trails can be found in nursing homes, where the aged may live out their days without seeing a single person from their "tribe."[3] Many a hard worker has given years to a company, loyally producing, only at the end to be handed a watch and be put on the shelf, trail, or ice floe of retirement. In yet other cases, older Americans have been Norman Vincent Peale's, Grandma Moses, Bernard Baruch's, and have otherwise either retained or achieved places of honor. They have been blessed with sufficient health to stay out of the nursing homes, retain their independence, and lead joyous, and yes, productive lives. The Gray Panthers have urged older folks to get off the shelf and live and also reminded the larger society that they are still a very lively group who are not about to be counted out.[4]

Our Concerns

The panegyric seems necessary in the youth culture of our day, an emphasis that is not limited to the American scene by any means.[5] Yet our basic concern in this book remains bioethics, medical ethics, the ethics of health care. Society's attitude toward the aged will affect the allocation of scarce resources. Many of the older people are women, including many singles (widows, divorced, never married), because, on the average, women live longer than men. Thus, society's attitude toward women will affect allocation. Many unnecessary surgeries are done on women. Attitudes toward menopause ("it's all in your head") affect the kind or quality, if

not the quantity, of medical care. Postmenopausal women may be seen as unproductive and hence useless, if medical personnel take the Freudian perspective that a woman is only a uterus surrounded by a supportive mechanism.

Our second concern will be death and dying. Adequate health care and the allocation of resources may affect the death and the dying of the aged. We will look at such things as ordinary and extraordinary means of keeping people alive and the ethics of euthanasia. Death with dignity is being achieved in a movement called *hospice*. It is worth a long look.[6]

ALLOCATION OF RESOURCES

Statistically, the health needs of the aged are greater than those of the younger. The last year of life may cost as much as all the earlier years put together.[7] Hospitals have built intensive care units and cardiac care units. These are costly to operate. There are those who question whether we should put that much money into old people who may not live very long anyway. The strict utilitarian approach here may be that the money would do more good providing for the born well, but now nutritionally deprived children of the world. Just as the old nomad sits down and lets the tribe travel on, using its resources for the younger, so some suggest our aged should do the same. Others point out that the Western world, at least, is not a society of scarcity. Judging by the money we spend on baseball, lipstick, alcohol, vacations, pleasure vehicles, and the military, we are certainly not lacking in resources. Those opposed to defense spending point out that for a few less bombers and battleships, obsolete before they were manufactured, we could supply our aged with most, if not all, their health needs. But it has also been pointed out that it would be naive to think that spending less on war would mean more for health. Our national priorities simply do not run in that direction.[8]

The fight for health dollars may be more a matter of political pull than the ethics of life. A sanctity of life doctrine insists that all are equal. A just distribution of goods on this basis would suggest an equality of distribution among all segments, regardless of sex, socioeconomic status, race, creed, color, or age. A utilitarian approach might say dollars spent on youth will improve or maintain the health of the future, whereas money spent on the aged will soon be gone. The utilitarian exception, of course, could be the rewards concept noted previously.

Clashing Views

In two recent discussion groups, this contrast between generations came out very strongly. One concerned professionals in public health. Given a choice between spending money on children or the chronically diseased, they chose the children and did not seriously consider the other group whom they assumed to be old. Nor did they consider a third category who happened to be women, on the theory that the women could take care of themselves, but the children could not or, at least, might not.

Of course, it is not only the aged who may have chronic disease, just as it is not only older people who die. But the emphasis in our culture is for youth. A second discussion group consisted of lay people studying death and dying in relation to ICU's. The unit in question was small and the beds were filled. One contained a comatose old man whose prognosis was limited. He might live for months, but death was more likely to come in a matter of days. An eighteen-year-old motorcycle accident victim was brought to the emergency room. He needed a bed in the ICU. The ethics of care include a covenant, a promise, not to abandon the patient once the care has begun. Pulling the plug on the old man would bring certain, if not instant, death. We will discuss euthanasia later. Here the conflict was saving the life of the teen-ager in contrast to letting the older citizen die. In the group discussion was a seventy-eight-year-old woman who thought the old man should at least be given consideration. The rest of the group were younger and, for them, there was no question but that the young person should be saved. The only slight doubt was a question about the motorcycle—was this a hoodlum? We noted the question of social worth in Chapter Seven in relation to dialysis. Questions of productivity, of course, are also questions of social worth.[9]

ORDINARY/EXTRAORDINARY MEANS

The ethics of care in death and dying are a main topic today. Partly that may be a matter of the increasing age of American society. More of it seems to come from the increasing technology that we have noted earlier. Once more it is the *success* of modern medicine that raises new and old questions.[10] Sophisticated machinery may be able to keep blood circulating and lungs breathing far beyond the time in which nature might take its course. One of the many ways in which we "play God" is to keep people "alive" long after they might have died a natural death. The debate here tends to focus on the ordinary/extraordinary combination noted earlier, and on acts of omission and commission. These, in turn, are involved in passive and active euthanasia.[11]

Pope Pius XII is often quoted from his 1957 speech in which he suggested that extraordinary means need not be used to maintain life. Ordinary means *must* be used.[12] Extraordinary means *may* be used but do not have to be. He was speaking of the later years primarily. As noted in earlier chapters, the doctrine has been applied to various ages, including the neonate. Again, the problem often turns on the interpretation of *ordinary*. For the doctors in the Quinlan case, the respirator was ordinary. For her father, it was extraordinary, but the intravenous was ordinary.[13] What is ordinary to one may not be to another. What is ordinary to one area may not be to another. The ICU may be ordinary only because it's there. In an area where there is none, or only one limited one, it may be extraordinary.

Dr. Paul Ramsey wants to drop the terms because he thinks these words have been used to let people die when they were not actually dying.[14] In the broad sense, of course, we are all dying.[15] So perhaps the real problem of semantics is at what point do we say the patient is "dying." In an earlier day, the person was dead when he stopped breathing or when the heart stopped.[16] In recent years, a number of laws have been passed accepting "brain death" (a flat EEG) as a sign of death.[17] One part of this has been the freeing up of the body for the removal of heart or kidneys for transplant. Another part of it has been to allow medical personnel to turn off the respirator or the machinery that was keeping the heart going.[18]

Living Will

Some older people have decided they do not want to be maintained on machinery once they go beyond a reasonable quality of life, or become comatose.[19] One solution has been the *living will*.[20] They prepare a document ahead of time, indicating their wishes. There are very few places where authorities *have* to follow the living will, but it indicates the wishes of the individual should they become comatose and if their wishes can be considered.[21]

The living will implies that we have a "say" in what happens to us. We avoided the use of the term "right" in that sentence. For some, we have a right to determine what happens to us. Others say no. We are stewards, rather than owners of the life we have from God or nature.[22] The ANA *Code for Nurses* Interpretive Statement starts out with the patient's self-determination.[23] If the patient is comatose, a living will might indicate his/her wishes at some earlier stage of life. Otherwise, the next of kin might be consulted. When the patient is awake and competent, his/her own opinion or desire can be checked. Even so, some would insist that self-determination does not extend to the refusal of treatment, especially if the treatment is life saving. When death is imminent and the treatment is only life-prolonging, the ethical dilemma is whether a person can do what he/she will with his/her own life. Medical practice through the ages has often realized there comes a time when the practice of medicine moves from cure to care. If we cannot "rescue the perishing," we can at least "care for the dying."[24]

Refusal of Care

There is greater acceptance today for the competent patient to refuse medical procedures that only prolong the dying.[25] The acceptance of active suicide is more widespread today, but is still largely proscribed in both morals and law. At one stage in the history of Christianity, the afterlife was pictured so vividly that many people committed suicide. Life was so wretched and the afterlife was so glorious that they saw no point in waiting.[26] Leaders of church and state took a dim view of this loss of membership, army recruits, and slaves for the mines. By A.D 310, Augustine was speaking out strongly against suicide, and it has been prohibited ever since. Church leaders decreed that anyone commiting suicide would go to the horrible tortures of hell rather than the glories of heaven.[27]

Suicide is an active taking of one's own life. The taking of someone else's life may be murder, which has always been prohibited, although its definition has varied from culture to culture. Occasionally, medical people have been charged with murder for pulling the plug on modern life-prolonging machinery.[28] The failure to insert the plug or to restore a life-prolonging procedure that has stopped or run out is a less active form of "letting die." The active act of commission that results in another's death is usually against the law, except for self-defense or in time of war.[29] The failure to do something that might keep another alive is more problematic in law. Generally, if there is a relationship, as in families, or between health personnel and patient, the omission is more questionable than if there is no relationship. If we are walking along the lake and see someone fall through the ice, there are those who say we do not have to risk our lives to save that person. If we do, it's an act of heroism. If our own child is in danger, or if it's our own patient, and we do not do all we can to protect or save that child or patient, we have violated what some refer to as the *covenant relationship*. Sometimes this relationship is vague. An individual walked into an emergency room at 3 A.M. This "stranger off the street" was first checked for ability to pay and then put in a bed. Some eighteen hours later, the head nurse contacted the doctor on call to remind him of this patient. An emergency midnight operation saved a life. If the patient had died, it's an open question whether heirs could have held the hospital liable. There was no covenant relationship. Death would have resulted from a failure to act, an omission, rather than an act of commission.[30]

EUTHANASIA

The legal niceties here are not our prime concern. Those will be discussed in Chapter Nine on "rights." The ethical concern is a question of the direct versus the indirect. Direct killing is generally held to be wrong and even called murder. Indirect killing might be called neglect, or an accident, or simply an act of God, or the Natural Law.[31] "Letting die" is sometimes related to passive euthanasia. Direct killing is related to active euthanasia. The latter is seen as wrong in most ethical systems. The euthanasia societies around the world, however, are more concerned with a "good death" (the meaning of the Greek word) than getting rid of people or killing them off.[32]

The former head of the British Euthanasia Society toured the facilities of St. Joseph Hospice.[33] He observed that if people in general could be assured of such a good death, the Society could be disbanded.

Hospice Movement

The Hospice movement started in England and has since spread to other countries.[34] The United States will soon have more than 200 units.[35] Some of these are extensions of hospitals. Some are separate places. The concept is to accept the dying person as dying. Instead of hooking them up to all the machines that can prolong their dying, they are encouraged to spend their final days at home.[36] With help from visiting nurses and volunteers, these days can be made more comfortable and even joyous, as the dying person lives in familiar surroundings with family, friends, and even pets.[37] When or if the patient's condition deteriorates to the point where she/he can no longer be cared for at home, the hospice building is designed to maintain a home atmosphere that avoids the cold white walls of the traditional hospital.[38]

A crucial aspect of the program is the covenant relationship, so the person does not need to fear abandonment. That may mean having someone there twenty-four hours a day. A second major facet, and an extension of the covenant, is that the patient is the whole family, rather than the individual who is dying.[39] That means, among other things, psycho-logical support for the family during the dying process and afterward until there is mutual agreement that the grief process has been worked through and is under control. Sometimes, ongoing groups of spouses are formed to provide a support community. The movement has a strong emphasis also on the team approach to care, with nurses and doctors, clergy, social workers, psychologists, and volunteers working together for the good of the patient, rather than the convenience of the institution.[40]

Although there are expenses involved, of course, these can be less than the traditional hospital care.[41] Thus, the hospice movement might be seen not only as death with dignity but as another form of the allocation of scarce resources. The extensive use of volunteers in the program also extends the scarce resource of medical personnel. In many geographical areas, personnel and time are a scarce resource, but personnel who have worked through their own feelings about death are an even scarcer resource.[42]

Talking About Dying

Health personnel working with the dying face problems similar in a way to those working in NNICU's and ICU's and with dialysis patients. The intensity and emotional involvement raise a number of problems. Ethically, there are problems of providing optimum care for the patients while dealing with one's own feelings, as noted for the role of the nurse in dialysis. Attitudes toward death are, of course, a part of our larger culture.[43]

Several decades ago, the hush-hush attitude changed, and death came out of the closet. Now we can talk about it. The voluminous literature on the subject suggests we may be talking the subject to death.[44] A great deal of the earlier work was done by Dr. Elizabeth Kübler-Ross.[45] She has worked to train health personnel and lay people alike to face death, their own and that of those they love, as well as their patients. Her work with the families of the dying as well as with the dying patients parallels in some ways that of the hospice movement. There is an emphasis upon home care out of the hospital context. Her books and her work can be highly recommended to those who work in the ICU's, the nursing homes, the hospice settings, and wherever people are dying. For some, death remains the final enemy. For others, it is a friend. For some, it is not death that is the enemy, but the health care that prolongs their agony in irony of an ancient code that says "do no harm."[46]

THE ISSUES

The issues in ethics for the aged come near to the whole gamut of bioethical concerns. We highlighted here the allocation of scarce resources, death and dying, and death with dignity. Related to these issues are principles of equality and the dignity of the individual, cost-benefit analysis, mercy, quality of life as compared to or contrasted with sanctity of life, or existence. Self-determination and autonomy versus dependency is a major thread in issues related to the aged. Lack of resources may drastically cut self-determination. Autonomy may be determined by ability to care for oneself, but institutional policy and the attitude of health care personnel may require dependency (a Child or Under Dog status) for people who might be able to do more for themselves.

The right to control one's body, even to the point of suicide, is a major concern. Some relate the refusal of health care to suicide. Others relate it to passive euthanasia, the letting die that is becoming more well known in our society today. Active euthanasia, actually helping or hastening the dying process, remains far less acceptable. The main exception is medication that relieves pain in terminal cases. Even if this hastens death, it may be allowed for there are times when mercy takes precedent over the value of sheer existence.

The quality of life may be the greatest of all issues involved in the quality of our dying. Some speak harshly against any QOL element in ethical decision making. That is especially important when someone makes a decision about someone else's death. But in the end, many people would prefer to die if life is no longer tolerable. The Hospice movement is one way to help people live until they die, a standard that may be worth considering for all, even if biological death is many years away.

NURSES AND CARING FOR PEOPLE IN THEIR LATER YEARS

Nurses provide the majority of care for the aged and dying, whether in hospital, nursing home, hospice, or patient's home.[47] Nurses who work with the elderly become involved with decisions about or carrying out the decisions on the allocation of scarce lifesaving resources. An extension of the decision on who should receive these resources is the idea of under what circumstances are these lifesaving techniques considered ordinary treatment and when are they extraordinary or possibly not indicated for use? This latter idea leads us to discussion of the nurse's role and responsibilities in euthanasia, as well as in caring for adults who are dying and for whom care is palliative and supportive, not cure-oriented.

As noted in previous chapters, the roles of nursing run the gamut of decision maker to the person who carries out another's decisions, responsibly. Each of these roles will be discussed in relation to the allocation of scarce resources to the elderly, ordinary versus extraordinary treatment including the concept of euthanasia, and caring for people who are dying. The ethical issues raised by each of these situations, including truth telling, will also be included.

Nurses and People Receiving Lifesaving Resources

Nurses who work in intensive care units, either surgical, medical, or coronary, daily, if not hourly, face the ethical dilemma of deciding which patient will be given a bed in such a unit. These units are generally limited in numbers of beds and highly skilled professional staff, not to mention being very costly, and care in such units is aimed at preserving life.[48] This limitation of space and staff implies that not everyone who may need the care provided here will be able to get it— hence, it becomes a scarce resource.

Decision Making

Chapter Seven discussed the various aspects of deciding who will get limited or scarce resources and on what basis such decisions are or should be made. This same topic is discussed here more fully to explain how nurses are involved in such decisions, particularly in the intensive care units. It is often the older adult who is in need of such services and yet these people may often be denied services in favor of a younger person with "more potential" for life. It is easy to see the value-laden component of deciding on the allocation of scarce ICU beds on the basis of age, and it is a common practice in our culture.

Nurses provide the majority of minute-to-minute care of patients in intensive care units. They are the professionals whose knowledge and judgment in interpreting various monitor printouts and patient's reactions are depended upon by physicians in order to plan and update treatment regimens. It is also the nurse in constant attendance who notes when a patient shows signs of improvement or deterioration, the data often used to decide whether the patient should remain in the unit or be transferred to another level of care, such as recovery or terminal care units.[49]

Responsibility: Nurses who work in the critical care units often more openly recognize their decision-making responsibilities in the care of patients. Because of the limited space and clientele, nurses and physicians seem to work much more readily as a team, a collegial relationship, based on mutual respect and autonomous clinical judgment when indicated for the welfare of the patient. This placement of the patient's welfare at the center of activities is the ideal in nursing and medical practice, although, in reality, decision on the allocation of scarce resources may *not* benefit the individual patient who will not receive or continue to receive life-support therapy in favor of another person. Nurses working in such situations are often the first to be vocal about continued treatment for a given person who shows limited or no signs of recovering. Many authors note that to require nurses and other personnel to continue life-support machines and repeated CPR activi-

ties on patients who show little obvious evidence of responding to treatment serves only to prolong the dying for the patient and to demoralize the staff.[50] Skillman goes on to note that continuation of intensive care when it is clear that a patient has no chance of recovery is a mockery of the intense physical and emotional efforts of nurses.[51]

Let Others Decide?

For some nurses who work in critical care units, the involvement in decisions on which patients will receive care is minimal. In these situations the nurses may respond in a variety of ways. One response is relief for the nurse who is more comfortable letting others (usually the physician) assume responsibility for deciding who gets the scarce resources.[52] This is a rather traditional nursing response—passing the buck when the responsibility stakes are high—but may not be in the best interests of the people in the care of the nurse.[53] Other nurses would like a recognized voice in decision making but are thwarted in their efforts. This may lead to high rates of staff turnover in the unit or progressive loss of interest in working in such a place with concomitant alienation from the patient. Another somewhat typical nursing response when overt decision making is not possible is the nurse's resorting to covert decision making. Because of the continuous nature of nursing contact with critically ill patients, there are many opportunities for the nurse to put into action his/her decision of whether to initiate or continue life-support treatment. The most obvious situation is how fast or slow the nurse initiates or calls for the CPR team the next time the patient arrests.[54] Each of these response patterns has ethical implications, and how the nurse chooses to respond when open participation in decisions on treatment is not allowed can result in unethical versus ethical nursing practice.[55]

Nurses and Termination of Life-Support Therapy

An extension of the discussion of deciding who should receive life-sustaining treatment resources is the examination of the decision to discontinue such treatment. We have noted earlier in this chapter the distinction between ordinary and extraordinary treatment in medical care and the variance in definitions, depending on who is defining the concept. Even among nurses, the specifics of which treatment modalities (IV, respirator, oxygen, antibiotic) constitute extraordinary care differ.[56] Consensus among team members, patient, and family may be one approach to defining "ordinary" care for a given patient. If consensus is not achieved, many would say that the patient has priority in the decision on whether to continue treatment.[57] If the patient is incompetent (for example, comatose), the family is usually second in priority. We have noted earlier the wide divergence of opinions on this, including the view that treatment always continues, no matter how "extraordinary."

Self-Determination

A part of the position that the competent adult patient should have priority in deciding whether life-support measures should be continued involves the concept of self-determination. The ANA *Code for Nurses* Interpretive Statement Item 1[58] discusses the nurse's responsibility for allowing clients to determine what care they will receive. Nurses' value systems that support the concept of self-determination often result in nursing actions that promote self-determination in competent, adult patients. These activities include the provision of information needed by the patient in order to make an informed decision about his medical care. Some of the ethical issues that may arise in the provision of information to patients include decisions on what or how much information should be given, and by whom. All are value-laden decisions. The issue of informed consent will be dealt with in more detail in Chapter Nine.

Control of Information: Payton[59] states that when professionals seek to control the information shared with patients, for whatever reasons, there is raised the ethical issue of loss of autonomy. In other words, there is no such thing as patient self-determination if health professionals choose to control the amount of information given about the patient's condition and options for treatment. Most nurses have controlled information, consciously or unconsciously, in nursing practice and for a variety of reasons. Some suggest that withholding information from clients results from the professional's uncertainty of knowledge, striving for status that is defined by the possession of a "unique" body of knowledge, or conditioning that one must have *all* the answers or else don't provide information that might raise questions you can't answer.[60] Another reason given is to protect the patient. However, if patients are to be able to fully participate in the decision about whether life-support measures are to be continued, they must know the full details of their disease, condition, options for treatment, and chances for survival. On the basis of this information, a patient may choose to discontinue treatment. Professional respect for the client's right to choose to terminate treatment requires a commitment to care for the patient until death occurs.[61] This aspect of nursing care will be discussed in the next section of this chapter, as will more detail on truth telling.

The Nurse and Euthanasia

Sometimes when patients and/or professionals decide to terminate life-supporting, extraordinary treatments in anticipation of death, the patient may request a hastening of death. As noted earlier, the concept of euthanasia originally meant "good death." It has now come to mean a hastening of death—active or passive, voluntary or involuntary. Beauchamp[62] notes that nurses receive far more requests from patients for euthanasia than do physicians, and he implies that nurses are actively involved in decisions on euthanasia whether they choose to be or not. One possible explanation of why patients ask the nurse to help them die (pull the plug, give the lethal dose of analgesic) rather than the physician, is the depth of trust invested in the nurse-patient relationship. That is, the nurse is a caring friend who has the means to provide for the final patient request—death.[63] How the nurse responds to this request will depend on many factors. One may also note that the nurse's decision to not act on the patient's request *is* a decision. Those nurses who believe in the quality of life may base their reason for allowing or hastening death on the prevention of unnecessarily cruel treatment and prolonged pain and suffering plus support of the competent adult's request. Those nurses who choose not to accede to the patient's request may believe in the sanctity of life, or fear their role as "executioner"—either emotionally or legally. We encourage nurses on both sides of the euthanasia question to remember that they are not the only ones who will bear the consequences of their decision.

Many medical care institutions have formulated guidelines for deciding when treatment should stop or euthanasia be employed.[64] These guidelines are helpful to the nurse who believes in the concept of euthanasia, but of minimal use to nurses who oppose euthanasia for any reason. Active euthanasia usually takes the form of overdosing the patient, and passive euthanasia usually involves "no treatment" decisions—no further surgery, no CPR, no IV. Passive euthanasia is more widely accepted by health workers, possibly because of the legal implications (murder) of active euthanasia.[65]

Decisions: Nurses are in a unique position to assist in the decision on whether extraordinary treatment measures should be discontinued. They have the most constant contact with the patient and family, and know much about their reactions to the patient's current condition and the prospect of death. The nurse often relays this information to the physician responsible for care and/or to the review team that will assume responsibility for making the final decision on treatment. The relaying of such information involves good communication patterns among team members as well as the provision of complete information. The nurse has the opportunity to influence how the decision goes by the choice of information relayed, which may support the nurse's unconscious decision already made. Sensitivity to this possible control of information as well as team decision making may help to ensure that ethically sound decisions are made in the best interest of the patient.

Dilemmas: Another dilemma for nurses working with patients who choose to termi-

nate life-support therapy or on whom the decision has been made occurs when the nurse cannot personally support such a decision.[66] How is the nurse who does not believe in euthanasia or termination of life-support machines to work responsibly with the persons who are the recipients of such decisions? It is not always possible to assign another nurse to provide the terminal care, and the Code for Nurses implies that the nurse is responsible for continuous care with "respect for the nature of the health problem."[67] In some situations, nurses can call for a team review of the decision with opportunity to explain their reasons for thinking the decision to terminate treatment was inappropriate.[68] In other situations, nurses may wish to terminate their employment in settings where such decisions are made. We would also suggest that nurses examine closely the basis for their beliefs—is it a religious motive (sanctity of life), a genuine disagreement with the decision for a particular patient, or a fear of death (their own)? How the individual nurse responds in such situations will depend a great deal on her personal beliefs and value of life. Ethical practice is based on knowledge of personal and professional responsibilities as well as values so that a nurse does not unknowingly impose personal values on patients.[69]

Nurses and the Dying

The majority of nursing care issues raised in working with adults in their later years eventually lead the nurse to examination of her/his feelings, anxieties, and reactions to the final stage of living—death. Elizabeth Kübler-Ross[70] has provided a classic work on understanding the stages of dying, and many authors support the idea that people who work with the dying often go through the stages of dying themselves as they begin to accept death as inevitable.[71] Many have been culturally conditioned to believe in one's infiniteness, so that working with the dying seems alien and unnatural. How nurses carry out their professional responsibilities to provide care and support of the elderly and dying is often directly correlated with their own level of personal acceptance/rejection of death as a natural part of life.[72]

Some specific examples of the preceding

statement may help to sensitize the nurse to her own reactions to caring for the dying. When nurses fear death, or have not come to terms with their own death, they often deny that another person is dying or simply avoid taking care of that person. Either response leaves the dying person without the personal closeness helpful in facing death.[73] Another possible situation that the nurse can promote with her own fear of death is to become angry at the demands for attention and comfort from the dying, and then avoid the patient even more. Some nurses allow their fear of death to form a callous exterior, with the nurse-patient relationship taking on a superficial quality. It does not necessarily follow, however, that nurses who have come to grips with their own finality are the only ones who can provide the sensitive, supportive care needed by those who are dying.[74] All can learn new ways of relating and meeting clients' needs.

Truth Telling

An aspect of working with dying patients that nurses find troublesome at times is the issue of truth telling. For purposes of discussion here, we will limit the scope of truth telling to patients with incurable diseases, although the principles apply to all of nursing practice. One common interpretation of the issue of truth telling is that it is the physician's responsibility to decide when, how much, and to whom the truth will be given. This is a particularly naive view for health professionals to hold today, because the majority of care of the dying is provided by nurses who also have the most extended contact with the patient and family.[75] It usually follows that the nurse also receives the most requests for information about the patient's condition.[76] To have to constantly reply, "You'll have to ask your doctor" to a patient's request for information does little to support the foundations of the nurse-patient relationship so important to helping the dying *live* until the moment of death. This type of response also hints of nursing incompetence, because few patients (or nurses) believe that the nurse does not know the condition of the patient she is caring for.

Another perspective on whether a patient should be told the truth about his incurable condition is based on whether the patient requests such information. Elizabeth Kübler-Ross suggests that denial is an important stage in the dying process, and if a patient chooses to deny his impending death, care givers should support this denial by not telling about the extent of disease.[77] She goes on to note that this same individual may later on be ready to discuss his condition and death, and the care giver should then respond to requests for information with the truth. Yarling also supports the notion that patients have a moral right to information about themselves, but they have no obligation to have this information. He goes on to note that if a patient has a moral right to such information and exercises his right by requesting same, the professional has a moral obligation to provide the information requested.[78] He adds that this moral obligation to provide patients with information rests equally and inescapably upon any person who has the needed information and the ability to tell it correctly once the patient requests it. It would seem that nurses who support the notion of the patient's right to self-determination would also be in a position to provide this truth when asked.

One of the basic conflicts among professionals occurs when they disagree on whether the patient should be told the truth, usually in response to the family's request that the patient "be spared." It would seem, however, that the majority of professionals would wish to respond truthfully to direct questions from their patients rather than lie, no matter what the family or others decide. Several authors suggest that lying to a patient for whatever reason only serves to destroy the trust and confidence needed for effective supportive care giving. Lying in such cases of terminal disease also denies the patient freedom of self-determination in dealing with and preparing for death.[79]

The last issue in the discussion of truth telling deals with how the truth is disclosed. Generally, it can be assumed that the patient has selected the most trusted person (family, friend, or professional) from whom he/she seeks the truth. If all were to agree that they are morally obligated to speak the truth when asked, one still may speak in many ways. Several writers suggest that the bearer of grim news does not have to speak grimly or brutally, but with sensitivity, understanding, warmth, and directness.[80] This action also implies that the nurse or whoever is sharing the truth would also be prepared to sit quietly with the patient, encourage expression of feelings, and listen sympathetically while the patient is processing the information.

Care of the Dying

Caring for the dying patient requires a great emotional investment from professionals and family alike, in addition to the patient. To be able to laugh when the person laughs and cry when the person is crying can be a demanding, but enriching experience for the nurse.[81] To be able to listen and accept the anger and hostility of people who are dying without shying away from them and producing the isolation most feared by the dying often is a daily challenge for the nurse. To be able to deal with one's own fear of death and grieving as a favorite patient is dying and still care for that patient objectively can be a growing experience for nurses. These types of situations also carry risks, especially the risk of the nurse's alienation from anyone else who might be dying.[82]

The principal goal of care for the dying patient is to keep the person as comfortable and alert as possible while supporting his/her and the family's efforts in working toward acceptance of death. The care of the dying is a process involving the needs of patients, families, and care givers. To deny any one of these person's needs is to be less than supportive of the dying person. This care is also based on treating the person with respect. It requires a multidisciplinary team approach as spiritual and economic needs as well as medical and nursing ones are evident.[83]

Hospice Care: One of the unique aspects of providing care for the terminally ill is the nurse's role in creating as personal and home-like a setting for death as is possible when a patient chooses to die outside his/her own home.[84] The hospice movement in this country is beginning to take hold, and is built on the concept that dying is a natural event and a family affair.[85] Nurses who work in hospices experience great satisfaction in pro-

moting meaningful life in people until the moment of death. One of the important treatment modalities to come out of the hospice movement in Europe is the idea that pain in terminal illness can be controlled and often prevented. Nurses found that regular use of analgesics often prevented the occurrence of pain, and once the patient realized he could be pain-free, he relaxed and less medication was needed to control the lessened pain.[86] Nurses have also realized that diversion may be the best pain-killer of all, and use their creativity to provide a variety of activities for the dying person.

Communication: Other aspects of the nurse's role in caring for the dying include seeking ways to communicate with those who want to talk about death and dying, and support of those who do not.[87] The nurse can decrease fear and mistrust by explaining procedures and treatments simply, by being a reassuring presence for the patient when requested, and supporting family members in their grief process.[88] It is important to note that for care of the dying to be successful in terms of being responsive to the needs of the dying person, it should be geared to and built around the patient's needs and desires, and not the institution's or staff's. This is a challenge to nurses who may have placed responsibility to employer and institution above responsibility to individual clients in the system, in the "interest of efficiency."

Working with the dying requires knowledge of self and a willingness to remain a person while also carrying out professional responsibilities. Through work with the dying, nurses often learn how better to live and support meaningful life in others.[89] Acceptance of death as a natural ending to life is helpful in working with the dying person, but not essential. Nurses who work with dying persons quickly realize that grief is only one side of death; hope and courage is the other.

CASE STUDIES

The following case studies are offered to illustrate and stimulate discussion on the various ethical dilemmas of nurses caring for the aged and the dying. We encourage your use of the *Guidelines* found in Chapter One as you study and reflect upon the cases.

Patient's Right to Die

T. R. is a student nurse caring for Mr. B., a sixty-nine-year-old retired farmer, who was admitted to the hospital with a severe heart condition three weeks ago. Since that time, Mr. B. has had two cardiac arrests and was revived with some difficulty. As T. R. sits with Mr. B., he confides to her that he is ready to die and has asked the doctor to "let him go" the next time his heart stops. He goes on to talk about his contentment with the life he has had. T. R. leaves for a short while to check if Mr. B.'s request for a 'no code' has been written, and is told by the head nurse that "everyone is coded on this unit; it's an unwritten policy." As T. R. returns to Mr. B.'s room, trying to think about what to say about his request, she notes that he is nonresponsive, with no heartbeat, although his body is still somewhat warm.

In addition to the *Guidelines,* please consider the following questions:

1. What options for action are available to the student nurse?
2. Discuss each option in relation to ethical issues raised and value decisions required.
3. What action(s) would you take as the nurse in this situation? Give the rationale for your decision.
4. When is it justifiable, if ever, to refuse a patient's request for no treatment when you need to go against institutional policy?

Truth Telling

T. T. is the nurse assigned to care for B. J., a fifty-seven-year-old woman with a newly revised diagnosis of histiocytic lymphoma. B. J. has been hospitalized for three weeks with a high fever and was informed a week ago that the doctors thought she had Hodgkin's disease. The final lab studies have just been returned, and the doctors have changed their diagnosis. During the morning conference, the doctors requested help from the nursing staff to keep the new diagnosis from the patient until they were "completely sure" of the results of the tests. The nurses agreed, although somewhat uncomfortably, because they knew B. J. would be asking questions about the tests. Sure enough, during the day B. J. asked T. T. what her tests showed about Hodgkin's disease. The nurse responded, "The tests are back but the doctors are not sure what they mean yet." At this, B. J. cried out, "What do you mean, they don't know? You people are supposed to know what's wrong with sick people." At that point, she turned her face into her pillow and sobbed, "I knew it—I'm going to die. You people are lying to me."

Consider the following questions, applying the *Guidelines:*

1. What options for response to B. J.'s first question did the nurse have?
2. In the strictest sense, the nurse was telling the truth. Would you have done the same, and why?
3. How would you have responded to B. J.'s last comments?
4. Are there other ways of sharing the truth in this situation?

Death with Dignity

Ms. P. is an eighty-six-year-old nurse who has recently retired to her hometown. A month ago, she was knocked down in a revolving door of a large department store, and broke both legs. She was being cared for in a small rehabilitation unit in this city. She appeared to be doing well until one morning the attendant found her very confused and unable to speak coherently. The preliminary diagnosis was some type of cardiovascular accident (CVA) and she was transferred to a local Catholic hospital for care. A young physician decided to operate after locating a cerebral blood clot, and did so twice in one week (the second for recurrence of an embolus). Ms. P. was left paralyzed on her left side after the surgery, and when she could speak a couple of words, she said to a friend, "Why? It's so cruel. Why don't they let me die?" There was no family involved, but a close friend of Ms. P. relayed the questions and concern to the nursing staff, stating that she felt Ms. P. had the right to die. The nurses quickly responded, "Oh no, Miss. She has the 'right' to live, and we're going to do all we can to keep her alive."

Consider the following questions, applying the *Guidelines:*

1. What values are evident in the physician's choice of action?
2. What values are evident in the nurses' statements?
3. What values are evident in the patient's request, and what responsibility does the nurse have to respond to these?
4. Because Ms. P. did not have a choice in the hospital to which she was sent in a semicomatose state, what options does she have now that she is there and alert?
5. What role does the nurse have in informing Ms. P. of these options?

Allocation of Life-saving Resources

You are the nurse in charge of the intensive care unit of a local hospital. The beds are filled presently, and an accident victim arrives in the emergency room. The accident victim is a seventy-year-old woman with severe head injuries and in need of intensive care. The physician calls to request a bed for her and suggests that you move out the man in a coma who has been there for two weeks (he's forty years old).

Consider the following questions, applying the *Guidelines:*

1. What factors would you want to take into consideration before making such a decision?
2. What values seem evident in the physician's request? Can you support these values?
3. What values will determine how you might decide who gets or keeps a bed in the ICU?

NOTES AND REFERENCES

1. Elisabeth Kübler-Ross reports that an old Eskimo may simply get up from dinner, say goodbye and go outside to die. *Questions and Answers on Death and Dying* (New York: Macmillan Publishing Co., Inc., 1974), p. 153, and pp. 33–37, "Dying Among Alaskan Indians: A Matter of Choice," by Murray L. Trelease. Edmund Cahn, *The Moral Decision* (Bloomington: Indiana University Press, 1955), pp. 216–217. Margaret Mead, "The Cultural Shaping of the Ethical Situation," pp. 4–23, in *Who Shall Live?* ed. by Kenneth Vaux (Philadelphia: Fortress Press, 1970). David Landy, "Death I: Anthropological Perspectives," *Encylopedia of Bioethics* 1:221–229. The Encyclopedia is cited hereafter as *EB*. Drew Christiansen, "Aging and the Aged III: Ethical Implications in Aging," *EB* 1:58–65. Phillipe Ariès, "Death Inside Out," pp. 10–24, and, Ivan Illich, "The Political Uses of Natural Death," pp. 25–42, in *Death Inside Out*, ed. by Peter Steinfels and Robert M. Veatch (New York: Harper & Row, Publishers, 1974).

2. Theoretically, the law follows this "equal worth" concept, which we noted in neonatology and the allocation of scarce resources. If there is any preference, it would be for the dependent (weak, helpless, child, comatose, incompetent, including temporarily incompetent). Thomas C. Oden, *When Shall Treatment Be Terminated?* (New York: Harper & Row, Publishers, 1976), p. 13–14. The Institute of Situational Ethics set up an ethical aptitude test for applicants to professional schools and for government jobs. Asked what establishes the value of human life, most people answered, "potential productivity." Leonard C. Lewin, "Ethical Aptitude Test," *Harper's Magazine*, no. 1517 (Oct. 1976), **253**:20–21. Lewis P. Bird, "Dilemmas in Biomedical Ethics," pp. 131–155, in *Horizons of Science*, ed. by Carl F. H. Henry (New York: Harper & Row, Publishers, 1978). Gerald J. Gruman traces this "productive" concern to the economic theory of Mercantilism (1498–1714) and secondarily to social Darwinism. According to the latter, the old and ill, as well as women after the reproductive years and the uneducated are inferior and parasitic. "Death and Dying: Euthanasia and Sustaining Life I: Historical Perspectives," *EB* 1:261–268. Darwin's evolution through "survival of the fittest" is now seen as only a partial truth at best. Our concern is hardly limited to mere survival. The cockroach has done that. See further, Anthony G. N. Flew, "Evolution," *EB* 1:479–484. Christiansen, op. cit., pp. 58–59, traces the productive concept to the Protestant work ethic about the same time as mercantilism. The older people most admired, he says, are those who continue the work roles of adult life.

3. The homes have also been compared to concentration camps. Once people get in there, it may be difficult to get out, sometimes simply because they're forgotten, sometimes because government regulations require their poverty. "The Nursing Home Gulag," *Psychology Today*, no. 2 (July 1979), **13**:22. Jeffrey Wack and Judith Rodin, "Nursing Homes for the Aged: The Human Consequences of Legislation-shaped Environments," *The Journal of Social Issues*, no. 4 (1978), **34**:6–21. They say there are 1.5 million elderly in 20,000 nursing homes. For most of these people, this will be the last place they live, "one of the most debilitating environments available." Abandonment, autonomy and self-determination, consent, personal dignity, the treatment of people as people rather than things, and distributive justice are moral/ethical issues in this situation. Ernlé W. D. Young, "Aging and the Aged IV: Health Care and Research in the Aged," *EB* 1:65–69, says the sick aged (bedfast and housebound) are more than three million. The $9 billion nursing home industry, which often involves neither home nor nursing, is a "ripoff," a victimization of the elderly. Federal programs have helped make commercial homes profitable, partly by lax auditing and lax enforcement of standards.

We balance the perspective by noting there are good nursing homes and only 5 percent of those over sixty-five are in long-term care institutions. Of the other 95 percent, 54 percent are with a spouse, 19 percent live with others, and 27 percent live alone. See Peter E. Dans and Marie R. Kerr, "Gerontology and Geriatrics in Medical Education," *New England Journal of Medicine*, no. 5 (1 Feb. 1979), **300**:228–232. The Journal is cited hereafter as *NEJM*. There are also programs to upgrade care. See Ginette A. Pepper, Robert Kane, and Barbara Teteberg, "Geriatric Nurse Practitioners in Nursing Homes," *The American Journal of Nursing*, no. 1 (Jan. 1976), **76**:62–64. The Journal is cited hereafter as *AJN*.

4. Christiansen, op. cit., p. 60, refers to the segregationists (the elderly should disengage) and the integrationists (those who think the elderly should continue to participate). Ethically, here we are talking about the quality of life (QOL) rather than mere existence. This is a basic concern of the later years, including the last days of the dying. See Hospice and Kübler-Ross following. Daniel Maguire points out that the new technology puts us in a qualitatively different situation today. Technology has carried us beyond the old legal and ethical positions; that is, to speak of sanctity of life without regard to QOL is to be out of touch with reality. On the other hand, to speak only of QOL without concern for the sanctity of life raises the question, where do we draw the line? Do we "let die" or "mercy kill" the aged, the retarded, the unproductive? "The Freedom to Die," pp. 171–180, in *Bioethics*, ed. by Thomas A. Shannon (New York: Paulist Press, 1976). Oden, op. cit., p. xi. David Belgum, *When It's Your Turn to Decide* (Minneapolis: Augsburg Publishing House, 1978), pp. 57–58, calls QOL the difference between human and animal existence. Others have used the term *vegetative state* when talking about the comatose patient kept alive by machinery. That might be extended to the shelved person who is environmentally encouraged to be nothing. We note also that productive, useful lives are not limited to producing consumer goods for Gross National Product figures. A good QOL might be cultivating a garden or simply enjoying the grandchildren. See Kübler-Ross following. The Catholic Hospital Association says a person's worth comes from relationship to God, rather than one's effectiveness or usefulness to society. Belgum, op. cit., p. 63. Hamilton Southworth points out that the humane physician is as concerned with QOL as with length of life. "Commentary," *Man and Medicine*, no. 3 (Spring 1977), **2**:184–186. Leonard Hayflick reminds us that maximum productivity can occur throughout the life-span. He sees most people as more interested in QOL than in mere longevity. Without enjoyment, the length of life doesn't mean much. He recalls research from the 1930s that shows how to increase longevity as much as 50 percent. It is simply a low-calorie (slightly undernourished), nutritious diet (no malnutrition). It is so simple, but has had few takers. "Aging and the Aged I: Theories of Aging and Anti-Aging Techniques," *EB* **1**:48–53.

5. Kübler-Ross, *Death, The Final Stage of Growth* (Englewood Cliffs, N.J.: Prentice-Hall, Inc., 1975), p. x. Dans and Kerr, op. cit., p. 231. Christopher Lasch, "Aging in a Culture Without a Future," *The Hastings Center Report*, no. 4 (Aug. 1977), **7**:42–44. The Report is cited hereafter as *HCR*. Young, op. cit., p. 66, claims younger people get better hospital care than the aged.

6. Chistiansen, op. cit., pp. 61–62, sees a moral confusion and ambivalence about the aged in modern society. He relates it to the balance or imbalance in work and leisure, freedom and dependence, attitudes toward sickness, and social life. From this, he draws three areas of ethical concern for the elderly: dependency and autonomy (the first increases as the latter decreases), family justice (who is going to support old Mom), and medical care. He thinks health policy and personnel should encourage as much autonomy as possible, perhaps including part-time employment and continuing psychological and spiritual growth for the elderly. Health maintenance through nutrition and exercise and reliance on simpler technologies could ease costs. He is concerned that life-extending technologies should lead to a fuller life and not merely prolong illness. As a special feature of the autonomy-dependency issue, Young is concerned with research on the aged. As a "captive audience," their consent might not be free. They might not be clearly informed. Op. cit., p. 68.

7. In fiscal 1977, people over sixty-five (11 percent of the United States population) spent $41.3 billion, about 30 percent of the American total. (The reader may recall that 20 percent goes for neonatology.) The over sixty-five per capita expenditure is $1,745 compared to $661 for those aged nineteen to sixty-four, and $253 for those under nineteen. Public funding amounted to 67 percent for those over sixty-five, and 29 percent for those nineteen to sixty-four. The elderly go to the hospital twice as often and stay twice as long. Young, op. cit., p. 65. In 1900, there were 3

million Americans over sixty-five (4 percent of the population). This has increased to 23 million (11 percent). In fifty years, by present trends, it will be 55 million. Dans and Kerr, op. cit., p. 228. Their concern is the extent to which medical schools should teach care of the aged. This, too, is an allocation of scarce resources—study time, teaching time, and so on. Robert M. Veatch, *Death, Dying, and the Biological Revolution* (New Haven: Yale University Press, 1976), pp. 3–4. Bernice L. Neugarten notes the division of young-old (ages fifty-five to seventy-five; over 15 percent of the United States population; relatively healthy and vigorous) and the old-old (seventy-five and up; less than 4 percent of the population; disproportionately disadvantaged in health, economics, education). "Aging and the Aged II: Social Implications of Aging," *EB* 1:54–58. Ivan Illich, "The Political Uses of Natural Death," pp. 25–42, in Steinfels and Veatch, op. cit.

8. In real life, the poor tend to be terminated first, and the aged poor first of all. Young, op. cit., p. 66. Oden, op. cit., pp. 57–58, reminds us that costs and financial burden are part of the definition of extraordinary. The 1976 cost of $400 a day for ICU eliminates most of the uninsured poor. Arthur Dyck, "Beneficent Euthanasia and Benemortasia: Alternate Views of Mercy," pp. 117–129, in *Beneficent Euthanasia*, ed. by Marvin Kohl (Buffalo: Prometheus Books, 1975), pp. 126–127. Paul Ramsey, *Ethics at the Edges of Life* (New Haven: Yale University Press, 1978), p. 201. Raymond S. Duff and A. G. M. Campbell, "Moral and Ethical Dilemmas in the Special-Care Nursery," *NEJM*, no. 17 (1973), **298**:890–894. John G. McEllhenney, *Cutting the Monkey Rope* (Valley Forge: Judson Press, 1973), p. 107.

9. R. B. Schiffer and Benjamin Freedman, "The Last Bed in the ICU: A Medical or Moral Decision?" *HCR*, no. 6 (Dec. 1977), **7**:21–22.

10. We've noted this earlier in terms of technology. Modern medicine has overcome smallpox, bacillary and amoebic dysentery, salmonella, syphilis, gonorrhea, leprosy, malaria, cholera, meningitis, tetanus, tuberculosis, yellow fever, typhoid, polio, whooping cough, pellagra, plague, diphtheria, scarlet fever. We could add pneumonia, formerly known as the "old man's friend." Belgum, op. cit., p. 17. Veatch, op. cit., p. 16. Dallas M.

High, "Is 'Natural Death' an Illusion?" *HCR*, no. 4 (Aug. 1978), **8**:37–42. Gary Marotta, "The Enlightenment and Bioethics," pp. 62–65 in *Bioethics and Human Rights*, ed. by Elsie L. and Bertram Bandman (Boston: Little, Brown and Company, 1978). Eric J. Cassell, "Dying in a Technological Society," pp. 42–48, in Steinfels and Veatch, op. cit.

11. Julia and Harry Abrahamson, *Who Shall Live?* (New York: Hill and Wang, 1970), pp. 42–43. Joseph Fletcher, "Technological Devices in Medical Care," pp. 116–136, in *Who Shall Live?* ed. by Kenneth Vaux (Philadelphia: Fortress Press, 1970). Veatch, op. cit., pp. 105–107. "Pope Pius XII: Prolongation of Life," *The Pope Speaks* (1958), **4**:393–398.

12. Not always, notes Maguire, op. cit., p. 180. The distinction of means blurs. The ordinary in medicine may be extraordinary to the recipient in terms of pain, money, or other burden. Edwin F. Healy claims ordinary means may not be required when results are not of sufficient benefit. *Medical Ethics* (Chicago: Loyola University Press, 1956), p. 60. Bernard Häring notes the ordinary in wealthy countries is so extensive, it is not always required. *Medical Ethics* (Slough, England: St. Paul Publications, 1972).

13. Pope Pius XII also thought the respirator was extraordinary. Joseph and Julia Quinlan, *Karen Ann: The Quinlans Tell Their Story* (New York: Doubleday & Company, Inc., 1977). Ramsey, op. cit., pp. 268–299. Kübler-Ross, op. cit., pp. 81, 85, suggests that if the body is kept alive only by machine and the brain waves are flat, she would naturally stop the IV feedings. News reports were mixed on the nature of Karen Ann Quinlan's EEG readings. She was taken off the respirator and moved to a nursing home. As we write, her body continues to function. Tabitha M. Powledge and Peter Steinfels, "Following the News on Karen Quinlan," *HCR*, no. 6 (Dec. 1975), **5**:5–6, 28. Hans Jonas, "The Right to Die," *HCR*, no. 4 (Aug. 1978), **8**:31–36. "Comatose Patient's 'Right to Die'," *The Christian Century*, no. 15 (23 Ap. 1980), **97**:463.

14. Ramsey, op. cit., pp. 145–188. He also wants to drop from our vocabulary euthanasia, direct and indirect, passive and active, useful and useless, reasonable and unreasonable. These are all wrong. Yet, he is willing to let the dying die. He wants (p. 188) to tread a

middle ground between mercy killing and relentless treatment of the dying. This is basically Kübler-Ross' position also. Op. cit., p. 77. She suggests (pp. 56–57) that it is not our job to kill people but to help them live until they die a natural death. Oden, op. cit., pp. 18–19, also wants to drop the terms *ordinary/extraordinary* and *euthanasia*. They are too vague and have too many meanings, including Naziism. Others think the terms continue to have value. McEllhenney, op. cit., pp. 106–108. On the middle ground, he notes (p. 115) that it is best to neither artificially prolong the life of the dying nor artificially induce death in the living. Veatch, op. cit., pp. 77–115. Darrell W. Amundsen, "The Physician's Duty to Prolong Life: A Medical Duty Without Classical Roots," *HCR*, no. 4 (Aug. 1978), 8:23–30. The duty to prolong life appears with Francis Bacon (A.D. 1561–1626), who also saw active euthanasia for the relief of suffering as an essential medical skill. Gruman, op. cit., p. 262. Jonas, op. cit., p. 34. Thomas A. Shannon, "What Guidance From the Guidelines," *HCR*, no. 3 (June 1977), 7:28–30.

15. Elisabeth Kübler-Ross, *Death*, op. cit., p. xix. Veatch, op. cit., p. 3.

16. This, of course, is not as simple as it sounds. Catholics could conditionally administer the final annointing for two hours after death. Maguire, op. cit., p. 173. Some Jewish figures have insisted, contrary to custom, that burial should not take place for three days. Only putrefaction is a sure sign of death. Immanuel Jakobovits, *Jewish Medical Ethics* (New York: Philosophical Library, 1959), p. 128. Paul A. Byrne, "On Death," *Missouri Medicine* (June 1978), pp. 256–258, suggests a definition of death. It is the "dissolution of the organizational and functional unity of a unique individual." He sees death as a process also. The time of death is not known until the process is completed. Veatch, op. cit., pp. 21–76, includes a view of death as the loss of capacity for social interaction. On this basis, many people are "dead" long before they are officially so pronounced. Gaetano F. Molinari, "Definition and Determination of Death I: Criteria for Death," *EB* 1:292–296. Dallas M. High, "III: Philosophical and Theological Foundations," *EB* 1:301–307.

17. Ad Hoc Committee of the Harvard Medical School to Examine the Definition of Brain Death, "A Definition of Irreversible Coma," *The Journal of the American Medical Association* (1968), 205:337–340. The Journal is cited hereafter as *JAMA*. Leonard Isaacs, "Death, Where Is Thy Distinguishing?" *HCR*, no. 1 (Feb. 1978), 8:5–8.

18. "The Right to Die," *The Christian Century*, no. 26 (16–23 Aug. 1978), 95:759, reports on several cases in which courts allowed cessation of treatment. One was a comatose sixty-seven-year-old woman with no hope of recovery. Another was a seventy-three-year-old man's own request to disconnect the respirator. He had amyotrophic lateral sclerosis. See also, "Recent Court Decisions," *American Journal of Law and Medicine*, no. 4 (Winter 1979), 4:423–424. Several years ago, Mary McDermott Shideler suggested a panel of judges to make this type of decision. She thus anticipated such court decisions as these. "Coup de Grace," *The Christian Century*, (7 Dec. 1966), 83:1499–1502. See also, George J. Annas, "The Incompetent's Right to Die: The Case of Joseph Sackewicz," *HCR*, no. 1 (Feb. 1978), 8:21–23, and "After Saikewicz: No-Fault Death," *HCR*, no. 3 (June 1978), 8:16–18. He reports on a number of cases, some of which were allowed termination and some not. He notes that there has never (June 1978) been a criminal indictment for stopping treatment on a terminally ill adult. That's accepted as a medical decision. Stopping treatment on a defective newborn or a retarded adult is not a medical decision. There, the decision should go to court. This is a matter of QOL. Jonas, op. cit., p. 31. Saikewicz was sixty-seven and retarded (mental age less than three). He had leukemia. Treatment had serious side effects including pain. It would have meant a 30 percent to 50 percent chance of remission for three to thirteen months. The court ruled treatment was not required. He died peacefully four months and eighteen days after diagnosis. The decision turned on autonomy. See also, Paul Ramsey, "The Saikewicz Precedent: What's Good For an Incompetent Patient?" *HCR*, no. 6 (Dec. 1978), 8:36–42. John Robertson, "Legal Criteria for Orders Not to Resuscitate," *Medicolegal News* no. 1 (Feb. 1980), 8:4–5, 26. Sissela Bok, "Death and Dying: Euthanasia and Sustaining Life II. Ethical Views," *EB* 1:268–278. Alexander M. Capron, "Definition and Deter-

mination of Death II: Legal Aspects of Pronouncing Death," *EB* **1**:296–301, notes that courts rely on precedents that do not apply in new situations.

19. In one sense, this chapter is about the quality of our dying. Kübler-Ross is interested in the quality of our living while we die. In her work and that of the hospice movement (see following), people do not ask for the right to die. Kübler-Ross and Mal Warshaw, *To Live Until We Say Goodbye* (Englewood Cliffs, N.J.: Prentice-Hall, Inc., 1978), p. 21. See also, John Knoble, "Living to the End," *Modern Maturity* (Aug.-Sept. 1977), pp. 63–64. Eric J. Cassell, "The Function of Medicine," *HCR*, no. 6 (Dec. 1977), **7**:16–19, says it is life that matters, not death, to medicine and to mankind. Lasch, op. cit., p. 44. Daniel Callahan discusses the idea that life itself is evil, so there's no sense in prolonging it. That seems a dismal view, which taken literally, would welcome death. "On defining a 'natural death,' " *HCR*, no. 3 (June 1977), **7**:32–37. See also n. 4.

20. Euthanasia Educational Council, 250 W. Fifty-seventh St., New York, N.Y. 10019. Thelma M. Schorr, "The Right to Die," *The American Journal of Nursing*, no. 1 (Jan. 1976), **76**:53. The Journal is cited hereafter as *AJN*.

21. The California Natural Death Act (1976) provides for a living will with very careful protections against coercion and forgery, and for changes of mind. It applies only to terminal situations, as determined by the attending physician and at least one other physician. *Extraordinary means* was eliminated from the language of the bill, and was replaced by *life-sustaining*. Michael Garland, "Politics, Legislation, and Natural Death," *HCR*, no. 5 (Oct. 1976), **6**:5–6. Veatch, op. cit., pp. 176–186. High, *HCR*, op. cit., pp. 40–41. Karen Lebacqz almost got the bill vetoed. She thinks our moral traditions already provide for cessation of treatment. Because the bill covers very limited circumstances, it will become harder to die for those not covered by the bill. "On 'Natural Death,' " *HCR*, no. 2 (Apr. 1977), **7**:14. Callahan, op. cit., pp. 32–37, claims natural death is a social concept rather than a medical one. Ramsey, op. cit., pp. 318–332, believes living wills depersonalize by taking judgments out of the hands of physicians and families. For him, natural death acts are counterproductive, but the carefully worded California act protects against euthanasia. Ramsey seems to take away with one hand and give with the other. Oden, op. cit., pp. 16–18, doubts the legality of living wills. They are too vaguely worded. Another view is that living wills help self-determination. This would seem to personalize the patient. How it depersonalizes others is not clear. McEllhenny, op. cit., p. 111.

22. Ramsey, op. cit., pp. 146–147, says we have no right to refuse medically indicated treatment (ordinary versus extraordinary), anymore than we have a right to ruin our health. Doctors decide what is medically indicated (pp. 181–188). He admits (p. 156) that more and more extraordinary treatments have become ordinary, that is, medically indicated. Shannon, *Bioethics*, op. cit., p. 6, reminds us that scientific terminology does not mean the issue is value-free. Grumann, op. cit., p. 263, notes the point at which medicine changes from attempts to cure to letting die is based not on biology, but social considerations, including money. One could speculate that Ramsey has here shifted supreme authority from God, Pope, or Bible, to the physician, who has been called the high priest of modern society, a position which Jacques Barzun says is losing ground, "The Professions Under Siege," *Harper's Magazine*, no. 1541 (Oct. 1978), **257**:61–68. It's a position some doctors refuse or hold most uncomfortably. See Duff and Campbell, op. cit., p. 894. Belgum, op. cit., p. 18, finds many doctors relieved to be off the divine pedestal. Others continue to claim the authority Ramsey suggests. David H. Smith, "Fatal Choices: Recent Discussions of Dying," *HCR*, no. 2 (Apr. 1977), **7**:8–10. Shideler, op. cit., p. 1501, excludes doctors and clergy from the final decision to terminate treatment. They are, or should be, too personally involved. She says nothing about nurses, which is true of most of the literature. In the Quinlan case, the high court of New Jersey spread out doctors' responsibilities to colleagues and family, and a hospital ethics committee or the like. Jan Wojcik, *Muted Consent* (West Lafayette, Ind.: Purdue University Press, 1978), pp. 111–112. "In the Matter of Karen Quinlan, An Alleged Incompetent," New Jersey Superior Court 227 (1976), 57–58. See also, Helmut Thielicke, "The Doctor as Judge of Who Shall Live and

Who Shall Die," pp. 146–186, in Vaux, op. cit. After the Quinlan case, the state of New Jersey and New Jersey medical groups adopted rules for a committee of doctors to decide if the attending physicians could pull the plug. Tom Ferrell and Virginia Adams, "Ideas and Trends: N.J. Sets Up the Quinlan Guidelines," *New York Times* (30 Jan. 1977), E 7. Shannon, *HCR*, op. cit., 7:29. The American Medical Association Judicial Council Report (A–77) on "Terminal Illness" notes that it is the decision of the patient and/or the immediate family to decide on stopping extraordinary means. The advice and judgment of the physician is to be available. Jerry J. Griffin, "Family Decision," *AJN*, no. 5 (May 1975), **75**:794–796. Jonas, op. cit., p. 34, agrees that a patient can say "enough" but malpractice policy might make medical personnel cautious about hastening to comply. Shannon, *HCR*, op. cit., 7:28, cautions that the treatment refusal must be competent and not a temporary distortion from pain or medication. Only one of the four sets of guidelines he surveys acknowledges the competent patient. The others have decisions controlled by the physicians. Oden, op. cit., p. 91. McEllhenney, op. cit., p. 110, believes that life is a gift from God, and so is death. High, *HCR*, op. cit., p. 37. Robert M. Veatch, "Death and Dying: Euthanasia and Sustaining Life III. Professional and Public Policies," *EB* 1:278–286. "Kübler-Ross believes that in the end, it is our life, suggesting ownership of life rather than stewardship. *Questions and Answers*, op. cit., p. 148.

23. This is a key issue for Kübler-Ross also. Kübler-Ross and Warshaw, op. cit., p. 22. On p. 79, she notes the hostility of the medical staff to a patient's decision to *not* have chemotherapy. In her early work, she faced considerable hostility from her medical colleagues. This is attributed to the failure of nurses, doctors, and others to come to grips with their own feelings about death. For many, patients have no right to die. *Death*, op. cit., p. xix. She thinks that physicians have been trained to see dying patients as a failure by the doctor. *Questions and Answers*, p. 79. Richard Schulz and David Aderman found this to be the case with nurses and others, as well. "How the Medical Staff Copes with Dying Patients: A Critical Review," *Omega*, no. 1 (1976), 7:11–21. At least one survey suggested doctors and nurses plan together to not prolong life unnecessarily, as in deteriorating cancer patients who develop a fever. "Doctors 'Not Guilty' of Prolonging Life at Any Cost," *HCR*, no. 4 (Aug. 1979), 9:2–3.

Oden, op. cit., pp. 17, 30–31, argues strongly that self-determination is not an absolute right. There is no right to commit suicide. There is no constitutional right to die. Oden speaks from a Protestant perspective. Healy, op. cit., p. 10, notes a similar thought from a Roman Catholic perspective. Life belongs to God. One aspect of self-determination is informed consent and truth telling, that is, autonomy requires accurate knowledge. The patient's right to know is a moral issue and sometimes a legal one. Roland R. Yarling, "Ethical Analysis of a Nursing Problem: The Scope of Nursing Practice in Disclosing the Truth to Terminal Patients," Parts I and II, *Supervisor Nurse*, no. 5 (May 1978), 9:40–50, and no. 6 (June 1978), 9:28–34. Veatch, op. cit., *Revolution*, pp. 204–248. Häring, op. cit., pp. 127–131. Beatrice K. Kastenbaum and Rachel E. Spector, "What Should a Nurse Tell a Cancer Patient," *AJN*, no. 4 (Apr. 1978), **78**:640–641. Lucie Y. Kelly, "The Patient's Right to Know," *Nursing Outlook*, no. 1 (Jan. 1976), **24**:26–32.

24. Nurses do much, if not most, of this caring. Dr. Samuel C. Klagsbrun says they have to because doctors run from the dying. Quoted by Schorr, op. cit. The review of Schulz and Aderman, op. cit., suggests the whole staff "runs." Thus, there is a real challenge in Joy K. Ufema's words, "Dare to Care for the Dying," *AJN*, no. 1 (Jan. 1976), **76**:88–90.

The modern hospital, committed to cure, faces a real problem here. Death is an embarrassment, a threat to professional roles. Kübler-Ross, *Death*, op. cit., p. 7, and pp. 7–24, "The Organizational Context of Dying," by Hans O. Mauksch. Ramsey, op. cit., p. 151. He claims (pp. 300–318) that we have no right to withhold treatment from others if the treatment is lifesaving, whether the others are minors, incompetent (retarded), or in a coma. It is only when the patient is truly dying that we move from cure to care. His position seems to be that when in doubt, treat. The QOL is *not* to be considered. Veatch, op. cit., *Revolution*, pp. 103–104,

116–163. High, *HCR*, op. cit., p. 42. Cassell, op. cit., pp. 16–19, concludes on the basis of patient autonomy, when in doubt, treat. His position is similar to Kübler-Ross' at this point.

25. European law is moving toward a similar right to terminate treatment but still denies direct or active euthanasia. Clarence Blomquist, "A New Era in European Medical Ethics," *HCR*, no. 2 (Apr. 1976), **6**:7–8. "Swiss Guidelines on Care of the Dying," *HCR*, no. 3 (June 1977), **7**:30–31.

Cassell, op. cit., pp. 16–19, suggests that treatment refusal depends on the situation. A dialysis patient or a religious believer is probably known to the medical staff; that is, the patient is a known quantity. Thus, such patients are more likely to be accepted as autonomous, refusing treatment and knowing what they are doing. An unknown person is more of an unknown factor. The refusal of treatment may be judged temporary incompetence from pain, shock, or medication. When in doubt, treat.

Elderly patients who refused treatment have been called suicidal. Kübler-Ross, *Questions and Answers*, op. cit., pp. 147–148, suggests checking on the stage of dying. If the patient is depressed, get him/her out of the depression and ask again. If the patient still refuses treatment, it is one's right. It is one's life and body. Oden, op. cit., pp. x, 12, also raises the depression angle and adds that patients may not know what is best for themselves. David L. Jackson and Stuart Youngner discuss the complications with a series of case study examples, illustrating the range of difficulties in "Patient Autonomy and 'Death with Dignity,' " *NEJM*, no. 8 (23 Aug. 1979), **301**:404–408. See also, Steven S. Spencer, " 'Code' or 'No Code': A Nonlegal Opinion," *NEJM*, no. 3 (18 Jan. 1979), **300**:138–140. One approach here is the Golden Rule: "Do unto others as you would have others do unto you."

Therapy that continues life, that is, the patient is not dying but needs the therapy to live, is even more problematic. The patient, possibly faced with a low QOL (agonizing pain, for example), may refuse the therapy. Medical personnel are here in an even vaguer area of ethics and legality. They are protected legally if they continue treatment. Ethically, it may violate the Hippocratic "do no harm" concept and the religious/philosophical concepts of mercy. Nevertheless, some say self-determination and consent are limited principles and medical people (Parent) have a right to do what they think is necessary for the good of the patient (Child). See Wojcik, op. cit., p. 93. In the Quinlan case, the first court decision gave the doctors, rather than the parents, the right to decide. Oden, op. cit., pp. 11–12, notes that refusal of treatment will work better if the patient does not enter the hospital. It's harder to get out than in. Although theoretically you can refuse treatment and leave, your very entrance gives consent that you may not get back. He finds (pp. 33–35) parallels between treatment refusal and suicide, and suggests a guideline: the greater the opportunity for continued meaningful life, the more traditional morals and ethics stand against treatment termination, as against suicide and murder. See Bok, op. cit., pp. 270–272. Leroy G. Augenstein, *Come, Let Us Play God* (New York: Harper & Row, Publishers, 1969), p. 52. The Patient's Bill of Rights (American Hospital Association) claims patients can refuse treatment to the extent permitted by law. Belgum, op. cit., p. 19. Steven S. Spencer claims a mentally competent patient always has the right to say no. The opinion of the incompetent person's family does not have the same weight. He agrees that "who decides" is a moral question rather than a medical one. "Sounding Board: 'Code' or 'No Code': A Nonlegal opinion," *NEJM*, no. 3 (18 Jan. 1979), **300**:138–140. Shideler, op. cit., p. 1501, and "What Recourse for the Hopelessly Ill?" *The Christian Century*, (1 Mar. 1967), **84**:272–273, insists that life is social. As in marriage and birth, society needs to be a part of a decision to die. In contrast, the Quinlan case and some other legal decisions have turned on the individual's right to privacy. See also, Robert B. White and H. Tristam Engelhardt, Jr., "A Demand to Die," *HCR*, no. 3 (June 1975), **5**:9–10, 47. Hugo A. Bedau, "The Right to Die by Firing Squad," *HCR*, no. 1 (Feb. 1977), **7**:5–7.

26. Legally, it appears that one does not have a constitutional right to die. In a case involving religious freedom (*J.F.K. Memorial Hospital* v. *Heston*), the court gave the hospital permission to give a blood transfusion to a

member of Jehovah's Witnesses. One is free to believe, but not necessarily to practice a belief. Oden, op. cit., pp. 15, 30–33.

Although the glories of heaven attracted early Christians, McEllhenney, op. cit., p. 116, warns against suicide talk on psychological grounds. The more we talk about it, the more people will try it—the old power of suggestion. How true this is is not clear, but he quotes the statistic that if anyone in a child's immediate world commits suicide, the chances the child will also increase 75 percent. Veatch, *Revolution*, op. cit., pp. 237–238, reports very little or no suicidal tendencies in studies of the terminally ill. Yet, one of the common excuses for not telling the terminally ill how sick they are is the idea that the patient will give up hope. One wonders if at this point staff members are talking to themselves rather than the patients.

27. Bok, op. cit., pp. 274–277. More than eighty Americans kill themselves every day. Between 6 and 7 million Americans have tried it. Of these, 25 percent will try again and succeed. Two to three times more women than men try it, but men are more successful (guns are surer than pills). Maguire points out that the first moral/ethical concern should be the correction of the causes. Rather than talking about life as a gift, he sees suicide as a loss of hope and, hence, the sin of a lack of faith. Although self-killing is murder, he follows Protestant Dietrich Bonhoeffer in reserving judgment. Saul (I Samuel 31:5) and Samson (Judges 16:30) in the Bible killed themselves with no apparent protest by the biblical writers. Maguire notes that virgins have committed suicide to avoid rape. The Israelis honor the nearly 1,000 people who committed murder and suicide at Masada rather than be captured by the Romans. In this country, people have committed suicide to protest social and military policies of the government. Robert E. Neal, *The Art of Dying* (New York: Harper & Row, Publishers, 1971), pp. 49–70, claims that suicide statistics are understated. Many suicides are reported as accidents. If we add indirect suicides (car accidents, drunkenness, smoking in the face of lung cancer, overeating, and so on), the numbers increase even more. Cahn, op. cit., p. 237, points out the self-determination or choice in such deaths as Socrates, Jesus, and

the Christian martyrs. These deaths, of course, were not suicides in the face of despair, but death for a purpose. Not all would agree with the purpose. Amundsen, op. cit., p. 26, notes that in the ancient Greco-Roman world, the free man had an inherent right to dispose of his life. Few voices were raised against this until the Classical period waned and Christianity rose in influence. Interestingly enough, Augustine was heavily influenced by the Stoics, but he ignored their aproval of suicide. James Gutman, "Death III: Western Philosophical Thought," *EB* 1:235–243.

28. "Murder Charges Dropped in 'Mercy' Deaths," *New York Post* (30 Mar. 1979), 65.

29. Oden, op. cit., pp. 36–68, reports on the Drew ad hoc committee on Treatment Termination (Drew University, Madison, N.J.). The committee concluded that there are three levels of influencing factors for treatment termination: primary indicators, secondary influences, and special considerations. There are five primary factors: permanently impaired cognition, patient consent, family consent, medical consent, imminent death. There are three secondary factors: discomfort, unsalvageable physical disability, limited equipment or medical resources. There are four special considerations: age and life expectancy, degree to which life support invades the body, cost, moral and religious values. All primary factors need to be present before treatment termination, or the other factors need to be especially strong if any primary indicator is absent.

30. Bok, op. cit., pp. 269–270. This same hospital later notified a friend of her husband's death. The notification was by telephone with a command to get the body out of there. Kübler-Ross objects to this. Notification should be by the physician or designated representative, in a quiet room where the family can have support from nurses, clergy, and others. *Questions and Answers*, op. cit., p. 63. This is a wise strategy. Sometimes one can distinguish strategy and ethics, and sometimes they are interwoven or overlap. The ethics in notification of death might be seen in terms of human dignity, the covenant concept of medical care, the Golden Rule of Hillel and Jesus, the biblical concept of love thy neighbor as thyself, Kant's principle of

universality (what would the world be like if everyone did this?), or just plain human decency. Paul Ramsey, *HCR*, no. 6, **8**:37, claims competent and incompetent patients have a right not to be neglected to death, purposefully or inadvertently.

31. An indirect case that is also an act of commission is giving pain-killers that may or will hasten death. If the intent is to relieve pain, the side effect may be acceptable. Once more, we have the principle of double effect, as in removing a cancerous uterus when the woman is pregnant, thus secondarily performing an abortion. Bok, op. cit., p. 273. Oden, op. cit., p. 24. Belgum, op. cit., p. 60, notes that a living will can be written to include medication, even if the medication hastens death in terminal illness. Veatch, op. cit., pp. 82–93, lists five distinctions between actions and omissions in causing or allowing death: 1) they are psychologically different; 2) active or direct killing conflicts with the physician's role (and the nurse's role, we might add); 3) the intent is different; 4) long-range effects differ (Veatch refers here to the fear of promoting Nazi-type exterminations); and 5) the cause of death differs.

32. Euthanasia has been around for a long time. The Hippocratic Oath forbids giving a deadly drug. This is sometimes interpreted as against euthanasia and suicide, as well as against murder. In the sense of mercy killing, the term goes back to William E. H. Lecky in 1869. Jewish laws and most traditional Christians forbid direct euthanasia, as does most civil law. Letting the dying die is accepted in Jewish law and by some Christians. It is one interpretation of the Pius XII statement on extraordinary means. Jakobovits, op. cit., pp. 123–125. Joseph Fletcher, "Ethics and Euthanasia," *AJN*, no. 4 (Apr. 1973), **73**:670–675, claims passive or negative euthanasia is a normal thing. Daily, hundreds are allowed to die. The only issue is positive euthanasia, helping the dying die. He argues that because the consequences are the same as in passive euthanasia, this, too, may be appropriate. It is the humane and good that determines which we will do. Ramsey, op. cit., p. 324, notes that mercy killing is carefully forbidden in the California Natural Death Act. Keith I. Pohl reminds us that there is a wide spectrum in belief. For some, euthanasia and suicide may be wrong, but they could be the lesser of the two evils when one is faced with horrible suffering. "The Good Death: When, If Ever?" *The Circuit Rider*, no. 4 (Apr. 1979), **3**:6–7. Veatch, *Revolution*, op. cit., p. 77–115. Kübler-Ross, *Questions and Answers*, op. cit., p. 75, calls letting someone die his own death the good death of euthanasia. She opposes direct or mercy killing. She recognizes that real life situations are not that simple. The Judicial Council of the AMA, Report A–77, "Terminal Illness," speaks against mercy killing.

Sometimes the Nazis are accused of practicing euthanasia. Their policies were neither "good death" nor "mercy killing," but systematic murder that was unmerciful. Peter Steinfels, ed., "Biomedical Ethics and the Shadow of Nazism," *HCR*, no. 4 (Aug. 1976), special supplement, **6**:1–18. St. Thomas More's book *Utopia* (1516) first outlined an organized system of euthanasia for the terminally ill. Gruman, op. cit., p. 263.

A case might be made for mercy in medical treatment. That could be a principle or rule as in the deontological approach to ethics. Unmerciful treatment would thus be wrong, but the utilitarian approach would allow this if the expected consequences are good, that is, the health or betterment of the patient, or new experimental knowledge that could help others. This is an example of the old charge against the utilitarians that they proclaim an ethic in which the "end justifies the means." This is a charge made against the Nazi regime. When a terminal patient is going to die regardless of the treatment, no matter how merciful or unmerciful the treatment, the "end" may be the practitioner's curiosity or research interest, which puts him or her into the Nazi tradition. Mercy would favor the welfare of the patient rather than serving the ends of the practitioners. Bok, op. cit., pp. 268, 274, claims every society has tried to set limits on killing but the limits may collide with the demand for mercy in a time of intolerable suffering. To continue treatment under hopeless conditions may constitute assault and battery.

33. Hospice people note that euthanasia is not a problem. People who are living until they die do not ask for termination. Ramsey, op. cit., pp. 152–153. Dr. Cicely Saunders

began the modern hospice movement about 1950. She is Medical Director of St. Christopher's Hospice in London, England. Cicely Saunders, "Living with Dying," *Man and Medicine* 1, no. 3 (Spring 1976), pp. 227–244. Austin H. Kutscher, "Commentary," *Man and Medicine* 1, no. 3 (Spring 1976), pp. 245–246, notes she was trained as a nurse and then as a social worker before becoming a physician. In her own person, she represents the multidisciplinary approach to caring for the terminally ill. Janet Plant, "Finding a Home for Hospice Care in the United States," *Hospitals* (1 July 1977), **51**:53–62. "A Better Way to Care for the Dying," *Changing Times*, no. 4 (Apr. 1979), **33**:21–23. Knoble, op. cit., p. 63, notes that hospice personnel are trained to treat patients as persons rather than things. This view might be related to Kant's idea that people are an end in themselves rather than a means to an end.

34. Kübler-Ross attributes the word to the Swiss mountain passes where the monks with the famous St. Bernard dogs rescued and cared for travelers in the Hospice of St. Bernard. Kübler-Ross and Warshaw, op. cit., p. 137. The National Hospice Organization (765 Prospect Street, New Haven, Conn. 06511), also notes the origin in medieval Europe by religious orders. They suggest the word means a community for sojourners along the way, a place of care and refreshment. "Hospice in America," p. 2.

35. "A Better Way . . ," op. cit., p. 21, reports for April 1979 seventy-five hospices providing care and another 150 in the planning stages. The first in this country was in New Haven, Conn. The second was in Boonton, N.J., which is the first to have a separate in-patient facility. It's a ranch-style home set in rolling acres. A sunken living room provides visiting area for patients and families. It overlooks a pond with ducks and a wooded picnic area. Other hospices are in Kentfield, California; Tucson, Arizona; New York City; Los Angeles, and Cincinnati.

36. When asked why she had no ICU, Dr. Saunders said that all they had there was intensive care. Ramsey, op. cit., pp. 152–153. No machinery is used in hospices. Kübler-Ross, *Questions and Answers*, op. cit., p. 75, claims that the questions that come up in this country do not occur there. They apply "the true art of medicine." Patients are surrounded with love, faith, and excellent medical-emotional support. Patients live until they die.

37. One aspect of the comfort is the elimination of shots, which the family may not be able to administer. Pain medication can be given orally. One type is the famous Brompton mixture, which includes morphine or heroin. Some ethicists have objected to addiction-producing drugs. Others say drug addiction is scarcely a problem for the terminally ill. Kübler-Ross says that in all the years she and her colleagues have used the Brompton mix, they have never had an overdose or drug addiction. Kübler-Ross and Warshaw, op. cit., p. 63. A. Jann Davis, "Brompton's Cocktail: Making Goodbyes Possible," *AJN*, no. 4 (Apr. 1978), **78**:610–612. *A Primer on the Brompton Cocktail* (Indianapolis: Methodist Hospital of Indiana, 1979, 2nd. ed. (mimeographed; $1 for costs and postage: 1604 N. Capitol, Indianapolis, Ind. 46202.) The report is based on treatment of more than 1,200 patients. The name is from the Brompton Chest Hospital in London. Home care is being extended in other ways, too, so this is not limited to the hospice concept. Lynne S. Ostrow, "Intensive Respiratory Care: From ICU to Home," *AJN*, no. 1 (Jan. 1976), **76**:111–112.

38. The AMA House of Delegates approved the concept of hospice in June 1978. "Hospice in America," op. cit., p. 5. Kübler-Ross and Warshaw, op. cit., p. 22, note that 75 percent of our population die in hospitals. The hospice movement is helping more people to stay home or at least have family and friends with them when they die. Knoble, op. cit., p. 22. Belgum, op. cit., p. 58, notes that children do not catch cancer or old age. Some people try to shield children from death rather than letting it be part of life.

39. This concern appears elsewhere in the life cycle, too. Susan A. Yates, "Stillbirth—What Staff Can Do," *AJN*, no. 9 (Sept. 1972), **72**:1592–1594, reports on concern for the mothers of stillborns.

40. The holistic approach to health care can be applied throughout the life cycle. That includes treatment for older people. Niel Fiore, "Fighting Cancer—One Patient's Perspective," *NEJM*, no. 6 (8 Feb. 1979),

300:284–289, reminds us that the patient's attitude is important and the practice of medicine is more than removing a tumor. He does not mention nurses in his health teams. In reality, they carry a major responsibility in health care. See also, Sally Guttmacher, "Whole in Body, Mind, and Spirit: Holistic Health and the Limits of Medicine," *HCR*, no. 2 (Apr. 1979), **9**:15–21.

41. At this stage in the movement, costs are hard to pin down. Home care costs less. The in-patient facility costs are equivalent to the ICU (Plant, op. cit., p. 61). Generally, hospice does not use X-ray, diagnostic tests, chemotherapy, or extensive surgery. One claim is for 50 percent less than general hospital care. Knoble, op. cit., pp. 63–64. "A Better Way," p. 23 notes $147 a day (Apr. 1979) in Washington, D.C., for in-patient care. A six-month demonstration project in Rochester, N.Y., suggested costs of 50 percent or less. The home-hospice program involved two stages. Stage I (mostly family care) averaged $40 a day, and Stage II (24-hour a day nursing care) averaged $117 a day. Anthony Amado, Beatrice A. Cronk, and Rich Mileo, "Cost of Terminal Care: Home Hospice vs. Hospital," *Nursing Outlook*, no. 8 (Aug. 1979), **27**:522–526. In some situations, care to the patient is free. Costs are covered by contributions, the American Cancer Society, and some health insurance programs. Hospice in New Haven is building a unit financed in part by government funds. As we write, government funding is under consideration for operations as well. Kübler-Ross and Warshaw, op. cit., pp. 137–147. We might add the reminder that dollars are only part of the costs in medical care. Hospice lowers the costs of isolation and its psychological effects. Constant medication lowers the debilitating costs of pain. The quality of life is raised for those patients who live while dying.

42. The hospice movement is by no means universally accepted. Some fear competition for health dollars in the allocation of scarce resources. Some see hospice as nothing new, simply good medical care that must be kept within the mainstream. What's more, because we can't build enough hospices, we should not build any. This view is strikingly similar to the empty lifeboat ethic that says because we cannot save all, we must save

none. Plant, op. cit., p. 62. Cahn, op. cit., p. 71. Henry O. Heinemann describes this history of hospitals as moving from care to cure with the help of scientific medicine. The latter is not designed to care for the terminally ill in his view. "Incurable Illness and the Hospital of the Twentieth Century," *Man and Medicine*, no. 4 (Summer 1976), **1**:281–285.

43. Death as the enemy has long been a standard. Fiore, op. cit., p. 285. Sidney Callahan and James F. Childress, "Regulating an Anti-Aging Drug," *HCR*, no. 3 (June 1978), **8**:19–20. Veatch, *Revolution*, op. cit., pp. 284–286. Ramsey, op. cit., p. 147. A Roman Catholic thinker, Dr. Gerald P. Ruane, notes that life is a gift, but how we face death determines our view of that gift. He finds that death provokes the whole gamut of emotions: fear, anger, resentment, frustration, futility, joy, acceptance, peace, resignation, hope, faith. He sees it as a second birth to the Judeo-Christian concept of heaven. There is no evidence that his view has encouraged suicide as in an earlier day. *Birth to Birth: The Life-Death Mystery* (New York: Alba House, 1976). Brian P. Copenhaven, "Death IV: (4) Ars Moriendi (The Art of Dying)," *EB* **1**:254–255, notes that in the Middle Ages death was seen not as an end, but the beginning. There was no need for heroic measures to postpone it. Kübler-Ross also see attitudes toward death as influencing attitudes toward life. We can only truly live when we come to terms with our own death. *Questions and Answers*, op. cit., p. 156. We have not learned how to live if we have not learned how to die, says anthropologist Ashley Montagu, *Immortality, Religion, and Morals* (New York: Hawthorne Books, Inc., 1971), p. 46. Lasch, op. cit., p. 44, claims the pro-longevity movement is neurotic, lacking an adequate view of life. Amundsen, op. cit., pp. 23–30, notes the rise of pro-longevity as a medical concern in the late sixteenth century. Daniel Callahan, *HCR*, no. 3, op. cit., **7**:34–35, comments on the prolongation as evil, but death is also evil. See also his observation on the range of attitudes in the Preface, pp. xiii–x, in Steinfels and Veatch, op. cit. Many religions have traditions that life was originally immortal. Death came through carelessness or as punishment for sin. Others see death as present from the beginning or as the "natural" end of

life. Both traditions appear in the Judeo-Christian and Islamic traditions. The well-known story of Adam and Eve represents the punishment motif, but throughout the Hebrew Scriptures is the attitude that death is normal, symbolized by the phrasing, "gathered to his fathers" (II Samuel 7:12). Frank Reynolds, "The Lizard, the Chameleon, and the Future Buddha," *HCR*, no. 3 (June 1977), **7**:38–44. Gutmann, op. cit., p. 239, notes Ecclesiastes 3:2, "a time to be born and a time to die." Lloyd Bailey, "Death IV: Western Religious Thought (1) Death in Biblical Thought," *EB* **1**:243–246. McEllehenney, op. cit., p. 109, suggests that what God has overcome we can welcome as a friend. Again, the biblical view varies from peace (Genesis 15:15) to enemy (I Corthinthains 15:55). One major facet of this is the concept of life after death, common to many religions and believed by people who are not otherwise religious. In some cases, death is still an enemy, but it is overcome or transcended by life after life (Wisdom of Solomon 1:13; Daniel 12:1–3; I Corinthaians 15:53–54). Traditional views include heaven for the faithful and punishment for the unfaithful. The latter may increase the fear of death for those who expect such punishment, but hope for heaven has brought reassurance and peace. Montagu, op. cit., pp. 40–43, 52. Ruth I. Stoll, "Guidelines for Spiritual Assessment," *AJN*, no. 9 (Sept. 1979), 1574–1577. Raymond Moody, Jr., *Life After Life* (New York: Bantam Books, 1976). John H. Hick, *Death and Eternal Life* (New York: Harper & Row, Publishers, 1977). Michael Marsh, "Beyond Death: The Rebirth of Immortality," *HCR*, no. 5 (Oct. 1977), **1**:40–42. Saunders, op. cit., p. 244. Seymour Siegel, "Death IV: Western Religious Thought (2) Post-Biblical Jewish Tradition," *EB* **1**:246–249. Richard A. Kalish, "Attitudes Toward Death," *EB* **1**:286–291.

McEllehenney, op. cit., p. 111, quotes the Euthanasia Educational Fund's living will as saying people do not fear death. They fear the indignity of deterioration, dependence, and hopeless pain. Ulfema, op. cit., p. 89, reminds us that inhumanity is the enemy rather than death.

44. Until recently, death as a topic of conversation was rather deadly, about as popular as sex in Victorian England. Funerals continue the old process of pretending it's not there. The greatest comment is, "He looks so natural." Goeffrey Gorer, *Death, Grief, and Mourning* (London: The Cressett Press, 1965), pp. 169–175. Maguire, op. cit., p. 171. Häring, op. cit., p. 128. David H. Smith, op. cit., p. 8. Gutmann, op. cit., p. 242. Peter Steinfels recognizes that death may not become as popular as sex but, as a discussion topic, it's doing all right. "Introduction," pp. 1–6, in Steinfels and Veatch, op. cit.

45. She says her work really began in postwar Poland. While doing relief work, she saw the concentration camp of Maidanek, death scene for hundreds of thousands of Hitler's six million Jewish victims. A Jewish girl who had lost her entire family was busy helping with the relief work. She taught Kübler-Ross that one can face death without bitterness. Her first lecture on death and dying was in 1964 in Denver, Colorado, where she was teaching psychiatry. Kübler-Ross and Warshaw, op. cit., p. 18. On page 152, she describes Shanti Nilaya, "Final Home of Peace," her own growth and healing center. It opened in November 1977 in the mountains above Escondido, California. In her work, she has found five stages of death: denial (not me), anger (why me?), bargaining, depression, and acceptance. The stages vary in order and may occur simultaneously. *Questions and Answers*, op. cit., pp. x–xii, 123–125. See also, Kübler-Ross, *On Death and Dying* (New York: Macmillan Publishing Co., Inc., 1969).

46. Kübler-Ross' concern is to help the dying live. A group with a similar aim is called "Make Today Count," founded by Orville Kelly, 218 S. Sixth Street, Burlington, Iowa. There are now MTC units throughout the country. Members share one another's burdens and live by the biblical injunction: "This is the day which the Lord hath made, let us rejoice and be glad in it." (Psalm 118:24). Shideler, "Coup . . ." op. cit., p. 1502, notes that we are ready to die to the degree that we are able to live.

47. P. E. Dans and M. R. Kerr, "Gerontology and Geriatrics in Medical Education," *NEJM*, no. 5 (1 Feb. 1979), **300**:231. D. L. Berg and C. Isler, "The Right to Die Dilemma: Where Do You Fit In?" *RN*, August 1977, p. 53. Betty L. Hopping, "Nursing Students' Attitudes Toward Death," *Nursing Research*, no.

ETHICS AND THE LATER YEARS **207**

6 (Nov./Dec. 1977), **26**:443. Anne Davis and Mila Aroskar, *Ethical Dilemmas and Nursing Practice* (New York: Appleton-Century-Crofts, 1977), Chapter Seven, "Dying and Death," pp. 111–135.

48. J. J. Skillman, "Ethical Dilemmas in the Care of the Critically Ill," *Lancet*, (14 Sept. 1974), 634–637. Jack Tinker, "General Intensive Therapy," *Nursing Times* **74**:266–268.

49. Skillman, op. cit., p. 635.

50. Tinker, op. cit., p. 268. Skillman, op. cit., p. 634. A. M. Parkam, "Last Rights—Letter to the Editor," *NEJM*, no. 20 (11 Nov. 1976), **295**: 1139. R. Roettinger, "Letter to the Editor," *NEJM*, no. 20 (11 Nov. 1976), **295**:1140. V. A. Bishop, "A Nurse's View of Ethical Problems in Intensive Care and Clinical Research," *British Journal of Anesthesia* **50**:515 (1978).

51. Skillman, op. cit., p. 636.

52. Dale Wittner, "Life or Death?" *Today's Health*, March 1974, 48–53. Berg and Isler, op. cit., p. 50. J. Beauchamp, "Euthanasia and the Nurse-Practitioner," *Nursing Forum*, no. 1 (1975), **14**:49.

53. M. A. McGuire, "Have You Ever Let a Patient Die by Default?" *RN*, Nov. 1977, p. 58.

54. Berg and Isler, op. cit., p. 49.

55. McGuire, op. cit., p. 58. Berg and Isler, op. cit., p. 53.

56. David Popoff, "What Are Your Feelings About Death and Dying? Part II," *Nursing*, no. 10 (Oct. 1975), **5**:41. Wittner, op. cit., p. 61.

57. Popoff, op. cit., pp. 40, 42. Beauchamp, op. cit., p. 61.

58. ANA *Code for Nurses With Interpretive Statements* (Kansas City: ANA, 1976).

59. Rita J. Payton, "Information Control and Autonomy," *Nursing Clinics of North America*, no. 1 (Mar. 1979), **14**:23–33.

60. Ibid., p. 25.

61. Berg and Isler, op. cit., p. 52. Priscilla Johnson, "The Gray Areas—Who Decides?" *AJN*, no. 5 (May 1977), **77**:856–858. Sylvia C. Gendrop, "The Order: No Code," *Linacre Quarterly*, no. 4 (Nov. 1977), **41**:312–319.

62. Beauchamp, op. cit., p. 70.

63. See also, Michele Anne Cawley, "Euthanasia: Should It Be A Choice?" *AJN*, no. 5 (May 1977), **77**:859–861. Chapter Six, "Helping the Patient to Die," in Loretta S. Bermosk and Raymond J. Corsini, *Critical Incidents in*

Nursing (Philadelphia: W. B. Saunders Company, 1973), pp. 54–65.

64. Payton, op. cit., p. 63. N. H. Cassem and H. Pontoppodan, "Letter to the Editor," *NEJM*, no. 20 (11 Nov. 1976), **295**: 1142.

65. Popoff II, op. cit., p. 40. Elsie Bandman and Bertram Bandman, "The Nurse's Role in Protecting the Patient's Right to Live or Die," *Advances in Nursing Science*, no. 3 (Apr. 1979), **1**:21–35.

66. Chapter Fourteen, "The Doctor Lets the Patient Die," in Bermosk and Corsini, op. cit., pp. 127–133.

67. *Code for Nurses*, op. cit., p. 5.

68. Norman Fost and J. Robertson, "Letter to the Editor," *NEJM*, no. 20 (11 Nov. 1976), **295**:1141.

69. Kim L. Kelleher, "Go Gentle," *Nursing*, no. 7 (July 1979), **9**:96. Myra E. Levine, "Nursing Ethics and the Ethical Nurse," *AJN*, no. 5 (May 1977), p. 847. Bandman and Bandman, op. cit., p. 34.

70. Kübler-Ross, *On Death and Dying*, op. cit., pp. 38–137.

71. Kübler-Ross, *On Death and Dying*, op. cit., pp. 1–37. Joan C. Murphy, "Communicating with the Dying Patient," *AJN*, no. 6 (June 1979), p. 1084. Hopping, op. cit., p. 443.

72. Hopping, op. cit., p. 443. David Popoff, "What Are Your Feelings About Death and Dying? Part I," *Nursing*, no. 8 (Aug. 1975), **5**:15–21. Kelleher, op. cit., p. 96. David Popoff, "What Are Your Feelings About Death and Dying? Part III," *Nursing*, no. 10 (Oct. 1975), **5**:45–48.

73. Hopping, op. cit., p. 443. J. C. Quint, "Awareness of Death and the Nurse's Composure," *Nursing Research* **15**:49–55 (Winter 1966). Mary F. McLaughlin, "Who Helps the Living?" *AJN*, no. 3 (Mar. 1978), **78**:422–423.

74. Popoff, Part I, op. cit., p. 16. Murphy, op. cit., p. 1084.

75. Elsie Bandman, "How Much Dare You Tell Your Patient?" *RN* (Aug. 1978), 39–41. Yarling, Part II, op. cit., p. 31.

76. Yarling, Part II, op. cit., p. 31.

77. Kübler-Ross, *On Death and Dying*, op. cit., p. 39.

78. Yarling, Part I, op. cit., pp. 45, 47.

79. Yarling, Part II, op. cit., p. 29. Martin Shephard, *Someone You Love Is Dying* (New York: Harmony Books, 1975), pp. 32–33. Fiore, op. cit., p. 286. Chapter Nineteen, "Dig-

nity in Dying," in Bermosk and Corsini, op. cit., pp. 160–170.

80. Shideler, op. cit., pp. 1375–1378. Shephard, op. cit., p. 33. J. D. Thullen, "When You Can't Cure, Care," *Perinatology/Neonatology*, Nov./Dec. 1977.

81. Kübler-Ross, *On Death and Dying*, op. cit., Preface. Beauchamp, op. cit., p. 70. R. W. Buckingham and others, "Living with the Dying: Use of the Technique of Participant Observation," *Canadian Medical Journal* 115:1211–1215 (18 Dec. 1976).

82. Murphy, op. cit., p. 1084. McLaughlin, op. cit., pp. 422–423. A. T. Stanley, "Is It Ethical to Give Hope To A Dying Patient?" *Nursing Clinics of North America*, no. 1 (Mar. 1979), 14:69–80.

83. International Work Group in Death, Dying, and Bereavement, "Assumptions and Principles Underlying Standards for Terminal Care," *AJN*, no. 2 (Feb. 1979), pp. 296–297.

84. Stanley, op. cit., p. 72.

85. Marian Osterweis and Daphne Champagne, "The U.S. Hospice Movement: Issues in Development," *American Journal of Public Health*, no. 5 (May 1979), 69:492–496. Amado, Cronk, and Mileo, op. cit., p. 522–523.

86. Cecily Saunders, "Control of Pain in Terminal Cancer," *Nursing Times* (July 22, 1976), pp. 1133–1135.

87. J. Brimigion, "Living With Dying," *Nursing*, no. 9 (Sept. 1978), pp. 76–79. Murphy, op. cit., p. 1084.

88. Brimigion, op. cit., p. 79. Loy Wiley, ed., "The Other Side of Death," *Nursing*, no. 12 (Dec. 1978), pp. 40–45. Cecily Saunders, "A Death in the Family—A Professional View," *British Medical Journal* (6 Jan. 1973), pp. 30–31. Mary J. Klepser, "How Long Does Grief Go On?" *AJN*, no. 3 (March 1978), 78: 418–420.

89. Victoria J. Lannie, "The Joy of Caring for the Dying," *Supervisor Nurse*, no. 5 (May 1978), 9:66–72.

Chapter 9

Legal Aspects of Patients' Rights and Unethical Practice*

Lucie Young Kelly, Ph.D.

Whether it is a consequence of the civil rights movement, the consumer movement, or simply a new era in society, everyone now seems to be concerned with people's rights. As might be expected, health care has also been affected.

Until recently, people have felt helpless in their patient role—and small wonder. Stripped of their individuality as well as their belongings, they are thrust into an alien environment with little control over what happens to them. They are surrounded by unidentified faces and unidentifiable equipment. Their privacy is invaded. Their dignity is lost. They hesitate to complain or criticize because of fear of reprisals from the staff. They are reluctant to press for answers to their questions because a "busy" message is communicated loud and clear. Underlying all this is fear for their health, and even their life.

There is evidence, however, that consumers are no longer willing to put up with this state of affairs, will no longer accept the traditional role of "good" patient: the one who does as he's told, asks no awkward ques-

* Adapted from Lucie Young Kelly, *Dimensions of Professional Nursing*, 4th ed., Macmillan Publishing Co., Inc., 1980.

tions, and doesn't make waves. The frequent denial of their fundamental rights—among them, to courtesy, privacy, and, most of all, information—has brought about the ultimate form of patient rebellion: malpractice suits. As the HEW Secretary's Commission on Medical Malpractice has noted, the quality of the relationship between the patient, on the one hand, and the doctor or hospital, on the other, may make the difference between filing or not filing a malpractice suit. The commission adds it "believes that to ignore these and other rights of the patient is both to betray simple humanity and to invite dissatisfaction that may lead to malpractice suits."[1]

PATIENTS' RIGHTS

Perhaps the saddest fact is that most of the rights about which patients are concerned are theirs legally as well as morally and have been so established by common law. They are also stated in the codes of ethics of both physicians and nurses (although much is by implication and thus open to considerable personal interpretation). And, since the well-publicized American Hospital Association's "A Patient's Bill of Rights" (page 212) was presented in 1972, a spate of such "rights" statements has followed: for the disabled, the mentally ill, the retarded, the old, the young, the pregnant, the handicapped, the dying.

A Patient's Bill of Rights

1. The patient has the right to considerate and respectful care.
2. The patient has the right to obtain from his physician complete current information concerning his diagnosis, treatment, and prognosis in terms the patient can be reasonably expected to understand. When it is not medically advisable to give such information to the patient, the information should be made available to an appropriate person in his behalf. He has the right to know, by name, the physician responsible for coordinating his care.
3. The patient has the right to receive from his physician information necessary to give informed consent prior to the start of any procedure and/or treatment. Except in emergencies, such information for informed consent, should include but not necessarily be limited to the specific procedure and/or treatment, the medically significant risks involved, and the probable duration of incapacitation. Where medically significant alternatives for care or treatment exist, or when the patient requests information concerning medical alternatives, the patient has the right to such information. The patient also has the right to know the name of the person responsible for the procedures and/or treatment.
4. The patient has the right to refuse treatment to the extent permitted by law, and to be informed of the medical consequences of his action.
5. The patient has the right to every consideration of his privacy concerning his own medical care program. Case discussion, consultation, examination, and treatment are confidential and should be conducted discreetly. Those not directly involved in his care must have the permission of the patient to be present.
6. The patient has the right to expect that all communications and records pertaining to his care should be treated as confidential.
7. The patient has the right to expect that within its capacity a hospital must make reasonable response to the request of a patient for services. The hospital must provide evaluation, service, and/or referral as indicated by the urgency of the case. When medically permissible a patient may be transferred to another facility only after he has received complete information and explanation concerning the needs for and alternatives to such a transfer. The institution to which the patient is to be transferred must first have accepted the patient for transfer.

8. The patient has the right to obtain information as to any relationship of his hospital to other health care and educational institutions insofar as his care is concerned. The patient has the right to obtain information as to the existence of any professional relationships among individuals, by name, who are treating him.

9. The patient has the right to be advised if the hospital proposes to engage in or perform human experimentation affecting his care or treatment. The patient has the right to refuse to participate in such research projects.

10. The patient has the right to expect reasonable continuity of care. He has the right to know in advance what appointment times and physicians are available and where. The patient has the right to expect that the hospital will provide a mechanism whereby he is informed by his physician or a delegate of the physician of the patient's continuing health care requirements following discharge.

11. The patient has the right to examine and receive an explanation of his bill regardless of source of payment.

12. The patient has the right to know what hospital rules and regulations apply to his conduct as a patient.

No catalogue of rights can guarantee for the patient the kind of treatment he has a right to expect. A hospital has many functions to perform, including the prevention and treatment of disease, the education of both health professionals and patients, and the conduct of clinical research. All these activities must be conducted with an overriding concern for the patient, and, above all, the recognition of his dignity as a human being. Success in achieving this recognition assures success in the defense of the rights of the patient.

In some cases, these statements have even been the basis for new statutory law, as evidenced by the Minnesota legislature's adoption of a variation of the AHA Patient's Bill of Rights.

A follow-up by the Minnesota Hospital Association on the effectiveness of this legislation one year later indicated that several of the hospitals and nursing homes surveyed reported patients *were* receiving better explanations about care, staff awareness of patients' rights and the importance of confidentiality *had been* heightened, and, in some cases, patient advocates had been appointed. However, a major flouting of the law was noted in relation to patient consent to observation of care by nonessential personnel; more than half of the respondents did not obtain such consent.

The vagueness of the AHA statement and the inability to force compliance without legal intervention have made it a butt of some bitter humor. George Annas, an attorney in the health field, quotes a commentator who likened the document to a fox telling the chickens what their rights are. Nevertheless, commenting on the required posting of the Minnesota bill in hospitals, Annas notes that the "trend toward publishing rights is important because it not only reminds people that they have rights, but also encourages them to assert them and to make further demands."[2] It might also remind the staff, for there is some evidence that they, too, are unaware of patients' rights, even legal rights.

By the end of the 1970s, variations of the Patient's Bill of Rights became law in many states. Some legislatures passed specific bills incorporating either the AHA statements or a similar version; state or municipal hospital codes took similar action, sometimes including mental institutions and nursing homes. In 1974, new Medicare regulations for skilled nursing facilities included a section on patients' rights. Just how disgraceful the violation of rights of this captive group was might be judged by reviewing the rights: the right to send and receive mail; the right to share rooms with spouses if both are patients, or to privacy for visits; the right to have restraints used only if authorized by the physician and only for a limited time; the right to use one's own clothes and possessions, as space permits; and the right to require both written permission from the patient and accountings for the management of his/her funds. And, as in other laws, the patient had to be informed of his rights.

Most patients have not known that they had any rights once they entered a health care institution. These rights are still being violated, but probably less so since there are now legal sanctions. Patients or their advocates can prevent violations, remedy them, or seek civil redress in such cases as lack of informed consent.

TRENDS IN INFORMED CONSENT

For years, when patients have been admitted to hospitals, they signed a frequently unread, universal consent form that almost literally gave the physician, his associates, and the hospital carte blanche in determining the patient's care. There was some rationale for this, because civil suits for battery (unlawful touching) could theoretically be filed as a result of giving routine care, such as baths. Patients undergoing surgery or some complex, dangerous treatment were asked to sign a separate form, usually stating something to the effect that permission was granted to the physician and/or his colleagues to perform the operation or treatment. Just how much the patient knew about the hows and whys of the surgery, the dangers and the alternatives, depended on the patient's assertiveness in asking questions and demanding answers and the physician's willingness to provide information. Nurses were taught *never* to answer those questions, or little else either, and to suggest, "Ask your doctor." Health professionals, and especially physicians, took a "we know best and will decide for you" attitude.

The majority of patients probably still enter into treatment and undergo a variety of tests and even surgery without a clear understanding of the nature of their condition or what can be done about it. Although they may be receiving care that is medically acceptable, patients have no real part in deciding what that care should be. Most physicians

have believed that anything more than a superficial explanation is unnecessary, for the patient should "trust" the doctor. Kalisch has elaborated this point, calling it *Aesculapian authority*.[3] Yet, the patient has always had the right to make decisions about his own body. A case was heard as early as 1905 on surgery without consent, and the classic legal decision is that of Judge Cardoza (*Schloendorff* v. *The Society of New York Hospital* (211 NY. 125, 129–130, 105 NE 92, 93-1914), "Every human being of adult years and sound mind has a right to determine what shall be done with his own body."

A noted hospital law book states the following:

> *It is an established principle of law that every human being of adult years and sound mind has the right to determine what shall be done with his own body. He may choose whether to be treated or not and to what extent, no matter how necessary the medical care, nor how imminent the danger to his life or health if he fails to submit to treatment.*[4]

The patient's need for and right to this kind of knowledge are highlighted by the increasing number of malpractice suits that involve an element of *informed consent.** For many years, in such suits, courts have tended to rule that the physician must provide only as much information as is general practice among his colleagues in the area, as determined by their expert testimony. Some recent decisions, however, are changing this approach, most of them hinging on informed consent.

There was, for instance, the case of the physician who repeatedly persuaded patients to have unnecessary laminectomies, and then performed them poorly. One facet of the case against him and the hospital was lack of informed consent (actually, coerced consent). Both were found liable.[5] The landmark decisions, however, have involved situations in which the surgery was not done ineffectively, but in which patients sued because of complications or results about which they had not been warned. In one such case, a patient, who had numerous complications after surgery

* Some lawyers are advocating the use of the term *authorization for treatment*, implying patient control.

for a duodenal ulcer, had been informed of the risks of the anesthesia but not the surgery. He won a verdict against both hospital and surgeon.[6] In another case, a woman of Korean ancestry won because the physician had not explained that with the dermabrasion she agreed to, the risk of hyperpigmentation (which she developed) was greater in those of Oriental background.[7]

In these and other cases, judges disallowed the right of the medical profession to determine how much the patient should be told; rather, they said, the patient should be told enough, in understandable lay language, to make a decision. The materiality of the risk or fact to be disclosed by the physician "is to be determined by applying the standards of a reasonable man, not a reasonable medical practitioner."[8]

There continue to be similar judgments and some legislation supporting the same concept. Annas states that the trend now is for the courts to view the doctor-patient relationship as a partnership in decision making, rather than as a medical monopoly.[9] These trends have moved hospitals into reviewing and revising their consent forms. The catchall admissions consent had already been ruled as "almost completely worthless" for more than avoiding battery complaints, because it does not designate the nature of the treatment to be given.[10] What has emerged are forms that contain all the required elements for the informed consent process, usually individualized by the physician for each patient, somewhat like those developed by Alfidi[11] and Hershey.[12] In many cases, they are available in the foreign languages most prevalent in the area.

Consent is defined as a free, rational act that presupposes knowledge of the thing to which consent is given by a person who is legally capable of consent. Informed consent is not expected to include minutiae, but to delineate the essential nature of the procedure and the consequences. The disclosure is to be "reasonable," without details that might unnecessarily frighten the patient. The patient may, of course, waive the right to such explanation. Consents are *not* needed for emergency care if there is an immediate threat to life and health, if experts agree that it is an emergency, if the patient is unable to consent and a legally authorized person can't

be reached, and when the patient submits voluntarily. Criteria for a valid consent are (1) it must be written (unless oral consent can be proved in court); (2) it must be signed by the patient or person legally responsible for him/her (a person cannot give consent to his/her spouse in a nonemergency situation); (3) the procedure performed must be the one consented to; and (4) it must contain the essential elements of an informed consent.[13] Those elements include (1) an explanation of the condition; (2) a fair explanation of the procedures to be used and the consequences; (3) a description of alternative treatments or procedures; (4) a description of the benefits to be expected; (5) an offer to answer the patient's inquiries; and (6) freedom from coercion, unfair persuasions, and inducements. The last has special significance, because the concept of informed consent really became viable with the Nuremberg Code, originating from the trials of Nazi physicians, convicted of experimenting on prisoners without their consent. The principles were then formalized in the Declaration of Helsinki, adopted by the Eighteenth World Medical assembly in 1964, and revised in 1975. HEW accepts the same principles and requires adherence to them in human research.[14]

The right to consent or not consent is one of the evolving issues in informed consent. The competent patient has the right to refuse consent, but a hospital can request a court order to act if the refusal endangers the patient's life. If a patient is considered physically incapable, legally incompetent, or a minor, a guardian has the right to give or withhold consent. The trend in court decisions seems to be that the patient, unless proven totally incompetent, has the right to refuse. For example, a Jehovah's Witness refuses a blood transfusion, even though it might mean his life, because taking such transfusions is against his religion. The rulings have been in favor of allowing him to make his own decision; in fact, the Witnesses and AMA in 1979 agreed upon a consent form that requests no blood or blood derivative be administered, and releases medical personnel and the hospital of responsibility for untoward results caused by that refusal.[15] If a minor child of a Witness needs the blood and the parent refuses, a court order requested by the hospital usually permits the transfusion.

This is based on a legal precedent when a judge ruled that parents had a right to be martyrs if they wished, but had no right to make martyrs of their children. On the other hand, if the child is deemed a "mature minor," able to make an intelligent decision, regardless of chronological age, the child has been allowed to refuse the treatment. In another case, a seventy-nine-year-old diabetic refused to consent to a leg amputation. Her daughter petitioned to be her legal guardian so that she (the daughter) could sign the consent. The judge ruled that the woman was old but not senile, and had a right to make her own decision. In a slightly different situation, an alcoholic derelict was found unconscious on the street and taken to a hospital. When he became conscious, he refused to have his legs amputated for severe frostbite. The court order sought by the hospital was denied because, although the man was alcoholic, at the time of making his decision he was competent. (As it happened, he lost only a few toes from his frostbite.) In still another case, a young man on permanent kidney dialysis decided he did not want to live that way and refused continued treatment. He was allowed to do so and he died within a short time. Other cases can also be cited.[16] Thus, the right of a competent patient to refuse treatment seems more firmly established than ever but, when the patient is unconscious, other legal questions arise.

The Nurse's Role in Informed Consent

Some physicians do not believe it is feasible to obtain an informed consent because of such factors as lack of interest or education and high anxiety level, in which case a patient might refuse a "necessary treatment or operation."[17] There are physicians and others who believe that despite the increasing number of rulings favoring patients' full knowledge, most patients are not given information so that they really understand (and the courts really don't do enough about it.)[18] The physician may also use "therapeutic privilege" in which disclosure is not required because it might be detrimental to the patient. Or, information about certain alternatives may be withheld because the physician

believes they are too risky, unproven, or not appropriate.[19] Because it is generally agreed that nurses do not have the primary responsibility for getting the informed consent, what does the nurse do, if she/he believes the patient has not been adequately informed? The nurse could, first of all, take the initiative to question the patient about what she/he understands, as well as to be alert to signs that the patient is not clear about what is to be done. The physician should then be informed. The question most nurses face is how much can be told, especially if the physician chooses not to reveal further information. The dramatic Tuma case, which resulted in an important state supreme court decision, is a case in point. In Idaho, in 1977, Jolene Tuma, an instructor in an associate degree program, went with a student to the bedside of a terminally ill woman to start the chemotherapy that had been ordered, supposedly with the patient's "informed" consent. When the patient asked Ms. Tuma about alternate treatments for cancer, she was told about several. The son, upset because the mother stopped the chemotherapy, told the physician, who brought charges against Ms. Tuma. Subsequently, she was not only fired, but her license was suspended for six months by the Idaho board of nursing for unprofessional conduct, because her actions "disrupted the physician-patient relationship."[20] The case aroused a national nursing furor.[21] Ms. Tuma took her case through the courts, and on April 17, 1979, the Idaho Supreme Court handed down a decision that Ms. Tuma could not be found guilty of unprofessional conduct, because the Idaho Nurse Practice Act neither defines unprofessional conduct nor sets guidelines for providing warnings. The judge also questioned the ability of the hearing officer, who lacked the "personal knowledge and experience" of nursing to determine if Ms. Tuma's behavior was unprofessional.[22] Unfortunately, the court did not address itself to Ms. Tuma's actions, which leaves the nurse's right to inform the patient in some question—at least in Idaho.

If a nurse believes it is an ethical duty to inform patient and family against the direct wishes of the attending physician, she/he may be taking a personal risk, as did Tuma. However, should the nurse decide to give further information, it should be totally accurate, carefully recorded, and shared with the physician and others. Nurses have found ways to make the patient aware of knowledge gaps so they ask the right questions, but it is unfortunate that most are still employed in situations where it could be detrimental to them to be the patient's advocate. More are taking the risk, and changes may very well occur. Of course, if the patient is coaxed or coerced into signing without such an explanation, the consent is invalid. Moreover, if the patient withdraws consent, even verbally, the nurse is responsible for reporting this and seeing that the patient is not treated. This is a legal responsibility, not only to the patient but also to the hospital, which can be held liable.

Hospitals are beginning to send a clerk to witness the consent form after the physician makes his explanation, on the theory that only the signature is being witnessed, not the accuracy or depth of the explanation. Other hospitals ask the physician to bring another physician, presumably to validate the explanation. Where nurses still witness the form, it should be clear *what* they are witnessing—signature or explanation.[23] Hospital policy can clarify this.

The nurse's own and specific responsibility is to explain nursing care, including the whys and hows. Nurses are still reluctant to do so and feel threatened by a physician who demands that only limited or no explanations be given.

THE RIGHT TO DIE

Perhaps because improved technology has succeeded in artificially maintaining both respiratory and cardiac functions when a person can no longer do so, the definition of clinical death as the irrevocable cessation of heartbeat and breathing is no longer pertinent.* What of irreversible coma? In 1968, a faculty committee of the Harvard Medical School identified certain characteristics of a permanently nonfunctioning brain: (1) unreceptivity and unresponsivity, (2) no move-

* Physicians have the authority and responsibility to pronounce a patient dead. Even though a nurse may quite accurately do so, the law, thus far, has not caught up with that reality.

ments of breathing, (3) no reflexes, (4) flat electroencephalogram. Others developed variations of this definition.[24]

In common law, there has been a strongly entrenched cardiac definition of death until, in 1977, in Massachusetts, the Supreme Judicial Court officially recognized the use of brain death criteria.[25] In 1970, Kansas was the first state to adopt a brain death statute, using the same Harvard-type criteria, thus offering two alternative definitions of death to be used at the discretion of the attending physician. A few states passed similar legislation. Other types of criteria were adopted by other state legislatures, but all were based on cessation of brain functioning.[26] A major point must be made about brain death. Black notes:

Patients with brain death are not merely perpetually unresponsive: they are patients whose brain destruction, including loss of respiratory and cardiovascular control, means that life of all kinds is soon to be lost as well.[27]

Still, there are many lay people and even health professionals who do not believe that brain death is an adequate definition of physiological death. (On the other hand, a variety of surveys indicate that most people are beginning to favor euthanasia, if there is a terminal illness.) Thus, the majority of states still use the classic definition, and questions arise about the status of patients maintained on respirators.

Two rulings on the terminally ill, incompetent patient, made by two different state supreme courts, were the Saikewicz[28] and Quinlan[29] cases. In the first, the court upheld a decision not to give a severely retarded sixty-seven-year-old more chemotherapy that would be unpleasant for the sake of a short, extended life-span. He died a month later of pneumonia. In the Karen Quinlan case, a twenty-two-year-old woman received severe and irreversible brain damage that reduced her to a vegetative state. Her father petitioned the court to be made her guardian with the intention of having all extraordinary medical procedures sustaining her life removed. The New Jersey Supreme Court ruled that the father could be the guardian and have the life-support systems discontinued with the concurrence of her family, the attending physicians, who might be chosen by the father, and the hospital ethics committee.[30] (After disconnection of the respirators, Karen continued to live, sustained by fluids and other maintenance measures, and was transferred to a nursing home.) Health law experts debate the congruity of these and similar cases, and it is expected that other supreme courts, faced by other unique circumstances, will make separate rulings.[31]

Part of the Quinlan judge's comments related to the belief that Karen would have made a similar choice, if able. Until 1977, a person could not be assured that she/he would be allowed to die if brain death existed. The Euthanasia Educational Council (now called Concern for Dying) has made available "A Living Will" that directs family, physician, and friends to withhold artificial means in case of inevitable death. Other versions also exist.[32] The will, although it can be revoked at any time, has no legal power, although presumably if the writer's intention were followed, those involved would not be judged guilty of murder. In 1977, California enacted a Natural Death Act, with carefully delineated and protective living will components. In the next year, Arkansas, Idaho, Nevada, New Mexico, North Carolina, Oregon, and Texas followed with similar statutes.[33],[34] All granted civil and criminal immunity for those carrying out living will requests. Although there were no reported difficulties, some attorneys believe because the right to refuse treatment already exists, such legislation only creates problems.[35]

The right-to-die issue is almost synonymous with euthanasia, a word of Greek origin meaning painless, easy, gentle, or good death. It is now commonly used to signify a killing that is promoted by such a humanitarian motive, such as the relief of intolerable pain. There are two major categories of euthanasia: voluntary and involuntary. The first usually involves two parties, the competent adult patient and a doctor, nurse, or both. (The patient could commit suicide alone.) It is voluntary euthanasia that the natural death laws seek to serve. Involuntary euthanasia, sometimes called mercy killing, is performed by someone other than the patient without the patient's consent, possibly because of unconsciousness. There are many pros and cons of euthanasia given, with arguments usually falling into secular or religious categories.[36],[37] Nevertheless, according to the law, euthanasia is murder. In cases in which a physician, nurse, or family member has "pulled the plug" or otherwise carried out involuntary euthanasia, and there appeared to be no ulterior motive, the jury has usually freed the individual, often on the basis of temporary insanity. In 1979, however, a Maryland nurse was indicted for murder for discontinuing life support systems of brain dead patients. She did not deny that she had done so, but based her not guilty plea on the fact the patients were brain dead GORKs (God only really knows), according to local terminology.[38] She was acquitted. (Although she was termed compassionate by her nursing colleagues, they felt obligated to report her actions when she would not stop.)

Orders Not to Resuscitate

Patients in irreversible coma may be under orders not to resuscitate (no-code, code blue, or other terms), with or without the consent and knowledge of the family. Is a nurse in legal jeopardy if she obeys? Is a nurse in trouble if she/he chooses not to? To a great extent these questions remain unanswered, because families may choose to let the patient die but do not want to say so, and many codes have been carried out with little discussion after the decision was made. Nurses who object on moral or religious grounds cannot be forced to participate (but for some people, it is just as wrong to resuscitate). However, without a specific hospital protocol, *not resuscitating* could be considered malpractice. Nonwritten orders could be a special problem for the nurse and should be questioned. If the orders are written, they should be in the context of the physician's judgment of the futility of resuscitation.[39] Some hospitals are following the Massachusetts General Hospital model, in which some patients are put into four categories from "maximal therapeutic effort" to "all therapy can be discontinued," with definitive protocols for each.[40] The arguments are strong that some policy should be set as a safeguard for all, including the patient.[41]

THE RIGHTS OF THE HELPLESS

Children, the mentally ill, the mentally retarded, and certain patients in nursing homes are often seen as relatively helpless, because they have been termed legally incompetent to make decisions about their health care for so many years. Often the rights overlap, as when a child or elderly person is mentally retarded (as in Saikewicz). Some of the rights of the elderly are being protected by the legalized bill of rights, and for mental patients, state laws and some high court decisions have served the same purpose. Both have focused on the mental patient's rights in the areas of voluntary and involuntary admissions; kind and length of restraints, including seclusion; informed consent to treatment, especially sterilization and psychosurgery; the rights of citizenship (voting for example); rights of privacy, especially as related to records; rights in research; and, especially, the right to treatment.[42],[43],[44],[45] Although rulings have varied, the trend is toward protection of rights. The landmark decision of *Wyatt* v. *Stickney* 325 Federal Supplement, Alabama, 1972 clearly defined the purposes of commitment to a public hospital and the constitutional right to adequate treatment.[46] Other legal decisions relate to sterilization of the retarded, which came to a head when it was found that black retarded adolescent girls were being sterilized without either their or their mothers having a clear notion of what that meant. Restraints were increasingly put on sterilization until in 1979 HEW tightened the regulations for federal participation in funding of sterilization procedures, which included requirements of written and oral explanations of the operation, advice about alternate forms of birth control to be given in understandable language, and a waiting period. In addition, it allowed no federal funding for sterilization of those under twenty-one, mentally incompetent, or those institutionalized in correctional facilities, or mental hospitals. However, this does not mean that a parent cannot have a retarded girl sterilized, but only that more precautions are being taken by courts and the government that the child's rights are not violated. There is general concern for the rights of young people in the mental health system,[47] but parents maintain considerable control. In 1979, the Supreme Court upheld the constitutionality of state laws that allow parents to commit their minor children to state mental institutions; thirty-six states have such laws.

The other rights of young people and children relate primarily to consent for treatment or research and abuse. (See legal reporting obligations later.) It is a general rule that a parent or guardian must give consent for the medical or surgical treatment of a minor except in an emergency when it is imperative to give immediate care to save the minor's life. Legally, however, anyone who is capable of understanding what he is doing may give consent, because age is not always an exact criteria of maturity or intelligence. Many minors are perfectly capable of deciding for themselves whether to accept or reject recommended therapy and, in cases involving simple procedures, the courts have refused to invoke the rule requiring the consent of a parent or guardian. If the minor is married or has been otherwise emancipated from his parents, there is likely to be little question about this legally. In addition, states cite different ages and situations in which parental permission is needed for medical treatment. The almost universal exception is allowing minors to consent to treatment for venereal disease, drug abuse, and pregnancy-related care.[48] Although it has been understood that health professionals have no legal obligation to report to parents that the minor has sought such treatment, a few states are beginning to add statutes that say the minor doesn't need parental permission, but parents must be notified.

The entire question of permission for contraception, abortion, and sterilization is in a state of flux. The key appears to be a designation of *mature minor;* emancipated minors are treated as adults. As recently as 1972, the U.S. Supreme Court ruled that state statutes prohibiting prescription of contraceptives to unmarried persons was unconstitutional because this would interfere with the right of privacy of those desiring them.[49] However, it did not rule on a minor's right to privacy in seeking or buying contraceptives. This was left to the states, and a number still set age limitations from fourteen to twenty-one. In many states, however, doctors and other health professionals may provide birth control information and prescribe contraceptives to patients of any age without parental consent.[50] Changes in federal and state laws also frequently require welfare agencies to offer family planning services and supplies to sexually active minors. In general, there is clearly a national trend toward granting minors the right to contraceptive advice and devices, and no case has been found where a doctor is liable for damage for prescribing contraceptives without parental consent.[51]

An even more dramatic change has occurred in relation to abortion. In 1976 the Supreme Court held that states may not constitutionally require the consent of a girl's parents as a condition for abortion during the first twelve weeks of pregnancy. In addition, then, parents cannot either prevent or force an abortion on the daughter who, in the eyes of the Court is now "a competent minor mature enough to have become pregnant." In the words of one federal court that overturned a parental consent statute:

> It is not they (the parents) who have to bear the child. . . . It is difficult to think of any self-interest that a parent would have that compared with those significant interests of the pregnant minor.[52]

Should the young woman decide against an abortion and elect to bear the child, she can receive care related to her pregnancy without parental consent in almost every state. (That a pregnant teen-ager can have an abortion without parental consent in some states, but not maternity services, is one of the peculiarities of law in a rapidly changing society.) It should be added here that this unwed "mature minor" may also consent to treatment of her child.[53] A number of groups, including the American Academy of Pediatrics, the Society for Adolescent Medicine, and the National Association of Children's Hospitals and Related Institutions, have taken stands on protecting the rights of minors in health care. For example, the AAP Committee on Youth has presented a model act for consent of minors for health services, recommended for enactment in all states. It states that a minor may give consent for care if she/he was ever married, had a child, graduated from high school, is separated from parents, or supporting herself/himself. Specified are treatment for any communicable disease, drug abuse, preg-

nancy, and mental illness. In these cases the physician is obliged to inform the parents only in extreme circumstances. On the other hand, self-consent for abortion or sterilization is excepted.[54] An alternative model act offered by the State Committee on Legislation Concerning Adolescents' Medical Care of the Society for Adolescent Medicine is somewhat more succinct but similar in most points. It differentiates between anyone over eighteen (who is treated as having achieved majority) and emancipated minors. It does not mention abortion or sterilization. It also makes the minor liable for payment of health services. Model laws are scarcely ever just that, nor are they generally accepted by every state, but they do point a direction, especially if developed by prestigious groups. The Pediatric Bill of Rights may also be a forerunner to legal action, as was the AHA Patient's Bill of Rights. (Unless such a statement is incorporated into law, the effect is only moral, a guideline to encourage protection of rights, with no enforcement powers.) The Pediatric Bill of Rights addresses the rights of young people in the areas of counseling and treatment for birth control, abortion, pregnancy, drug or alcohol dependency, venereal disease, confidentiality, and information about her/his condition, as well as protection if a parent refuses consent for needed treatment.[55]

Cases in which mature minors are being permitted to make life-and-death decisions are increasing, for example, a thirteen-year-old who chose not to have a bone marrow transplant because of religious beliefs and potential danger to her donor-sister. An interesting trend, however, is toward including very young children in making decisions about research in which they are asked to participate. In the past, as a rule, parents were asked whether they consented to their child's participation in research—medical, educational, psychological, or other. There has always been some concern as to whether the child should be subjected to such research if it was not at least potentially beneficial to him (for example, use of a new drug for a leukemic child). The child seldom was given the opportunity to decide whether or not to participate. New knowledge of the potential harm that could be done to the child, however innocuous the experiment, and appreciation of the child as a human being with individual rights have now resulted in recommendations that even a very young child be given a simple explanation about the proposed research and allowed to participate or not, or even withdraw later, without any form of coercion.[56,57,58] Given that choice, some children have decided not to participate.[59] Overall, though, the support for using healthy children in research, or being volunteered for procedures not beneficial to themselves is eroding.[60,61]

The question of whether parents may make a decision for a child, if the child's well-being is the parents' prime consideration, as in giving laetrile to a leukemic child, is not being decided with any consistency. (For that matter, neither has the legality of laetrile.)[62] Another unresolved issue is whether the grossly deformed neonate should be allowed to live. Few judges will rule to let it die, but often the decision is quietly made by parents and health personnel.[63] In other cases, the babies are used in research.[64] These situations are especially difficult for a nurse who may see the infant simply starve to death. More nurses and others are reporting such situations, but as in the right to die issue, ethical and moral considerations weigh strongly.

RIGHTS OF PATIENTS IN RESEARCH

The use of new, experimental drugs and treatments in hospitals, nursing homes, and other institutions that have a captive population—for example, prisons or homes for the mentally retarded—is extensive. Nurses are often involved in giving the treatment or drugs. As noted earlier, HEW regulations now require a very specific informed consent for research carried out under HEW auspices, with strong emphasis on the need for a clear explanation of the experiment, possible dangers, and the subject's complete freedom to refuse or withdraw at any time.

In addition, the National Research Act of 1974 established a commission to, among other things, "identify the requirements for informed consent procedures for children, prisoners, and the mentally disabled, and determine the need for a mechanism to assure that human subjects not covered by HEW

regulations are protected."[65] (Part of that Commission report was cited previously.) Actually, nurses were in the forefront of this move, with a statement in the ANA *Code of Ethics:* "The nurse participates in research activities when assured that the rights of individual subjects are protected," as well as an extensive ANA document on research guidelines.

When the nurse is participating in research, at whatever level, seeing that the rights of patients are honored is both an ethical and legal responsibility. Nurses should know the patients' rights: self-determination to choose to participate; to have full information; to terminate participation without penalty; privacy and dignity; conservation of personal resources; freedom from arbitrary hurt and intrinsic risk of injury; as well as the special rights of minor and incompetent persons previously discussed.[66] For instance, nurses have been ordered to begin an experimental drug when she/he knows that the patient has not given an informed consent. In that case, the nurse is obligated to see that the patient does have the appropriate explanation. This is one more case when institutional policy that sets an administrative protocol for the nurse in such a situation is helpful. Creighton cites a number of instances where nurses were among those who participated in research that violated patients' rights, such as the disgraceful Tuskegee Syphilis Study, conducted by the U.S. Public Health Service over a forty-year period.[67] Nurses can no longer absolve themselves from responsibility because they themselves are the researchers. If the nurse is the investigator, she/he must observe all the usual requirements, such as informed consent and confidentiality. Nurses are generally trusted by patients, and it has been found that there may be problems in getting the required consent; subjects will participate "for the nurse," but either refuse to sign the consent or not listen to an explanation as not necessary.[68,69] The quality of research in which human subjects are involved is particularly important. Peer review, such as that offered by a hospital review board, can be helpful,[70] although sometimes there are no nurses on the board at all. Unfortunately, these boards, required if the research is HEW-funded, have been found to not be as protective of patients' rights as they should be, especially in the areas of informed consent. There is usually no follow-up to determine whether the plans to preserve the subjects' rights that are presented in the proposals are really carried through.[71] The nurse, as primary investigator or participant, is in a position to see that these rights are not abrogated.

PATIENT RECORDS: CONFIDENTIALITY AND AVAILABILITY

All states have laws requiring hospitals, doctors, nurses, and, sometimes, other health workers to report on certain kinds of situations, because the patient may be unwilling or unable to do so. The nurse often has responsibility in these matters because although it may be the physician's legal obligation, the nurse may be the only one actually aware of the situation. Even if such reporting is not required by a law per se, regulations of various state agencies may require such a report. Common reporting requirements are for communicable diseases, diseases in newborn babies, gunshot wounds, and criminal acts, including rape and child abuse. In some states, there are penalties for *not* reporting such situations. There is also some evidence that other than these legal requirements, confidentiality of patients' records is frequently violated. Everyone has access except the patient.

The tremendous growth of computerized health data, the development of huge data banks, and the advancements in record linkage pose an enormous threat to the privacy of medical information, says a position paper on confidentiality adopted by the American Medical Records Association. The public is generally unaware of this threat or of the serious consequences of a loss of confidentiality in the health care system. Adequate measures to control medical privacy in the light of electronic information processing can and must be established. . . .[72]

A national study pointed out that from birth certificate to death certificate, the health and medical records of most Americans are part of a system that allows access by insurance companies, student researchers, and govern-

mental agencies, to name a few, and that the information is often shared illegally with others such as employers. The report's author recommended that

Health data systems should be created, altered, and periodically audited through public rather than closed procedures.

Every health data system should put limits on relevance and social propriety on the personal information it collects and records.

Every health data system should have clear rules and procedures to insure citizen rights.

Health data system managers should take special measures to protect the accuracy and the security of the data they keep.

Managers should follow special procedures to allow medical research, health care evaluation, and public oversight without impairing citizens' rights.[73]

Some thirty states have enacted laws to protect medical records, and the federal Freedom of Information Act (FOIA) denies access to an individual's medical record without that person's consent. Still, there are practical problems. If certain data are needed, as in following through on occupational health hazards,[74] can exceptions be made for research that would be beneficial to the well-being of people? The problem is not in aggregate figures, but when individual records must be scrutinized. (Researchers were quite concerned with enactment of the 1974 Privacy Act because HEW-funded research projects involving human subjects would be available to anyone, including participating subjects, by filing a request. Some of these cases are and will continue to go to court, but there seems to be a definite legislative and judicial trend toward safeguarding medical records and, in addition, giving patients access to their own records.

Most physicians and health administrators, however, have greeted this record sharing with open hostility. Some attorneys serving health care facilities tend to share the feeling, one group of authors writing that ". . . it is undesirable to allow patient or family to inspect the chart. [They] might find comments . . . which may be considered uncomplimentary or incorrect. The patient may then attempt to have the record changed or cause annoyance to the administration or the medical staff."[75] The writer was also concerned about the possibility of libel suits, and suggested the omission of "characterizations or other remarks which may offend . . ." in the abstract that could be given to the patient.

The time in which there is a choice in the matter of sharing the record may be ending. Although it is legally recognized that the patient's record is the property of the hospital or physician (in his office), the information that the record contains is not similarly protected. States and the federal government are legislating access, either direct patient access with or without a right to copy, or indirect access (physician, attorney, or provision of summary only). In 1979, nineteen states allowed patients direct access to their records: Colorado, Connecticut, Florida, Hawaii, Illinois, Indiana, Massachusetts,* Minnesota, Nebraska, Nevada, New Jersey,* New York,* Ohio, Oklahoma, Oregon, Tennessee, Texas,* Utah,* Virginia,* either through statutory or case law. Alabama,* Alaska,* California, District of Columbia,* Georgia,* Idaho,* Kansas,* Kentucky,* Louisiana,* Maine, Michigan,* Mississippi, North Carolina,* Pennsylvania,* Tennessee,* Utah, and Wisconsin give indirect access. States may differentiate between doctor's and hospital records and have other idiosyncratic qualifications.[76] Of course, one certain way in which the patient can get access is through a malpractice suit in which the record is subpoenaed, a costly process for both provider and consumer.

The Commission on Medical Malpractice noted the relationship between closed records and malpractice suits, but the commission members were split in their desire to open records to patients. A compromise recommendation suggested making records available to the patient's attorney (which may be more beneficial for the attorney's income than the patient's enlightenment), but a vigorous minority report, opposing this compromise, was included.[77] Westin's study recommended giving patients access, and he anticipated that this was an inevitability.[78] The

*Have mental health statutes that provide information to family, physician, attorney under certain circumstances, but not direct access.

Privacy Protection Study Commission, created by the 1974 Privacy Act, also included recommendations on patient access.[79] One federal step in this direction was the same FOIA and Privacy Act that prevented unauthorized access. Included are any records under the control of any agency of the federal government that contain an individual's name or any other identifying information. Medical records are specifically cited and would include those of patients in the Veterans Administration and other federal hospitals. Whether patients receiving medical care under Medicare are included is a subject of debate. Currently, the PSRO regulations allow patients access under certain circumstances. The law is highly controversial and interpretations are not altogether clear. For instance, there is some question as to whether contractors of a government agency, such as hospitals receiving federal funds for medical care or research, are included. If so, considering the ubiquity of federal aid, almost all patient records would be open to the patient concerned. Meanwhile, there is federal legislation being introduced to specifically include Medicaid/Medicare records, leading to inclusion of *all* medical records.

Although perhaps the majority of physicians and hospitals still object to the open record concept because the patient wouldn't understand, would be frightened, or might choose to treat himself, there is the beginning of a new philosophy—sharing the record with the patient so that both provider and consumer have an open relationship; deciding on the needed care together. A health care center associated with the University of Vermont states in its "Principles of Practice":

> The best care of the patient is assured when the patient is part of the team and he shares his medical records with the providers of care. This is best effected by assuring that the record is complete, well organized, and available to the patient so that he can review the record for reliability, the subjective data, and clarity of plans for treatment and education.[80]

Annas and others suggest that if the record is too technical, a knowledgeable patient advocate could be of assistance.[81] (Patient advocates are also recommended for other supportive purposes.)[82] Does the nurse have any legal responsibility to be that intermediary? The answer is more complex than just a yes or no. Certainly, a nurse would not simply hand a patient the chart at request, because that would be inappropriate. Most states, as well as health care agencies that permit access to records, have a protocol to be followed. This usually involves providing both privacy and an opportunity for the physician and/or another person to explain the content. (Many hospitals are now willing to have the patient see the record, because the administration realizes that if the patient is concerned enough to demand his chart and it is withheld, the next step is probably a malpractice suit; others simply agree that access is a right, or at least a trend, and are not waiting for legislation.) Both Annas[83] and Auerbach[84] give specific directions for obtaining records.

PRIVACY

Individuals who are in public life, such as politicians, royalty, and dignitaries, expect their every act will be of interest to the public, and they must, therefore, accept with good grace unfavorable news accounts and pictures as well as complimentary ones. Rarely can they successfully claim the citizen's right to privacy that is available to persons who are not of public interest.

Nurses who hold positions of importance may see unflattering pictures of themselves in newspapers and magazines that they might wish had never appeared in print. They would be unlikely to challenge the publication's right to carry them without permission, however, because the resulting publicity might turn out to be more unfavorable than the pictures. Under the law, they could instigate legal action if they wished because every citizen of our country can withhold from the public any information about himself—verbal, written, or depicted—if he so desires.

Nurses and others who work with sick patients must be especially careful to avoid invading the patient's right to privacy, which is identical to that of any other person. Consent to treatment does not cover the use of a picture without specific permission, nor does it mean that the patient can be subjected to repeated examinations not necessary to his therapy without his express consent. The information on a patient's chart is confidential and cannot be disclosed without the patient's consent.

Exceptions to respecting the patient's privacy are related to legal reporting obligations. The nurse may also be obligated to testify about otherwise confidential information in criminal cases.

Ethical practice prohibits the professional person from divulging any confidential information to anyone else, unless possibly to another physician or nurse who serves as a consultant. Neither does the ethical person engage in gossip based on this information, trivial and harmless though it may seem at the time. Moreover, the professional person has an obligation to set a good example for others in nonprofessional groups where persons may be less cognizant of their responsibilities in this respect.

Confidential information obtained through professional relationships is not the same as *privileged communication*, which is a legal concept providing that physician-patient, attorney-client, and priest-penitent have a special privilege. Should any court action arise in which the person (or persons) involved is called to testify, the law (in many states) will not require that such information be divulged. Not all states acknowledge that nurses can be recipients of privileged communications. The confidences exchanged between husband and wife are also considered privileged, and rarely is one spouse required to testify against another.

ASSAULT AND BATTERY

The terms *assault and battery* are used both in the context of criminal and civil law. *Assault* is an intentional act that threatens another; *battery* is touching without permission, possibly with force. Although assault and battery are often discussed with emphasis on the criminal interpretation, there is also a patient's rights aspect that is related to everyday nursing practice, especially when dealing with certain types of patients. Grounds for civil action might include the following:

1. Forcing a patient to submit to a treatment for which he has not given his consent either expressly in writing, orally, or by implication. Whether or not a consent was signed, a patient should not be forced, for resistance implies a withdrawal of consent.
2. Cutting a patient's hair or having it cut without his or her consent.
3. Lifting a protesting patient from his bed to a wheelchair or stretcher.
4. Threatening to strike or actually striking an unruly child or adult, except in self-defense.
5. Ejecting a visitor from a patient's room without the patient's consent.
6. In some states, performing alcohol, blood, urine, or health tests for presumed drunken driving without consent. There are some "implied consent" statutes in motor vehicle codes, which provide that a person, for the privilege of being allowed to drive, gives an implied consent to furnishing a sample of blood, urine, or breath for chemical analysis when charged with driving while intoxicated. However, if the person objects and is forced, it might still be considered battery. Several states, acknowledging this, have enacted legislation to insulate hospital employees and health professionals from liability.[86]

FALSE IMPRISONMENT

As the term implies, *false imprisonment* means "restraining a person's liberty without the sanction of the law, or imprisonment of a person who is later found to be innocent of the crime for which he was imprisoned." The term also applies to many procedures that actually or conceivably are performed in hospital and nursing situations *if they are performed without the consent of the patient or his legal representative.* In most instances, the nurse or other employee would not be held liable if it can be proved that what was done was necessary to protect others.

Among the most common nursing situations that might be considered false imprisonment are the following:

1. Restraining a patient by physical force or using appliances without written consent, especially in procedures where the use of restraints is not usually necessary. This is, or may be, a delicate situation because a nurse who does not use a restraint, such as side rails, to protect a patient may be accused of negligence, and if she/he does use them without consent, may be accused of false imprisonment. This would be a typical example of the need for prudent and reasonable action on the part of the nurse that a court of law would undoubtedly uphold.
2. Restraining a mentally ill patient who is neither dangerous to himself or to others. For example, patients who wander about the hospital division making a nuisance of themselves cannot legally be locked in a room unless they show signs of violence.
3. Using arm, leg, or body restraints to keep a patient quiet while she/he is being administered an intravenous infusion may be considered false imprisonment. If this risk is involved—that is, if the patient objects to the treatment and refuses to consent to it—the physician should be called. Should the doctor order restraints for the patient, the nurse should make sure it is in writing before allowing anyone to proceed with the treatment. It is much better to assign someone to stay with the patient throughout a procedure than to restrain her/him without authorization.
4. Detaining a patient in the hospital against his will. If a patient insists on going home, or a parent or guardian insists on taking a minor or other dependent person out of the hospital before his condition warrants it, hospital authorities cannot legally require him to remain. In such instances, the doctor must write an order permitting the hospital to allow the patient to go home "against advice," and the hospital's representative should see that the patient or guardian signs an official form absolving the hospital, medical staff, and nursing staff of all responsibility should the patient's early departure be detrimental to his health and welfare. If the patient refuses to sign, a record should be made of exactly what occurred.
5. Detaining for an unreasonable period of time a patient who is medically ready to be discharged. The delay may be because of the patient's inability to pay his bill or it

may be caused by an inordinate wait, at his expense, for the delivery of an orthopedic appliance or other service. In such instances, the nurse or nursing department may or may not be directly involved, but it is always wise to be cognizant of possible legal developments and to exercise sound judgment in order to be completely fair to the patient and avoid trouble for all concerned.

ABORTION, STERILIZATION, AND CONTRACEPTION

Abortion

Laws permitting abortion have varied greatly from state to state over the years. In early 1973 the Supreme Court ruled that no state can interfere with a woman's right to obtain an abortion during the first trimester (twelve weeks) of pregnancy. During the second trimester, the state may interfere only to the extent of imposing regulations to safeguard the health of women seeking abortions. During the last trimester of pregnancy, a state may prohibit abortions except when the mother's life is at stake.[87] (*Doe* v. *Bolton* and *Roe* v. *Wade*)* Theoretically, all hospitals then, are required to perform abortions within these statutes, and it is legal to assist with such a procedure; actually the rights cannot be withheld. However, because of religious and moral reasons, some institutions have delayed in complying with the law, and individual doctors and nurses have refused to participate in abortions. An individual professional or other health worker may make the choice, and there is legal support for them (conscience clause). (This does not preclude the right of the hospital to fire a nurse for refusing to carry out an assigned responsibility or to transfer a nurse to another unit. There have been some suits by nurses objecting to transfer, but rulings have varied.)

The Supreme Court has also addressed the issue of spousal consent and found that such

* Legislation on both the state and federal level, after this decision, let stand the woman's right to have an abortion, but gradually limited the conditions under which Medicaid would pay for abortions. The Supreme Court ruled that such decisions could be made by the states.

consent was not necessary. As mentioned earier, the courts are also moving in the direction of not distinguishing between female adults and minors on abortion rights.

Sterilization

Sterilization means termination of the ability to produce offspring. Eugenic sterilization is the attempt to eliminate specific hereditary defects by sterilizing individuals who could pass on such defects to their offspring. Approximately half the states have authorized eugenic sterilization of the mentally deficient, mentally ill, and others.[88] Legality where no law exists is questionable. Civil or criminal liability for assault and battery may be imposed on anyone sterilizing another without following legal procedure or specific legal guidelines. Both laws and regulations have been in the process of change. If the life of a woman may be jeopardized if she becomes pregnant, a therapeutic sterilization may be performed (with consent of the patient and sometimes the husband), although that is being challenged. If no statutes or judicial decisions state a policy against therapeutic sterilization, such operations may be considered as medically necessary. If there is no medical necessity, the operation is termed *sterilization of convenience* or *contraceptive sterilization*. In some states this is illegal; in others, arguable. (Seven states regulate therapeutic sterilization.) Here too, consents are often required from the individual and spouse and there may be a mandatory waiting period. The consequences of the operation must be made clear to all concerned, and often a special consent form is required. In some cases, patients have sued because pregnancy has resulted after sterilization. Interestingly enough, there is little legal concern about male sterilization, the vasectomy, which is being done with increasing frequency. The legal consequences of unsuccessful sterilization, both male and female, have resulted in suits.[89]

Laws on family planning also vary greatly. Some laws read as though they are absolute prohibitions against information about contraceptive materials, but courts usually allow considerable freedom. The Economic Opportunity Amendments of 1967 made family planning one of the eight national emphasis efforts and funded it accordingly. Family planning programs are growing under federal, state, and private aegis, because many individuals and groups see family planning as a basic human right. Nurses are particularly involved, for they do much of this counseling, either as specialists or as part of their general nursing role. Because there are still some state limitations, it is important for the nurse to keep up to date in this area.

Artificial Insemination

Artificial insemination, the injection of seminal fluid by instrument into a female to induce pregnancy, is evolving into an acceptable medical procedure used by childless couples. (Consent by husband and wife is generally required.) Homologous artificial insemination (AIH) uses the semen of the husband and appears to present no legal dangers for doctors or nurses. Heterologous artificial insemination (AID) uses the semen of someone other than the husband, and does raise the question of the child's legitimacy. On occasion the question of adultery also arises in the courts if the husband's consent has not been obtained. Few states have enacted statutes to deal with the AID situation.

Genetics

One relatively new legal aspect of human reproduction is the field of genetics, with which nurses, physicians, and lay genetic counselors must be concerned. Some of the issues have to do with AID, human genetic disease, genetic screening, *in vitro* fertilization (IVF), and genetic data banks. Confidentiality is of major interest; for example, if a genetic disease is discovered, the counselor should not contact other relatives, even if it would benefit those relatives, without the screenee's consent. Informed consent that enables the patient to make such serious decisions as having abortions, sterilizations, or artificial inseminations are also vital. The furor caused by the 1978 English test-tube baby is evidence enough that the legal and ethical issues are far from resolved. In addition, legislation such as the National Sickle Cell Anemia, Cooley's Anemia, Tay-Sachs, and Genetic Diseases Acts have encouraged or forced states to expand genetic screening to cover other disorders. Neonatal screening, for instance, will probably be expanded considerably and offers new opportunities and responsibilities for nurses. But with what is a still relatively new science, many legal questions will be evolving.[90]

DEALING WITH INCOMPETENT PRACTITIONERS

Because patients have a right to expect safe care, another issue is what a nurse should do about reporting incompetence or unprofessional conduct on the part of physicians or other health professionals. Because the nurse's code of ethics requires that she/he safeguard the patient, incompetent or unprofessional practitioners should be reported. One survey indicated that a large percentage of nurses would take some sort of action, usually speaking with the doctor, head nurse, or supervisors, if the patient were endangered by medical action. Few would report the physician to a peer review or licensing board.[91] Some nurses who have reported a physician at any time or place have either been dismissed from their jobs or made very uncomfortable and unwanted. All but six states (Massachusetts, New Hampshire, North Carolina, Oklahoma, South Dakota, and Vermont) have laws giving immunity from civil action to any person who reports to a peer review board, but this does not preclude being sued, even though legally the person must be cleared. In New York, a statute was enacted in 1977, requiring physicians to report other physicians' misconduct on penalty of being cited for unprofessional conduct themselves; nurses and others are encouraged to report such misconduct also.[92] (Some have interpreted the law as *requiring* such reporting by all licensed professionals). Similar statutes were already on the books in Arizona, Alabama, Connecticut, Idaho, Iowa, Maine, Montana, Ohio, Oregon, and Virginia.

Such reporting laws are focused on physicians, but there has been some discussion about similar legislation for reporting incompetent nurses for similar reasons; nurses do not report dangerous nurses any more frequently than other professionals report each other. Because nurses are licensed, the penalty for proven incompetence for unprofessional conduct includes revocation or suspension of the nurse's license or some other form of censure or discipline by the state board of nursing (the state agency that administers the nurse practice act).

The usual reasons for revoking a license are acts that might directly endanger the public, such as practicing while one's ability is impaired by alcohol, drugs, physical or mental disability; being habitually drunk or a habitual user of certain drugs; practicing with incompetence or negligence beyond the scope of practice. Other reasons are obtaining a license fraudulently, being convicted of a felony or crime involving moral turpitude, practicing while the license is suspended, aiding and abetting a nonlicensed person to perform activities requiring a license, and committing unprofessional conduct or immoral acts, as defined by the board. Recently, the refusal to provide service to a person because of race, color, creed, or national origin may also have been added. It may be noted that all these legal prohibitions also have ethical dimensions. Although this may seem to protect the public, data show that relatively few nurses have had licenses revoked or suspended. This is considered to be caused, in part, by the reluctance of other nurses to report and consequently testify to these acts by their colleagues before either the nursing board or a court of law. Nursing associations and state boards are now emphasizing the responsibility of professional nurses to report negligent practice.

The most common reason that nurses lose their licenses is the same as of physicians—drug use, abuse, or theft. It is rather shocking that not all states specify incompetence as a reason for professional discipline, and only a tiny fraction of a percentage of nurses lose their licenses for this reason. In some states, incompetence is subsumed under unprofessional conduct "as defined by the board." In 1977 and 1978, the New York State Board of Regents, which controls all health professional licensing boards, published a set of rules related to unprofessional conduct. Some particularly pertinent to nurses included abandoning, neglecting, harassing, abusing, or intimidating a patient; failing to

maintain accurate patient records; claiming professional superiority or special professional abilities or skills, unless so certified by an agency recognized by the Board of Regents; failing to exercise appropriate supervision over persons authorized to practice only under the supervision of a licensed professional; ordering excessive tests, treatment, or use of treatment facilities; claiming to use a secret method of treatment; failing to making available to a patient, at the patient's request to another licensed health practitioner, copies of records, reports, and so on; failing to wear an identifying badge, indicating the practitioner's name and professional status while practicing in a place where health care is given.

Not all states have such definitive regulations, as can be noted in the Tuma case. Nevertheless, there is an increasing public demand, frequently with subsequent legislative or regulatory action, that licensed practitioners fulfill the minimum mandate of their licensing privilege, providing safe and effective care. The corollary is the ethical/legal responsibility of all health professionals to see that incompetent practitioners are not permitted to practice.

THE RIGHTS OF NURSES AND EMPLOYERS

Nurses have rights, too, as human beings, citizens and professionals. Many of the legal rights of nurses are delineated in the nurse practice acts, an indication of the power and privilege given by society. Nevertheless, some of the rights nurses may assume they have, such as patient advocates, may conflict with the rights other professionals see as theirs or what employers see as inappropriate for employees.[93] There are even those who believe nurses should want no rights, because the concept of rights is interpreted as being given only to the powerless.[94] The nurse patient advocate who speaks for the patient can indeed have a problem; some nurses have been fired. At least one won a dramatic victory. She publicly criticized the care of patients in a state mental hospital, after leaving there in frustration because the administration neither listened to her nor made an effort to improve conditions. She was hired by another state institution, but dismissed shortly afterwards because of "incompetence." A newspaper printed her complaints about the first hospital, and this caused "staff anxiety." There was no grievance procedure, so eventually she instituted a lawsuit. Both the American Civil Liberties Union and the Pennsylvania Nurses' Association joined as *amicus curiae.* The court ruled in her favor, noting that incompetence was unproven and also an afterthought in her discharge and that the employer simply wanted to get rid of an outspoken employee; the nurse's First Amendment rights had been violated. She was reinstated and awarded back pay.[95]

Other nurses have fought sex discrimination on the job; they include nursing faculty who have suffered rank and salary discrimination. An unusual case was that of two Denver nurses[96] who were fired for having "outside interests," their private practice carried on outside of their hospital working hours. The nurses knew that it was common practice for men employed by the hospital to have second jobs or private patients. Sixteen months later, EEOC investigation found "reasonable cause" to believe that the nurses were victims of sex discrimination. When the hospital would not accept this arbitration, the nurses brought suit. Finally, the hospital settled out of court.[97]

It is clear that many nurse's rights issues are related to the nurse's employee status, and their resolution is the same as a similar situation with another employee, for example, hiring and firing incidents. One situation that has been gaining attention is fair treatment for nurses who cannot work on certain days for religious reasons. As might be expected, rulings have differed, so further EEOC and/or legal suits can be expected.

This is an example of an employer/employee rights conflict that has no clear-cut answer. Does the employer have a responsibility to patients that overrides an individual employee's personal needs, desires, or even moral commitment? As noted earlier, a conscience clause gives all health practitioners the choice not to participate in activities deemed "wrong" by them. But, what if such action results in understaffing or neglect of patients, however temporary? Does not an employer have the right to expect the employee to do his or her job (assuming that the components of the job were clear before employment)?

As with patients' rights, these issues have not been clearly decided, with or without legal intervention. There is no doubt that as medical and health care becomes more complex, whole new vistas of legal/ethical concerns will need to be dealt with.

NOTES AND REFERENCES

1. U.S. Health, Education and Welfare Department, *Secretary's Commission on Medical Malpractice* Report. (DHEW Pub. No. (OS) 73–88) (Washington, D.C., U.S. Government Printing Office, 1973), p. 71.

2. George Annas, "The Hospital: a Human Rights Wasteland," *Civil Liberties Rev.,* Fall 1974, p. 20. See also February 1980 *Medicolegal News* on "Patients Rights" no. 1 (Feb. 1980), **8:**4–13, and Leah Curtin, "Is there a Right to Health Care?" *American Journal of Nursing* 3 (Jan. 1980), **80:**462–465.

3. Beatrice Kalisch, "Of Half Gods and Mortals: Aesculapian Authority," *Nursing Outlook (NO)* **23:**22–28, (January 1975).

4. Emanuel Hayt and Jonathan Hayt, *Law of Hospital, Physician and Patient,* (Berwyn, Ill.: Physicians' Record Co., 1972), p. 479.

5. J. H. Hedgepeth, "Trial court finds hospital strictly 'liable' for physician negligence," *Hosp. Med. Staff,* (February, 1974).

6. Helen Creighton, "Law for the nurse supervisor: informed consent," *Superv. Nurs.,* **6:**9, 48–49 (January, 1975).

7. Ibid., p. 9.

8. Ibid., p. 48.

9. George Annas, *The Rights of Hospital Patients* (American Civil Liberties Union Handbook), (New York: Avon Books, 1975), p. 64.

10. Nathan Hershey and S. H. Bushkoff, *Informed Consent Study,* (Pittsburgh: Aspen Systems Corp., 1969), p. 3.

11. R. J. Alfidi, "Informed Consent. A Study of Patient Reaction," *JAMA,* **216:**1225–1329 (May 24, 1971).

12. Hershey and Bushkoff, op. cit.

13. David Warren, *Problems in Hospital Law*, 3rd ed. (Germantown, Md: Aspen Systems Corp., 1978), pp. 95, 138–141, 178.

14. Linda Besch, "Informed Consent: A Patient's Right," *NO*, **27**:33 (Jan. 1979).

15. "Consent Form for Jehovah's Witnesses Agreed Upon," *Medicolegal News*, **7**:12 (Summer 1979). Also in *Mod. Med.* (July 15–Aug. 15, 1978).

16. Helen Creighton, "Refusal of Blood Transfusion," *Sup. Nurse*, pp. 65–66.

17. H. L. Hirsch, "Informed Consent—Fact or Fiction," *J. Leg. Med.*, **5**:28 (Jan. 1977). See also Kathleen M. Fenner, *Ethics and Law in Nursing Professional Perspectives* (New York: D. Van Nostrand Company, 1980), Chapter 4, pp. 75–124.

18. Jay Katz, "Informed Consent—A Fairy Tale? Law's Vision," *University of Pittsburgh Law Review*, **39**:137–174 (Winter 1977).

19. Besch, op. cit., pp. 34–35.

20. "Professional Misconduct?" Letters. *NO*, **25**:546 (Sept. 1977). See also editorial, p. 561.

21. Follow-up letters in December 1977 issue, pp. 738–743; January 1978 issue, pp. 8–9; February 1978, p. 78; March 1978, pp. 142–143.

22. "Jolene Tuma Wins: Court Rules, Practice Act Did Not Define Unprofessional Conduct," *NO*, **27**:376 (June 1979).

23. Sue Reitz, "Signed Consent: Is It Really the Nurse's Responsibility?" (Letter to the Editor), *NO*, **27**:154–155 (March 1979).

24. Peter Black, "Criteria of Brain Death: Review and Comparison," *Nurs. Dig.*, **4**:71–73 (Summer 1976). Condensed and reprinted from *Postgraduate Med.*, **57**:69–74 (Feb. 1975).

25. Peter Black, "Brain Death," *New England Journal of Medicine (NEJM)*, **299**:398 (Aug. 24, 1978).

26. Ibid., pp. 398–399.

27. Ibid., p. 399.

28. *Belchertown State School* v. *Saikewicz*, 1977 Mass. Adv. Sh. 2461, 370 N.E. 2nd 417 (1977).

29. *In re Karen Quinlan*, 69 N.J. 399 (1976).

30. Daniel and Nancy Rothman, *The Professional Nurse and the Law*, (Boston: Little, Brown and Company, 1977), pp. 139–140.

31. George Annas, "Reconciling 'Quinlan' and 'Saikewicz': Decision Making for the Terminally Ill Incompetent," *Am. J. of Law & Med.*, **4**:367–396 (Winter 1979).

32. Sissela Bok, "Personal Directions for Care at the End of Life," *NEJM*, **295**:367–369 (Aug. 12, 1976).

33. Jane Raible, "The Right To Refuse Treatment and Natural Death Legislation," *Medicolegal News*, **5**:6–8 (Fall 1977).

34. Emily Friedman, "'Natural Death' Laws Cause Hospitals Few Problems," *Hospitals*, **52**:124–148 (May 16, 1978).

35. Dennis Horan, "Right-To-Die Laws: Creating, Not Clarifying, Problems," *Hospital Progress*, pp. 62–78 (June 1978).

36. Joyce Beauchamp, "Euthanasia and the Nurse Practitioner," *Nurs. Dig.*, **4**:83–85 (Winter 1976). Condensed and reprinted from *Nurs. Forum*, **14**(1):56–73 (1975).

37. Marya Mannes, *Last Rights* (New York: William Morrow & Co., Inc., 1974).

38. "Nurse, on Trial for Murder, Called Compassionate," *New York Times*, March 14, 1979, p. A 17.

39. "Terminal Patient and No-code Orders," *Regan Report on Nursing Law*, **14**:1 (Nov. 1973).

40. "Optimum Care for Hopelessly Ill Patients," *NEJM*, **295**:362–364 (Aug. 12, 1976).

41. Mitchell Rabkin and others, "Orders Not to Resuscitate," *NEJM*, **295**:364–366 (Aug. 12, 1976).

42. Robert Trotter, "Psychosurgery, the Courts and Congress," *Nurs. Dig.*, **2**:92–95 (Dec. 1973).

43. A. H. Bernstein, "Legal Rights of Mental Patients," *Hosp.*, **53**:49–52, 92 (March 1979).

44. E. Parker and G. Tennent, "The 1959 Mental Health Act and Mentally Abnormal Offenders: A Comparative Study," *Med. Science and the Law*, **19**:29–38 (Jan. 1979).

45. Walter Barton and Charlotte Sandborn, *Law and the Mental Health Professions* (New York: International Universities Press, 1978).

46. Charles Prigmore and Paul Davis, "Wyatt v. Stickney: Rights of the Committed," *Nurs. Dig.*, **3**:70–77 (Summer 1974).

47. John Wilson, *The Rights of Adolescents in the Mental Health System* (Lexington, Ma.: Lexington Books, 1978).

48. Marguerite Mancini, "Nursing, Minors, and the Law," *American Journal of Nursing (AJN)*, **78**:124,126 (Jan. 1978).

49. Alan Sussman, *The Rights of Young People*, an American Civil Liberties Union Handbook (New York: Avon Books, 1977), p. 26.

50. Ibid., pp. 224–226.

51. Ibid., pp. 27–28.

52. Ibid., p. 29.

53. Ibid., pp. 30–31.

54. "A Model Act Providing For Consent of Minors For Health Services," *Pediatrics*, pp. 293–296 (Feb. 1973).

55. The National Association of Children's Hospitals and Related Institutions, Inc., *The Pediatric Bill of Rights*, 1974.

56. "Research with Children: The Rights of Children," Editorial, *Child Psychiatry and Human Development*, pp. 67–70 (Winter 1973).

57. A. R. Jonsen, "Research Involving Children: Recommendations of the National Commission for the Protection of Human Subjects of Biomedical and Behavioral Research," *Pediatrics*, **62:**131–137 (1978).

58. "The Age of Consent," Editorial, *Am. J. Public Health*, **68:**1071–1072 (Nov. 1978).

59. Charles Lewis and others, "Informed Consent by Children and Participation in an Influenza Vaccine Trial," *Am. J. Public Health*, **68:**1079–1082.

60. Leonard Glantz, "Protecting Children and Society," *Medicolegal News*, **7:**2–3 (Summer 1979).

61. Edward Porcano, "Experimentation with Children: The Pawns of Medical Technology," *Medicolegal News*, **7:**4–9 (Summer 1979).

62. George Annas, "Legalizing Laetrile for the Terminally Ill," *Hastings Center Report*, **7:**19–20 (Dec. 1977).

63. John Kahring, "Conference Report: Seeking a Judicial Determination that Treatment May Be Withheld from a Seriously Ill Newborn," *Medicolegal News*, **7:**10–11 (Summer 1979).

64. Amatai Etzioni, "The Right to Know, to Decide, to Consent and to Donate," *Nurs. Res.*, **2:**43–50 (Oct. 1974).

65. R. S. Stone, "The Rights of Human Beings Participating as Subjects in Biochemical Research," Guest Editorial, *J. Lab. Clin. Med.*, **85:**184 (Feb. 1975).

66. "Protecting Research Subjects," *AJN*, **79:**1139–1140 (June 1979).

67. Helen Creighton, "Legal Concerns of Nursing Research," *Nurs. Res.*, **26:**337–341 (Sept./Oct. 1977).

68. Katharyn May, "The Nurse as Researcher: Impediment to Informed Consent," *NO*, **27:**36–39 (Jan. 1979).

69. Kathleen Kelly and Eleanor McClelland, "Signed Consent: Protection or Constraint?" *NO*, **27:**40–42 (Jan. 1979).

70. Ruth MacKay and John Soule, "Nurses as Investigators: Some Ethical and Legal Issues," *Nurs. Digest*, **5:**7–9 (Spring 1977).

71. Bradford Gray, "An Assessment of Institutional Review Committees in Human Experimentation," *Med. Care*, **13:**318–328 (Apr. 1975).

72. Marcia Opp, "The Confidentiality Dilemma," *Nurs. Digest*, **4:**17–19 (Fall 1976).

73. Alan Westin, *Computers, Health Records and Citizens' Rights*, NBS Monograph 157 (Washington, D.C.: U.S. Dept. of Commerce, National Bureau of Standards, 1977).

74. Carol Levine, "Sharing Secrets: Health Records and Health Hazards," *Hastings Center Report*, **7:**13–15 (Dec. 1977).

75. Hayt and Hayt, op. cit., p. 1094.

76. Melissa Auerbach and Ted Bogue, *Getting Yours: A Consumer's Guide to Obtaining Your Medical Record* (Washington, D.C.: Public Citizen's Health Research Group, 1978).

77. U.S. Department of Health, Education and Welfare, op. cit., pp. 76, 77, 109, 110, 127, 134.

78. Alan Westin, "New Era in Medical Records," *Hastings Center Report*, **7:**23–28 (Dec. 1977).

79. Auerbach and Bogue, op. cit., p. 14.

80. Given Health Care Center, *Principles of Practice* (Burlington, Vt.: University of Vermont, mimeographed), p. 1.

81. Annas, op. cit., pp. 112–120.

82. George Annas and Joseph Healey, "The Patient's Rights Advocate," *J. Nurs. Admin.*, **4:**25–31 (May/June 1974).

83. Auerbach, op. cit., pp. 34–36.

84. *The Rights of Hospital Patients*, pp. 116–118.

85. Mary Hemelt and Mary Ellen Mackert, *Dynamics of Law in Nursing and Health Care* (Reston, Va.: Reston Publishing Co., 1978), pp. 72–81.

86. Health Law Center, *Problems in Hospital Law* (Rockville, Md.: Aspen Systems Corp., 1972), pp. 95–96.

87. Hemelt and Mackert, op. cit., pp. 68–71.

88. Helen Creighton, *Law Every Nurse Should Know*, 3rd ed. (Philadelphia: W. B. Saunders Company, 1975), pp. 166–167.

89. Helen Creighton, "The Unplanned Child," *Sup. Nurse*, 3:7–8 (June 1972).

90. Philip Reilly, *Genetics, Law and Social Policy* (Cambridge: Harvard University Press, 1977).

91. Linda Stanley, "Dangerous Doctors: What To Do When the MD is Wrong," *RN*, 42:22–27, 29–30 (March 1979).

92. "Going Beyond the Hospital," *RN*, 42:28 (March 1979).

93. Elsie Bandman, "Do Nurses Have Rights? Yes," *AJN*, 78:84–86 (Jan. 1978).

94. Bertram Bandman, "Do Nurses Have Rights? No," *AJN*, 78:84–86 (Jan. 1978).

95. Helen Creighton, "A Nurse's Freedom of Speech," *Sup. Nurs.*, 5:45–48 (Apr. 1974).

96. Bonnie Bullough, "The Struggle for Women's Rights in Denver: A Personal Account," *NO*, 26:535–536 (Sept. 1978).

97. "Two Tenacious RNs Fight Hospital Over Sex Discrimination and Make It Pay," *RN*, 42:15–16 (March 1979).

Annotated Bibliography

Julia and Harry Abrahamson, eds., *Who Shall Live? Man's Control Over Birth and Death* (New York: Hill and Wang, 1970).

> This is a report prepared for the American Friends Service Committee. The Friends are frequently called Quakers. The report is liberal by some standards in dealing with the population explosion, birth control, quality of life and our control over death. It presents a good overview of the issues involved.

Paul Adams, Leila Berg, Nan Berger, Michael Duane, A. S. Neill, and Robert Ollendorf, *Children's Rights* (New York: Praeger Publishers, Inc., 1971).

> Subtitled, "Toward the Liberation of the Child," this collection of essays is concerned with the infant in relation to family and society, self-government for children in home, society, and school, and the child under the law. Not all agree with this approach but it's the wave of the present against the past. Whether it will be sustained in the future remains to be seen.

American Nurses' Association, *Code for Nurses With Interpretive Statements* (Kansas City: ANA, 1976).

> This document is the 1976 statement of the professional code of ethics for nursing practice. Although somewhat prescriptive, this revision of the 1950 code for nurses depends more on the accountability of the nurse to the client. The Interpretive Statements explain and expand in detail each of the eleven statements of the Code.

ANA, *Perspectives on the Code for Nurses* (Kansas City, Mo.: ANA, 1978).

The six papers that appear in this volume were originally presented at the ANA convention, June 1976. The perspectives on the code that are addressed include the historical, educational, practice, administration, research, and philosophical. Excellent background information for understanding the development and use of the current code for nurses.

George J. Annas, *The Rights of Hospital Patients: The Basic ACLU Guide to a Hospital Patient's Rights* (New York: Avon Books, 1975).

This is an American Civil Liberties Union Handbook. Rights overlap the legal field and morals and ethics. Some are written into law and others are matters of informed consent, self-determination, treatment refusal, transplants, and so on. A special chapter on children and another on women are most helpful. Although nurses do not get a lot of attention in the book, he notes (p. 15) that 99 percent of the time, patients are cared for by nursing staff.

Philippe Aries, *Centuries of Childhood* (New York: Alfred A. Knopf, Inc., 1962).

Not all will agree with the thesis that childhood was "discovered" in the Middle Ages. Yet all who work with children should read this volume, now available in paperback (Vintage V-286). The background will help our understanding on how parents can expect the children to act like adults and to be more mature than the parents themselves.

Leroy Augenstein, *Come, Let Us Play God* (New York: Harper & Row, Publishers, 1969).

Genetics and medical procedures now allow us to assume this role. In the face of the population explosion and increasing genetic defects, we should. Others say we have been playing God since the dawn of time, because all manipulation of our environment is "playing God." Augenstein is a very readable text that raises essential questions in an understandable way.

Jeanne Q. Benoliel and Jeanne S. Berthold, *Human Rights Guidelines for Nurses in Clinical and Other Research* (Kansas City, Mo.: ANA, 1975).

This booklet discusses the changing scope of nursing responsibilities, particularly in reference to the protection of human rights during research. Ethical guidelines are presented for the nurse, and mechanisms for the protection of rights are discussed. The interface of ethical and legal aspects of practice are also presented.

Elsie L. and Bertram Bandman, eds., *Bioethics and Human Rights* (Boston: Little, Brown and Company, 1978).

Short but insightful pieces by many authors on the nature of rights, genetics, abortion, euthanasia, rights of children, parents, nurses, patients, prisoners, and rights on the national and international levels. The views range from personal perspectives to well-documented studies.

Andrew Bauer, ed., *The Debate on Birth Control* (New York: Hawthorne Books, Inc., 1969).

The essays examine the pro and con of birth control, especially in the wake of the discussion following the Pope's encyclical, "Humane Vitae," which prohibited all forms of birth control except abstinence and the rhythm method.

Tom L. Beauchamp and LeRoy Walters, eds., *Contemporary Issues in Bioethics* (Encino, Calif.: Dickinson Publishing Co., Inc., 1978).

This is a very fine selection of essays covering ethical theory and its application as well as such traditional concerns as abortion, scarce resources, experiments, death, and dying. The editors give helpful introductions along the way.

David Belgum, *When It's Your Turn to Decide* (Minneapolis: Augsburg Publishing House, 1978).

A hospital chaplain offers helpful advice in how to talk to professionals, deciding on abortion, prolonging dying or living, having children, human experimentation. A guide to decision making brings order out of confusion.

Charles Birch and Paul Abrecht, eds., *Genetics and the Quality of Life* (Elmsford, N.Y.: Pergamon Press, Inc., 1975).

This is a series of papers from a 1973 conference in Geneva, Switzerland. The conference was sponsored by the World Council of Churches. Most of the papers state problems or ask questions without dealing with the underlying ethic or moral, or suggesting any direction.

Baruch Brody, *Abortion and the Sanctity of Life: A Philosophical View* (Cambridge, Mass.: The MIT Press, 1975).

The author changed views from pro-choice to pro-life. The emphasis is on the sanctity of life rather than quality of life.

Edmond Cahn, *The Moral Decision: Right and Wrong in the Light of American Law* (Bloomington: Indiana University Press, 1955).

An insightful and witty review of the interweaving of law and morals in United States history. It has been said we tend to write our morals into law. The result is sometimes confusing even as we claim we cannot legislate morality. Cahn looks at morals as a legal order, law as a moral order, and law in sex, business, and death as well as the sticky question of who decides.

Daniel J. Callahan, *Abortion: Law, Choice and Morality* (New York: Macmillan Publishing Co., Inc., 1970).

This liberal Catholic's massive study reviews the world situation up into the late 1960s. This reviews other religions and cultures as well as that of Roman Catholicism. Legally, he holds to a minimum of law, leaving it to various groups to influence their own members.

Daniel J. Callahan, ed., *The Catholic Case for Contraception* (London: Arlington Books, 1961).

The essays include pro and con, but the emphasis is on the case *for* contraception. Compare Healy, Noonan, Bauer, Spitzer and Saylor, Joseph Fletcher.

Eric J. Cassell, *The Healer's Art, A New Approach to the Doctor-Patient Relationship* (Philadelphia: J. B. Lippincott Company, 1976).

Cassell claims that the healer's art is not to treat disease but to treat patients. In this patient-centered approach, he tries to enter the world of the sick and see things from the patient's perspective. He is also concerned with overcoming the fear of death.

John Connery, *Abortion: The Development of the Roman Catholic Perspective* (Chicago: Loyola University Press, 1977).

Connery gives an historical survey to the mid-twentieth century. He claims a clear and consistent teaching against abortion from the moment of conception, even as he documents those Roman Catholics who thought otherwise.

Anne J. Davis and Mila A. Aroskar, *Ethical Dilemmas and Nursing Practice* (New York: Appleton-Century-Crofts, 1978).

Introductory chapters give an overview of ethics, and the second half of the book has chapters on such issues as abortion, mental retardation, public policy. A closing chapter gives examples of ethical dilemmas, although discussion of the role of the nurse is limited. A good beginning text for nurses.

Emily Taft Douglas, *Margaret Sanger: Pioneer of the Future* (New York: Holt, Rinehart and Winston, 1970).

This biography of Sanger also serves as a history of the modern birth control movement until her death in 1966.

Barbara Ehrenreich and Deidre English, *Witches, Midwives, and Nurses—A History of Women Healers*, 2nd ed. (Old Westbury, N.Y.: The Feminist Press, 1973).

One of a series of studies of the role of women who have been systematically excluded from the doctor role. Witches were burned, midwives banned, and nurses accepted only after they made it clear they were there to serve doctors and not challenge their authority or profits. Controversial consciousness-raising, worth a pause in the professionalization of women in the health field.

Encyclopedia of Bioethics, ed. by Warren T. Reich, four volumes (New York: The Free Press, 1978).

The 314 articles by 285 contributors cover issues, religious viewpoints, and related disciplines. Its price ($200) and size (almost 2,000 pages) make it more of a library acquisition than a personal item. Yet it is perhaps the most comprehensive single publication available in the field. Although more conservative than liberal, the articles generally present a fair and balanced overview of problems ranging from abortion to zygotes.

Ethical Dilemmas in Current Obstetric and Newborn Care, Report of the Sixty-Fifth Ross Conference on Pediatric Research (Columbus: Ross Laboratories, 1973). See Moore.

Ethical Dilemmas in Nursing—A Special AJN Supplement, AJN, vol. 77, no. 5 (May 1977), pp. 845–876.

An excellent selection of articles written about nurses and ethics. Insightful, provocative writing by Levine, Romanell,

Johnson, Cawley, Lestz, Yeaworth, the Bandmans, and Churchill with helpful anecdotal incidents interspersed throughout the main articles. A must for the nurse who is looking for direction in considering ethical dilemmas in nursing practice.

Joel Feinberg, ed., *The Problem of Abortion* (Belmont, Calif.: Wadsworth Publishing Co., Inc., 1973).

A collection of essays pro and con on abortion in morality and law, including a summary of the Supreme Court decision of 1973. The volume is part of a series in philosophy, and the discussion involves some of the esotericism of that discipline.

David M. Feldman, *Marital Relations, Birth Control and Abortion in Jewish Law* (New York: Schocken Books, 1978, original 1968).

This is the definitive work on Jewish ethics for this subject. The focus is on traditional positions, with discussion of the various opinions. Reform Judaism and Conservative Judaism tend to be more liberal than Orthodox Judaism.

Joseph F. Fletcher, *The Ethics of Genetic Control* (Garden City, N.Y.: Anchor Books, 1974).

Fletcher wants mankind to "end reproductive roulette" by taking charge of life from beginning to end. He writes from a secular, humanist position with a Protestant background. Some see him as logical, and others see him as an extremist liberal. For a balanced approach to the Protestant ethical perspective, one might read both Fletcher and Paul Ramsey, for example, Ramsey's *Fabricated Man.*

Joseph F. Fletcher, *Morals and Medicine* (Princeton: Princeton University Press, 1954).

In an early attempt to present a Protestant view, Fletcher acknowledges the work of his Catholic predecessors in ethics. He describes his own contribution as a personalist position, a regard for human personality as contrasted to an ethic of deontology (duty) or utilitarianism (consequences). He surveys rights, truth telling, contraception, and euthanasia.

Joseph F. Fletcher, *Situation Ethics* (Philadelphia: The Westminster Press, 1966).

This highly controversial work has gone through many printings. For Fletcher, love is the only norm. It justifies its means. Although his thesis is often denied in favor of traditional rules, his rule is itself a tradition in Judaism and Christianity.

Vincent J. Fontana, *Somewhere a Child is Crying: Maltreatment—Causes and Prevention* (New York: Macmillan Publishing Co., Inc. 1973).

After many years of work with battered and neglected children, the author shares experiences, his concern for the whole family, and recommendations on where we need to continue our efforts.

Vincent J. Fontana and Douglas J. Besharov, *The Maltreated Child*, 4th ed. (Springfield, Ill.: Charles C. Thomas, Publisher, 1979).

A follow-up and an update on the problem by people who work with neglected children.

R. F. R. Gardner, *Abortion, The Personal Dilemma* (Grand Rapids, Mich.: William B. Eerdman, 1972).

From the English scene, Gardner examines the moral, spiritual, psychological, medical, socioeconomic issues, with detailed discussions of history, techniques, pro and con alternatives. He writes after the liberal Abortion Act of 1967 in Britain. Gardner emphasizes a Christian viewpoint that is moderate Protestant; that is, abortion can be performed, but it is not a trivial matter. He cites numerous cases. Excellent review of the issues, including complications.

Joseph Goldstein, Anna Freud, and Albert J. Solnit, *Beyond the Best Interests of the Child* (New York: The Free Press, 1973).

Courts frequently focus on the physical aspects of child care. The authors focus more on the psychological, looking beyond a basic legal/ethical/moral principle of care for the abused or neglected child.

Robert E. Hall, ed., *Abortion in a Changing World*, vols. I and II (New York: Columbia University Press, 1970).

The proceedings of an international conference on abortion held 17 November 1968. Vol. I covers ethical, medical, legal, social, and global aspects. Vol. II covers topics such as animation, poverty, public health, mortality, birth defects, and women. The give and take of the discussants is interesting although it also interferes with continuity. Although over ten years old, this remains an important collection of thought on abortion.

Michael P. Hamilton, ed., *The New Genetics and The Future of Man* (Grand Rapids, Mich.: William B. Eerdman, 1972).

This book is a series of articles on new beginnings of life, genetic therapy, and pollution. A scientist presents the then current state of knowledge, which is then discussed from a legal, social, and ethical perspective.

Garrett Hardin, *Mandatory Motherhood: The True Meaning of "Right to Life"* (Boston: Beacon Press, 1974).

A strong, frequently humorous and incisive statement by a biologist who believes in freedom of choice. A woman should be able to have an abortion if she wants one.

Bernard Häring, *Ethics of Manipulation, Issues in Medicine, Behavior Control and Genetics* (New York: Seabury Press, 1975).

Father Häring shares his concern for manipulation—any use of technology that jeopardizes human freedom and dignity. He compares liberal and conservative Protestant ethics with traditional Roman Catholic teachings.

Bernard Häring, *Medical Ethics* (Slough, England: St. Paul Publications, 1972).

A review of the issues and official Catholic teaching, as well as the author's personal views. These are sometimes by fiat, so the reasoning behind his pronouncement that something is wrong is not always clear. He touches on genetics, birth, abortion, death, health, allocation of scarce resources, experimentation, professional secrecy, psychiatry, and so on.

The Hastings Center Report, a journal published by the Institute of Society, Ethics, and the Life Sciences, Hastings-on-Hudson, N.Y. 10706.

One of the finest resources available for bioethics. Articles deal with broad issues of policy as well as many specific issues. There are think pieces as well as reports on current happenings. An excellent way to keep up with a burgeoning field.

Edwin F. Healy, *Medical Ethics* (Chicago: Loyola University Press, 1956).

This book carries the imprimatur of Cardinal Stritch. To that extent, it can be said to carry the official teachings at the time for Roman Catholicism. Healy gives many case studies, illustrating the sometimes fine lines between such doctrines as ordinary and extraordinary, secondary effect, what is permissible, and what is not. A detailed guide for the time.

Ray E. Helfer and C. Henry Kempe, eds., *The Battered Child*, 2nd ed. (Chicago: The University of Chicago Press, 1974).

A series of essays focusing on the history, legal, medical, psychiatric, and social work aspects of child abuse. Still a very useful volume, although in part outdated.

Bruce Hilton, Daniel Callahan, Maureen Harris, Peter Condliffe, and Burton Berkley, eds., *Ethical Issues in Human Genetics* (New York: Plenum Publishing Corporation, 1973).

The papers here are from a symposium in 1971. The subjects include counseling, screening, legal and public policy issues, and the quality of life. A thorough coverage, including discussion of the pro and con on the issues.

Norman E. Himes, *Medical History of Contraception* (New York: Gamut Press, 1963).

This 1936 classic was reprinted in 1963. Alan F. Guttmacher's Preface gives an overview of the developments up to 1963. Himes reviewed the then current state of knowledge on primitive tribes, as well as ancient Egyptian, Greek, and Roman sources, the Bible, Talmud, Islam; China, India, and Japan, Europe in the Middle Ages, and the West to the modern period. He emphasizes the universal desire to control the number of offspring—neither too few nor too many.

Robert Hunt and John Arras, eds., *Ethical Issues in Modern Medicine* (Palo Alto, Calif.: Mayfield Publishing Company, 1977).

Republication can be very helpful at times, and that is the case here. The editors have gathered representative positions on genetics, abortion, euthanasia, informed consent, behavior modification, justice, and the allocation of scarce resources. The general introduction serves as an introduction to bioethics, and each section has an introduction outlining the issues. The collection is useful for introductory and advanced studies. Six of 44 authors are women.

Ivan Illich, *Medical Nemesis* (New York: Pantheon Books, Inc., 1976).

Illich takes off after medicine as he has education—with an ax. Get rid of it and go back to home remedies. Save money and be healthier. The concept of iatrogenic illness—illness having its origin in medical practice—is not new. An ancient prayer said, "God save us from the doctors." The message of "One Flew Over the Cuckoo's Nest" was "Save us from the Big Nurse." Illich will make one angry or make one think. We hope more the latter.

Immanuel Jakobovitz, *Jewish Medical Ethics* (New York: The Philosophical Library, 1959).

A review of the Talmud and traditional Jewish ethics bearing on medical practice as of the late 1960s. Compare Preuss, Rosner, and Feldman.

W. T. Jones, Frederick Sontag, Morton O. Beckner, Robert J. Fogelin, eds., *Approaches to Ethics: Representative Selections from Classical Times to the Present* (New York: McGraw-Hill Book Company, 1962).

Each reading has an introduction giving historical background to the material. The introduction to the book gives the background of ethical theory, main types, and problems in ethics. A helpful introduction to the field of ethics.

Albert R. Jonsen and Michael J. Garland, eds., *Ethics of Newborn Intensive Care* (Berkeley: University of California Press, 1976).

A welcome addition to the literature, the book reflects a 1974 symposium that considered clinical and social (including economics) concerns with suggestions for policy. Participants were generally agreed that at times it would be right to not resuscitate, or to withdraw life support. As a whole, the book thus leans to the more liberal side of the liberal-conservative spectrum.

Jay Katz, *Experimentation with Human Beings* (New York: Russell Sage Foundation, 1972).

This huge volume is more concerned with the legal sphere than the moral and ethical. Yet, as a reference, it is invaluable for anyone concerned with this area, one of increasing importance in the health field.

Lucie Y. Kelly, *Dimensions of Professional Nursing* (New York: Macmillan Publishing Co., Inc., 1980).

This is a comprehensive reference on the major trends and issues in nursing and health care. Chapter 10 on Ethics and Accountability and Chapters 17 to 22 on Legal Rights and Responsibilities are of special importance in reference to nursing practice and ethics. This is a well-written and documented text and an excellent reference. Our chapter 9 is an excerpt.

C. Henry Kempe and Ray E. Helfer, *Helping the Battered Child and His Family* (Philadelphia: J. B. Lippincott Company, 1972).

This is practical help for child advocates, following up Helfer and Kempe's original study of the battered child. This collection of essays is a companion volume to the editors' 1968, revised 1974, *The Battered Child*. Subsequent volumes change the word to "abused" to indicate a broader concern. These essays spell out help for parents and children, where it can be found, the relationship to the law, and an outline for a treatment center that was established in 1973. The volume is essential for anyone concerned with doing something to help the battered child.

David M. Kennedy, *Birth Control in America, The Career of Margaret Sanger* (New Haven: Yale University Press, 1970).

Through the medium of Ms. Sanger's life, the author reviews the enormous changes in social and legal attitudes toward birth control.

George H. Kieffer, *Bioethics: A Textbook of Issues* (Reading, Mass.: Addison-Wesley Publishing Co., Inc., 1979).

An excellent introduction to bioethics based on the author's theory of an evolution in ethics. The medical section covers genetics, reproduction, euthanasia, experimentation, and behavior control. Nonmedical issues include future generations, nature, population explosion, science, and society.

Evelyn M. Kitagawa and Philip M. Hauser, *Differential Mortality: A Study In Socioeconomic Epidemiology* (Cambridge, Mass.: Harvard University Press, 1973).

A classical study, showing that the mortality rate is more a matter of social and economic level than health care.

Marvin Kohl, ed. *Beneficent Euthanasia* (Buffalo, N.Y.: Prometheus Books, 1975).

A collection of essays on the ethical perspective on mercy killing, suicide, and euthanasia in general. Various points of view are presented but, as the title indicates, the editor is in favor of voluntary euthanasia.

Anthony Kosnik, William Carroll, Agnes Cunningham, Ronald Modras, and James Schulte, *Human Sexuality; New Directions in American Catholic Thought*, a study commissioned by the Catholic Theological Society of America (New York: Paulist Press, 1977).

The Bible, Church history, and the sciences are reviewed for attitudes and information on sexuality. A section on the theology of sexuality is followed by pastoral guidelines for human sexuality in marital, nonmarital, and homosexual relations. The attitude of this book is a major departure from traditional Roman Catholic attitudes toward sex. In no sense is so-called "free sex" approved but there is a new openness to sexuality beyond celibate abstinence. Compare Noonan, Healy, and Callahan.

Elisabeth Kübler-Ross, ed., *Death, The Final Stage of Growth* (Englewood Cliffs, N.J.: Prentice-Hall, Inc., 1975).

A series of essays on the positive aspects of death, including Jewish, Hindu, and Buddhist views, how to deal with grief, personal vignettes, and testimonies. Nurses can be helpful through creative listening (pp. 83–84), or they may hinder through commitment to insitutional roles (p. 18).

Elisabeth Kübler-Ross, *On Death and Dying* (New York: Macmillan Publishing Co., Inc., 1969).

This is the author's initial volume in which she spelled out the now classic five stages people go through in learning of pending death. Not everyone agrees, of course, but this volume remains a definitive work, exceptionally helpful to all who work with the dying or to those who face death in their own lives.

Elisabeth Kubler-Ross, *Questions and Answers on Death and Dying* (New York: Macmillan Publishing Co., Inc., 1974).

A rarity—the book is just what the title says it is. A good introduction to the thoughts of a person who has done more than anyone to help us face the issues. Not all will agree with her, but her answers will certainly stimulate discussion.

Elisabeth Kubler-Ross and Mal Warshaw, *To*

Live Until We Say Goodbye (Englewood Cliffs, N.J.: Prentice-Hall, Inc., 1978).

A photo essay book emphasizing Kubler-Ross' concern that people be allowed to die at home when the hospital can no longer really help. The hospice movement is included here, as well as her healing and growth center—Shanti Nilaya.

Law and Ethics of A.I.D. and Embryo Transfer, Ciba Foundation Symposium 17, new series (New York: American Elsevier Publishing Co., Inc., 1973).

This 1972 symposium in London is concerned with the biological, ethical, and legal aspects of artificial insemination and test-tube babies.

John Galen McEllhenney, *Cutting the Monkey-Rope* (Valley Forge: Judson Press, 1973).

The monkey-rope was a safety device used in whaling. In Moby Dick, Herman Melville claimed we are all bound to one another by invisible monkey ropes. The present book's subtitle is, "Is the taking of life ever justified?" McEllhenney calls this cutting the monkey-rope. He includes abortion and euthanasia in his concern and focuses on attitudes toward death and dying.

David R. Mace, *Abortion: The Agonizing Decision* (Nashville, Tenn.: Abingdon Press, 1972).

A very readable discussion of the issues, presented as a counselor and a woman wanting an abortion, but not quite sure, attending a conference in which the pro and con positions are presented. Although officially leaving the client to make up her own mind, Mace is very clearly against the extreme liberal position of abortion at will, without serious consideration of the issues in each case.

Ramona T. Mercer, *Perspectives on Adolescent Health Care* (Philadelphia: J. B. Lippincott Company, 1979).

Adolescence is a normal part of human development rather than a disease. But because the teen-ager is developing, special concerns remain. The authors look at the young person in terms of health, illness, sexuality, childbearing, and in relation to the health care system. This is a valuable book for health personnel working with teens.

James C. Mohr, *Abortion in America: The Origins and Evolution of National Policy*,

1800–1900 (New York: Oxford University Press, 1978).

Mohr presents historical data showing that abortion in the first trimester (before quickening) was not only common but openly advertised, even in religious magazines. He claims that "regular" doctors, seeking the development of the A.M.A., used the abortion issue to put the irregulars out of business by getting laws passed between 1825–1875 making abortion illegal. The Supreme Court decision of 1973 returned the country to the earlier position and put the "irregulars" (back alley abortionists) out of business. A controversial interpretation.

Tom D. Moore, ed., *Ethical Dilemmas in Current Obstetric and Newborn Care*, report of the Sixty-Fifth Ross Conference on Pediatric Research (Columbus, Ohio: Ross Laboratories, 1973).

The conference discussion ranged over pregnancy, abortion, and postnatal care, the complications encountered, the potential outcomes, the ethics of treatment in relation to outcome, who decides to do what and why, legal and administrative perspectives. Joseph Fletcher and Robert M. Veatch represent ethics and Dagmar Cechanek represents nursing.

James J. Nagle, *Heredity and Human Affairs* (St. Louis: The C. V. Mosby Company, 1974).

Written for the nonspecialist in genetics, Nagle reviews the processes of genetics with a clear overview of what happens. Along the way, he touches on social and ethical issues related to the present and the future.

Susan Teft Nicholson, *Abortion and the Roman Catholic Church*, JRE Studies in Religious Ethics II (Knoxville: University of Tennessee, 1978).

A careful and important critique. Nicholson does not approve of abortion on demand, but she also notes the justification for selected abortion, *from within* Catholic ethical theory. Controversial but crucial for people concerned with this area.

John T. Noonan, *Contraception: A History of Its Treatment by the Catholic Theologians and Canonists* (Cambridge, Mass.: Harvard University Press, 1965).

Noonan's overview shows the variety in what has sometimes been seen as a single viewpoint. He is not always consistent or, rather, on occasion he insists on an historical consistency that his own review shows did not exist. Compare Himes, Healy, Callahan, Spitzer and Saylor, and Joseph Fletcher.

John T. Noonan, ed., *The Morality of Abortion* (Cambridge, Mass.: Harvard University Press, 1970).

Contributors include Noonan, Paul Ramsey, J. J. Gustafson, Bernard Häring, and others. They give some of the historical and theological background for the issue of abortion from a Catholic and a Protestant perspective. The authors are either against abortion entirely or want to limit it to the most exceptional cases.

Thomas C. Oden, *When Shall Treatment be Terminated?* (New York: Harper & Row, Publishers, 1976).

Helpful guidance, developed by ethicists and lawyers, philosophers, and others after the Quinlan court decisions. The guidance is conservative, that is, in favor of the patient—when in doubt, prolong life—but not absolutist.

Jean Piaget, *The Moral Judgment of the Child* (New York: The Free Press, 1965).

Nurses working with children may find this very helpful. Piaget is hard to read for many people but is worth the struggle. Alternately, one of the introductions to Piaget can be reviewed for this section of his work. Not all child development people agree with his findings, but Piaget's influence continues to grow.

Julius Preuss, *Biblical and Talmudic Medicine*, transl. ed., Fred Rosner (New York: Sanhedrin Press, 1978, original 1911).

This is a classical study with traditional Jewish views that have bearing on the problems of today. Although applying most heavily to orthodox Judaism, the principles affect other Jews and Christians and the culture at large through such things as Supreme Court decisions. Compare Feldman, Jakobovits, and Rosner.

Paul Ramsey, *Ethics at the Edges of Life: Medical and Legal Intersections* (New Haven: Yale University Press, 1978).

The first edge of life Ramsey concerns himself with is abortion, and the last edge is death and dying, whether in defective neonates or the aged or ages in between.

Ramsey is opposed to quality of life judgments and uses his opposition to insist that we should not practice any form of euthanasia, passive or active. Yet, he also opposes relentless treatment of the dying. Thus he treads a narrow path between, a path that may be a bit vague at times. He reviews case law, Supreme Court decisions, and legislation as these relate to the edges of life.

Paul Ramsey, *Fabricated Man, The Ethics of Genetic Control* (New Haven: Yale University Press, 1970).

Ramsey does not like fabricated people. Women do not have a right to have a baby when it involves "in vitro" fertilization. That is a misuse of science. Science infringes upon nature and human rights in the genetic manipulation going on today.

Paul Ramsey, *The Ethics of Fetal Research* (New Haven: Yale University Press, 1975).

Basically he's opposed to fetal research. The fetus cannot give informed consent. Much of this research is not for the benefit of the individual fetus or it is very limited in benefit. If the fetus is an abortus, two wrongs do not make a right.

Paul Ramsey, *The Patient as Person: Explorations in Medical Ethics* (New Haven: Yale University Press, 1970).

Ramsey is a Protestant who represents a conservative position, sometimes described as more Catholic than present-day Catholics. His concern is to protect the patient without regard to the quality of life. Life is sacred. His discussion tends to be long, but it is important. The life you save may be yours. Protestant Joseph Fletcher and Catholic Richard McCormick present alternate views.

John Rawls, *A Theory of Justice* (Cambridge, Mass.: Harvard University Press, 1971).

A seminal study reviewing the concept of justice. Although Rawls does not give practical directions on what to do, his five principles have had a major influence in ethical theory. They are general, universal (compare Kant), public, orderable (can decide between conflicting claims), and final (higher than law or custom).

Philip Reilly, *Genetics, Law, and Social Policy* (Cambridge, Mass.: Harvard University Press, 1977).

Reilly's law background has helped him bring together the many strands in this field. Such things as genetic screening and counseling, confidentiality, genetic problems affecting particular ethnic groups, and public policy have moral and ethical implications. Both patients and health personnel need to know the legal as well as the ethical implications in the area of genetics. An important book for people working in this area.

Richard M. Restak, *Premeditated Man: Bioethics and the Control of Future Human Life* (New York: The Viking Press, Inc., 1975).

One of the great concerns about the new biology is our ability to control future generations. Who will do what? Restak's provocative discussion gives food for thought.

John Rock, *The Time Has Come* (New York: Alfred A. Knopf, Inc., 1963).

Rock sees the goal of Catholic and non-Catholic groups as being the same, that of responsible parenthood. Only the methods differ. He reviews some of the history of birth control, including public policy and theological perspectives. A Catholic president used federal funds for birth control; Catholic theologians see the natural law as eternal but subject to new interpretations.

Harold Rosen, ed., *Abortion in America: Medical, Psychiatric, Legal, Anthropological, and Religious Considerations* (Boston: Beacon Press, 1967).

A series of essays, most dating from the earlier form of the book in 1954.

Fred Rosner, *Modern Medicine and Jewish Law* (New York: Yeshiva University, 1972).

Rosner compares the Bible and the Talmud with today's issues, such as transplants, AID, euthanasia, contraception, abortion, smoking. A valuable update of Preuss (which he edited for the new edition). For birth and marriage issues, compare also Feldman.

Margaret Sanger, *An Autobiography* (New York: W. W. Norton & Company, Inc., 1938), reprint (New York: Dover Publications, Inc., 1971.)

Sanger (1883–1966) reflected on her life and her fight for birth control. There is much history on the latter and a fascinating glimpse of this American pioneer.

Jane Linker Schwartz and Lawrence H. Schwartz, eds., *Vulnerable Infants, A Psycho-*

social Dilemma (New York: McGraw-Hill Book Company, 1977).

High-risk pregnancies, premature births, mother-infant bonding, follow-up, critical issues in care for mothers and infants, including euthanasia for defective newborns are among the essays in this volume. The essays are reprints, but it's a valuable collection and good to have them conveniently in one place. An overall theme is to lower the vulnerability.

Thomas A. Shannon, ed., *Bioethics* (New York: Paulist Press, 1976).

Shannon introduces the tradition in Roman Catholic ethics. In the process, there is a reevaluation of this tradition. The articles continue this process but they are from across the field, dealing with the major issues as prominent scholars see them.

Harmon L. Smith, *Ethics and the New Medicine* (Nashville, Tenn.: Abingdon Press, 1970).

The author focuses on abortion, the meaning of parenthood, transplants, experimentation, and death and dying. He insists the Judeo-Christian ethic is crucial to an understanding of the ethical dilemmas we face today.

Walter O. Spitzer and Carlyle L. Saylor, *Birth Control and the Christian, A Protestant Symposium on the Control of Human Reproduction* (Wheaton, Ill.: Tyndale House Publishers, 1969).

The symposium was sponsored by evangelical Protestants, who are often seen as on the conservative side of the conservative-liberal spectrum. The twenty-seven men and one woman (a pediatrician), were among the participant geneticists, sociologists, legal, and medical people, as well as theologians. The general position favors abortion under restricted circumstances, such as health of the expectant woman, rape, and defective fetus.

Shirley M. Steele and Vera M. Harmon, *Values Clarification in Nursing* (New York: Appleton-Century-Crofts, 1979).

This readable text discusses the value elements of nursing decisions, many of which revolve around biomedical ethics and issues. The first three chapters discuss values and value clarification in detail, as well as medical and nursing codes of professional practice. With this background information, the rest of the book is set up as a workbook. Case situations and questions for self-study are included for the nurse. Areas discussed include quality of life, genetics and reproduction, euthanasia, and scarce resources.

Peter Steinfels and Robert M. Veatch, eds., *Death Inside Out* (New York: Harper & Row, Publishers, 1974).

A collection of essays on the new discussability of death, new concepts of death, new decisions being made about death, and the naturalness of death. Helpful for anyone working with the dying.

Barbara L. Tate, *The Nurse's Dilemma, Ethical Considerations in Nursing Practice* (Geneva: International Council of Nurses, 1977).

This book provides examples in nursing practice on an international scope. The book is organized according to sections of the *ICN Code for Nurses, Ethical Concepts Applied to Nursing, 1973*. Each illustrative situation is followed by some provocative questions that the reader is encouraged to use as a basis for discussion with others. A helpful set of questions for approaching each situation is offered on pp. x–xi.

Jacques P. Thiroux, *Ethics* (Encino, Calif.: Glencoe Press, 1977).

The first half of the book considers ethics in general, what it is, and its general concerns. Specific issues are then discussed, such as abortion and euthanasia.

Diane B. Uustal, *Values and Ethics: Considerations in Nursing Practice; A Workbook for Nurses* (South Deerfield, Mass.: D. B. Uustal, 1978).

This volume is a workbook with a variety of good exercises that one can use to identify one's own values and positions on certain situations that can arise in nursing practice. Unfortunately, there is minimal direction for use of the workbook or for understanding the context of values. Apparently intended for use in a workshop, it is not as helpful as it might be when used alone.

Kenneth Vaux, ed. *Who Shall Live?* (Philadelphia: Fortress Press, 1970).

Essays—Catholic, Protestant, deontological, utilitarian—compare technology and the ethics thereof. Margaret Mead points out how the culture shapes the ethical situation, and German theologian Helmut Thielicke offers theological foundations for ethics in modern medicine.

Robert M. Veatch, *Case Studies in Medical Ethics* (Cambridge, Mass.: Harvard University Press, 1977).

Veatch is Senior Associate of the Institute of Society, Ethics, and the Life Sciences (Hastings Center). *The Hastings Center Report* has regularly presented cases plus commentaries in bioethics. Here are 112 cases with introductions and comments. The book is a good introduction to bioethics, as well as an excellent teaching tool for those who use the case method. Values and principles are included as well as the topics of genetics, contraception, abortion, transplants, behavior modification, experimentation, consent, death and dying.

Robert M. Veatch, *Death, Dying, and the Biological Revolution: Our Last Quest for Responsibility* (New Haven: Yale University Press, 1976).

An essential text for anyone interested in death and ethics. Veatch reviews the problems of technical and natural death, euthanasia, truth telling, harvesting the dead for transplants, public policy. In all, he calls for responsible decision making.

Robert M. Veatch, *Value-Freedom in Science and Technology: A Study of the Importance of The Religious, Ethical, and Other Socio-Cultural Factors in Selected Medical Decisions Regarding Birth Control* (Missoula, Mont.: Scholars Press, 1976).

These decisions may pass as medical decisions, but they are not value-free. However, the values may be cultural rather than religious, and they are usually hidden rather than known, even from the decision makers.

Dr. and Mrs. J. C. Willke, *Handbook on Abortion* (Cincinnati: Hiltz, 1971).

In the abortion discussion, the Willkes represent an anti-abortion position. They present persuasive arguments against abortion and also call for responsible parenthood, which includes contraception and a concern for the world's population explosion.

Jan Wojcik, *Muted Consent* (West Lafayette, Ind.: Purdue University Press, 1978).

Muted consent refers to the many situations when informed consent is impossible or secondary: experimentation, genetics, abortion, behavior control, the comatose, and allocation of scarce resources. We, or those who come after us, may be subject to consentless medicine.

Nancy F. Woods, ed. *Human Sexuality in Health and Illness*, 2nd. ed. (St. Louis: The C. V. Mosby Company, 1979).

This is a solid overview of the subject of human sexuality with important sections on adolescent sexuality, pregnancy, and abortion.

Glossary

Abortion: The ending of a pregnancy prior to viability (usually 28 weeks gestation/500 Gms.). An induced abortion is brought on intentionally while a spontaneous abortion or miscarriage is due to natural causes or accident. Distinctions are also made between therapeutic abortions for health reasons and elective abortions to prevent the birth of a child.

Accountability: Responsible for one's actions. This may be a legal concept of being liable and subject to the law. It is also and, perhaps more often, a moral/ethical concept as when one is answerable to authority or responsible to a patient or a supervisor. One may *be* the authority who is held accountable.

Advocate: One who defends or speaks up for another. From the Latin "advocatus," which means counselor or lawyer. A patient's advocate represents the patient who is unable or limited in self-defense.

Affective: Expressing emotions or feelings, in contrast to cognitive thinking.

Allocation of Scarce Resources: The dividing up of something that there is little of. See "Justice."

Amniocentesis: The process of using a hypodermic needle to withdraw fluid from the amniotic sac. The fluid is then checked for evidence of birth defects. It can also be used to find out if the fetus is male or female. The Greek "amnion" comes from "amnus" or lamb, "kentesis" from pricking.

Amoral: Neither moral nor immoral.

Artificial Insemination: The insertion of sperm into the female vagina by artificial means. AIH refers to the husband as the source of the sperm while AID refers to a donor as the source of the sperm.

Ashkenazim: The Jews (and their descendents) who settled in Europe, especially Eastern Europe, contrasted to the Sephardim who settled in Spain.

Assault: A threat to do harm, whether it results in harm or not. Usually thought of as a violent physical or verbal attack.

Autonomy: Self-governing, self-determining, independent. From the Greek "autos" for self and "nomos" for law. The autonomy of the patient means not being subject to another's rules or having to do what one is told.

Battery: A legal term related to assault as in assault and battery. It refers to unauthorized touching, including touching with an instrument, without consent.

Beneficent: Something good or beneficial. The ethical principle of beneficence may be used interchangeably with the principle of the common good. See "Good."

Bioethics: The Greek "bios" means "life." In the broad sense, bioethics refers to ethics dealing with life or the life sciences. The *Encyclopedia of Bioethics* includes articles on the environment, behavior modification, man's religions, medical ethics, etc. The term is often used, however, in a more restrictive sense as medical ethics or biomedical ethics (as distinguished from traditional medical ethics which are now a matter of etiquette).

Birth Control: Anything that averts pregnancy. Technically, most birth control methods prevent conception. The IUD device prevents implantation.

Brain Death: As developed by the Harvard Ad Hoc Committee, brain death refers to a person having a flat EEG (electroencephalogram), without reflexes or voluntary breathing, and who is unreceptive and unresponsive. This concept of physiological death is becoming more prominent in contrast to cardiac death since the heart can be kept pumping artificially under certain circumstances.

Canon Law: Usually the laws or dogma decreed by a church council. The Latin "canon" means "rule" or "measuring line." Symbolically, it is that against which something is measured to see if the new principle is acceptable or correct. Because canon law is the law of the church, it is subject to change, in contrast to natural law which is unchanging (though interpretations may change).

Carrier: A person who does not suffer from a particular disease but can transmit that disease to another.

Categorical Imperative: A concept of the philosopher Immanuel Kant. He believed that all people have within them an impulse to do right. See "Universalism."

Cloning: Asexual reproduction by replacing the nucleus of an unfertilized egg with the nucleus of a cell from the organism to be reproduced. A genetically identical copy results. While cloning has been done with lower animals such as frogs, claims for the cloning of higher life forms remain to be confirmed.

Code of Ethics: A system of rules governing a group such as doctors or nurses. As used in this text, the code is based on the level of morals, the "shoulds" and the "oughts" of the profession. Ethics refer to the reasons behind the code, in such things as the ANA Interpretive Statements.

Cognitive: The thinking or verbal aspect of knowing, as contrasted with the affective or feeling aspect.

Commitment: A pledge, often of oneself, as in a professional commitment to care for a patient or uphold professional standards. See Covenant Fidelity." Latin "com" means together; "mittere" means to send. The sending or bringing together implies a relationship, often involving trust, as in the nurse—patient relationship.

Common Law: Law which is unwritten and is derived from custom, court decisions, and everyday experience, in contrast to legislated law which is officially pronounced as such.

Conceptus: A fertilized ovum at any stage of development, such as a fetus or an unborn baby.

Confidentiality: Something private or secret. In law, lawyers, clergy, doctors, and others cannot be required to divulge private or confidential matters. The concept is being extended to nursing and other fields such as journalism.

Consanguinity: Relationship by blood or common ancestor. Consanguinous marriages are often forbidden or carefully regulated in many societies.

Consequentialism: An ethical system concerned with the end result or consequences. Some ethicists use this term as the umbrella term while others see this term as part of a larger whole such as teleology (Greek "telos" or end) or utilitarianism. In this text, these meanings have been used interchangeably with utilitarianism the one most often used.

Cost-Benefit Analysis: The relationship between cost and benefit is studied. The usual concern is that benefits outweigh the cost, as in the utilitarian ethic of the greatest good for the greatest number. In economics, it means financial cost but in illness, it may be a matter of the emotional or physical cost of suffering for patient or family in relation to the benefit gained. Benefit is hard to define for some things mean more to some people. In kidney dialysis, one person might think the benefit is high while to another it is low.

Covenant Fidelity: Fidelity refers to faithful while covenant refers to agreement, usually a binding agreement. In the Hebrew Scriptures, the relationship between God and the Hebrew people is a covenant. In health care, the covenant may be a matter of contract but is more often an understood relationship, as when a person requests care and the provider agrees to give it. The agreement may be implied in the professional status of the provider.

Death: Usually physiological death, though the term is used in theology for alienation from God and we talk about the death of a relationship such as love. Traditionally, death has been judged by such vital signs as breathing and heart beat. More recently, "brain death" has been the criteria for death since machinery can keep the lungs and heart functioning. See "Brain Death."

Deontology: An ethical system of rules or duty. The Greek "deon" means rule or binding while "logos" means word or study.

Determinism: A belief in predestination. The philosophy or theology that man does not have freedom of will or choice.

Dignity: Worthy of respect. Expressed in the concept of respect for persons such as patients. Dignity is related to autonomy.

Distributive Justice: A division or sharing that is just, right, good, or equal. In health care, it's the idea that care should go to those who need it—without regard to their ability to pay—and that it be equally available to all.

Dominant: Prevailing over others. From the Latin "dominari," meaning to rule. In Mendelian law, the dominant characteristic will appear in the offspring when paired with a recessive.

Double Effect: An ethical concept that says a good means to a good end may result in a bad side effect but this can be acceptable because the intention and the means were good. The usual example cited in Roman Catholic ethics is the removal of a cancerous uterus even though the woman is pregnant. The abortion would not ordinarily be approved but in this case it is secondary and thus acceptable.

Down's Syndrome: A form of retardation ranging from mild to severe. It is often called mongolism. Technically, it is trisomy-21 because it is caused by an extra chromosome number 21. In the past, mongolism has been associated with pregnancy in older women but it is increasing in frequency in younger women as well.

Duty Ethics: This term is sometimes used as equivalent to deontology. It is associated with the philosopher Immanuel Kant who emphasized the importance of being moral out of duty—i.e., whether one feels like it or not.

Eclectic: A combination from different systems. In ethics, a person might draw from utilitarianism and deontology. Natural Law is sometimes seen as such a combination. Theoretically, one might expect to take the best from the various systems but it may be an unconscious selection and what is best may be a matter of opinion.

Egoism: Ego is the common term of Freudian language. It's original Latin refers to "I" or simply self. In ethics, the self is the standard of right and wrong. In Egoistic Hedonism, it is pleasure for the self. Thiroux describes universal ethical egoism as the idea that everyone should act in his or her own self-interest. One might also think in terms of one's group or nation.

Encyclical: A letter from the Pope, usually dealing with doctrinal or Church matters. A modern example is "Humanae Vitae" on birth control.

Equality Principle: The principle or idea that people should be treated equally. In health care, this may be applied to all living humans, i.e., whether comatose, defective, rich, or poor. Others see it primarily in terms of equal access to health care, regardless of ability to pay.

Ethical Dilemma: At times, there is a conflict between two goods. It may be the rights of society vs. the rights of the individual, or, the life of one person vs. that of another, as in dealing with scarce resources. The dilemma may also be between systems of ethics such as the utilitarian "greatest good for the greatest number" vs. the value of the individual. It may be between people such as patient vs. health researchers or religious groups, administrators vs. care givers, etc.

Ethical Pluralism: There is more than one right ethic or moral or ethical system. In practice, we often mix systems like utilitarianism and deontology. Some see natural law as a combination of all of these.

Ethical Theory: The Latin "theoria" means a looking at, a contemplation. Our theories often affect the way in which we view something. Ethical theory concerns how we look at ethics.

Ethics: From the Greek "ethos" meaning custom or character. In normal discussion, and for some ethicists, the word is interchangable with "morals." We have distinguished ethics as the study of morals, i.e., a concern with the reasons or the principles behind moral codes. Philosophical systems vary in word usages. Some see morals as normative ethics while the reasons are metaethics. Generally, we are talking about the way in which people relate to each other, themselves, and, for theists, a higher power usually called God.

Eugenics: The study of genetics to improve the genetic character of people, perhaps a nation, or one's group, or the human race.

Euthanasia: From the Greek "eu-" meaning well and "thanatos" meaning "death." Traditionally, it simply meant a good death. In more recent times, attention has been focused on passive euthanasia—"letting" someone die rather than artificially maintaining life with respirators or other machines. Active euthanasia, or mercy killing, involves doing something to hasten death.

Extraordinary Means: The term is said to originate from Pope Pius XII. In talking about caring for the aged, he suggested that it is not necessary to use extraordinary means to preserve life. If the person is dying, such attempts may mean prolonging the dying rather than prolonging life. Just what constitutes ordinary means and extraordinary means is debatable. In a wealthy country, some means of treatment are quite ordinary which in a poor country would be extraordinary. Scarcity, cost in money, or in suffering to the patient or family or society, unusual types of treatment, and such factors as the age of the person, potential benefit, prognosis, etc. are all factors in deciding whether a procedure is extraordinary or not. In ancient times, all surgery was extraordinary. In other words, the interpretation changes with the time, place, and circumstances.

Gene Therapy: The replacement of a disease-bearing or defective gene with a healthy one.

Genetics: The study of heredity. The gene (Greek "gen" means produce) is the smallest unit of heredity, with a definite position on the chromosome. Irregular placement results in genetic disease.

Genetic Engineering: Chemical change of genes to correct weakness, misplacements, etc. The artificial formation of a gene.

Genetic Screening: Checking large populations for genetic defects. Required by law for some defects in certain areas.

Good: The definition of this term is a basic concern of ethics. For some, the good is pleasure. For others, it is the will of God. Some see it as harmony with nature. While others see it as the right thing to do or justice.

Hedonism: From the Greek for pleasure or delight. In egoism, the good equals pleasure, that is personal pleasure. This may extend to one's group or even humanity. The utilitarian concept of the greatest good for the greatest number was originally interpreted in hedonistic terms. The ancient Greek philosopher Epicurur (342–270 B.C.) and the Austrian psychologist Sigmund Freud (1856–1939) are two of the more prominent figures in this tradition. The name epicurean comes from the former.

Hospice: A place of rest for pilgrims. The idea is sometimes traced back to the monks of St. Bernard and the famous St. Bernard dogs in the Alps. Dr. Cicely Saunders established a hospice for the dying at St. Christopher's in London. The idea has spread to the U.S. and several hundred are now in operation or under construction. Through home care or in a home like atmosphere, the dying are cared for, or rather, are helped to live until they die. This is in contrast to the use of extraordinary measures to prolong dying as long as possible.

Human Being: A member of the species "homo sapiens" meaning wise man. The question of who or what is human is a major issue in abortion and in issues related to the dying such as the comatose, as in brain death. Some prefer alternate terms like person or personhood. The "sapiens" suggests rationality as the human trait, leading some to say that the fetus has only potential humanness and that when the brain is dead, the person is dead, i.e., without rationality.

Human Dignity: Respect for human dignity, that is for the worth of persons, is a basic issue in health care. The present day health care system has been accused of robbing people of their human dignity by treating them as objects to be manipulated for the benefit of the system rather than the welfare of the patient.

Humanae Vitae: An encyclical of Pope Paul VI in 1968 in which he rejected birth control except for the rhythm method under certain circumstances.

Humanism: Basically any system or thought pattern concerned with humans. In ethics and philosophy, it tends to be a system of thought that excludes traditional religion or belief in a supernatural being. However, humanism is recognized as a religion by the U.S. Supreme Court.

Humanistic Ethics: An ethics that excludes the supernatural.

Incompetent: The "in-" means "not" while Latin "competens" means "able, sufficient." In contrast to "incapable" which describes the physically unable, incompetent refers to the "unqualified." With patients, it would mean unqualified to make decisions as in the case of a minor or infant, the comatose, severely retarded, or emotionally disturbed. With professionals, it would mean lacking the skills or knowledge to do what the professional supposedly is trained to do. It is also a legal term.

Infanticide: The killing of an infant. For those who believe the fetus is a child, abortion equals infanticide.

Informed Consent: A knowledgeable agreement. Consent is a growing concern in health care. A main side-issue is who can give consent for the incompetent. What constitutes "informed" is also of major importance. One definition is: "that amount of knowledge which is normally given to a patient." Legally, courts have often recognized this as sufficient but not always.

Intuitionism: In ethics, this is the idea that we know what is good or right without being taught. It is sometimes called subjectivism. It relies on feelings rather than reason. Its innate quality relates the concept to Kant's categorical imperative and Natural Law, as well as theories of child development which emphasize native ability rather than environment or training.

In Vitro Fertilization: Fertilization "in glass." It is sometimes referred to as test-tube babies and the "vitro" is more apt to be a flat dish called a petri dish. An unfertilized egg or ovum is removed from the female and fertilized in the laboratory. The fertilized egg is then implanted in the woman's uterus. This method of fertilization is used to help women with conception problems.

Justice: A legal term referring to unlawful. In ethics, it may mean being fair or impartial. The concept of equality is sometimes related to justice as in the just distribution of goods.

Liable: A legal term from the Latin "ligare" meaning to bind. The person who is liable is or can be held responsible or answerable for his or her actions.

Living Will: A will that a person can make out while still "being of sound mind and body," that directs family, doctors, lawyers, clergy, and other interested personnel not to use extraordinary means to prolong their dying, in the event they become comatose or otherwise incompetent to direct their last days.

Malpractice: Bad practice. As a legal term, it refers to unprofessional or incompetent care, advice, etc.

Medical Ethics: Originally, this referred to what today we might call etiquette, like how large the doctor's sign should be, how much the fee should be, etc. Today, it refers to the issues of bioethics and is often interchanged with biomedical ethics. As such, it refers to all health care. In the general sense in which morals and ethics are used interchangeably, medical ethics includes codes of ethics such as the ANA Code for Nurses and the Hippocratic Oath.

Mendel's Law: Gregor Mendel was an Austrian monk botanist who discovered laws of heredity such as the idea that each characteristic such as hair color, etc., is inherited separately and that some of these characteristics are dominant while others are recessive. If two parents each carry a recessive characteristic, their children will inherit that characteristic. On a statistical basis, one child will show the characteristic, two will be carriers of the recessive gene, and one will be free of it. In reality, none of their children or all of their children might be in one of the three categories.

Mercy Killing: Active euthanasia.

Metaethics: Greek "meta-" means above or beyond. As used in this book, metaethics is the analysis of ethics, as ethics is the analysis of morals. In some philosophical systems, metaethics is a second type of ethics, sometimes compared to other types such as normative ethics, which we have been using as equivalent to morals.

Morals: In Latin "moralis" means manners, customs. Currently used in relation to right and wrong in conduct. Some systems use the Latin morals as interchangeable with the Greek ethics. In this book, morals refers to the "shoulds" and "oughts" of life, i.e., what conduct should be carried out or what is prescribed, as contrasted to ethics that are concerned with the reasons behind the morals. On this basis, the code of ethics like the ANA Code for Nurses is a moral code, while the Interpretive Statements are an ethical analysis, i.e., they give reasons for the Code.

Natural Law: Law or rules of conduct or morals based on nature. They are derived from nature and can be discovered by reason as contrasted to spiritual revelation.

Negligence: Carelessness. In legal terminology, carelessness results in injury.

Neonatology: Greek "logos" means study while Greek "neos" means new. A neonate is a newborn so we have here the study of the newborn. In practice, it refers to all phases of care of the newborn. The term was coined in 1969 by Dr. Alex Schaffer.

Nonconsequentialism: Ethics based on principles rather than consequences. Equivalent to deontology. The supernatural revelations of Judaism and Christianity are examples. So are the duty ethics of Immanuel Kant.

Normative Ethics: An ethics concerned with norms. All prescriptive ethics such as egoism and utilitarianism are examples.

Obligation: Obliged to something or someone through promise or contract or by professional status. The Latin "ob" means before and the word "Ligare" means to bind. This implies a responsibility to which we are bound before it happens.

Ordinary Means: Ordinary means are the usual or common means. What is ordinary in a wealthy country may be extraordinary in a poor one. In the Quinlan case, the doctors thought of the respirator as ordinary treatment while Roman Catholic thought implied the opposite. See "Extraordinary Means."

Paternalism: The Latin "pater" means father. Here fatherhood has extended to a company or group, or to patients, who are treated like children. In the face of the rising tide of human rights, the term seems derogatory. The female equivalent, "maternalism," does not have the same derogatory meaning.

Personal Ethics: Individual ethics, which may or may not be different from the ethics of a group or others.

Personhood: Used to refer to the unborn fetus, the incompetent, or the comatose. Personhood is an issue in abortion and euthanasia discussions.

Pragmatism: A philosophy or attitude concerned with being practical.

"Primum non Nocere": "First Do No Harm."

Principle: From the Latin "principium" meaning beginning. It is the origin or cause of something, or more broadly, it is a basic truth or doctrine. The principles of ethics or ethical principles are basic truths, concepts, or reasons.

Privacy: The state of being away from observation. The right to privacy was instrumental in the Supreme Court decision allowing a pregnant woman to get an abortion in the first trimester without permission of others.

Professional Ethics: The ethics of professionals such as those in health care, lawyers, clergy, businessmen, engineers. The term professional is sometimes used as the equivalent of ethical while unprofessional equals unethical.

Quality of Life (QOL): Usually contrasted to Quantity of Life or Sanctity of Life. The idea that life itself is sacred or the highest good. QOL implies that sheer or mere existence is not enough. Life must be free enough of pain or disability to be meaningful or meaningful enough to overcome the pain or disability. The Living Will reflects a concern for the QOL. Some see severly defective children as lacking QOL. See "Sanctity of Life."

Recessive: In genetics, the characteristic that appears the least. The opposite of dominant. See "Dominant."

Relativism: Values vary among persons, groups, cultures, circumstances.

Respect: Esteem, honor, high regard, consideration for another.

Responsibility: That for which one is responsible, accountable, or liable.

Rights: That to which one has a claim, as in the right to health care. Some say that wherever there is a right, there is a corresponding obligation, i.e., if one has a right to health care, privacy, equal treatment, etc., then someone else has an obligation to provide such care, privacy, etc. Some say the "other" is merely obligated not to interfere, as in privacy, to leave the first party alone. Rights are debatable with widely differing opinions.

Sanctity of Life: Used interchangeably with Quantity of Life, and opposed to Quality of Life. The Sanctity of Life doctrine sees life as the highest good which must be protected and prolonged whenever possible. This is sometimes seen as sanctioned by deity. Many agree except in unusual circumstances such as protecting one's country or one's honor. It may mean artificially prolonging life regardless of the degree of defectiveness or incompetence.

Self-Determination: The individual can determine for her/himself whether to continue or discontinue treatment.

Slippery Slope: Equivalent to the wedge argument in ethics. If one exception is allowed, as in abortion, then one slips down the slope to where all abortions must be allowed. The argument then is that not even one exception can be allowed, regardless of circumstances or consequences.

Situation Ethics: An ethic originated by Joseph Fletcher who calls it "act utilitarianism." No moral rule applies except the rule of love. Apart from that, one is guided by the situation. Some have pointed out that most rules originated in a situation or a context, rather than in a vacuum.

Social Ethics: Ethics for society such as justice or feeding the hungry. These concerns may be the same as or different from individual or personal ethics. Some see the latter as a matter of privacy, e.g., sexual relations between consenting adults. Others think that all ethics are social, i.e., of concern to society. Still others believe that justice and such things as health care for the poor are of no concern to the individual. If every individual acted morally or ethically, there would be no need for social concern because society would then be ethical.

Statutory Law: Law set up by official bodies such as legislatures.

Talmud: A collection of Jewish writings or laws. The Mishnah (about 200 A.D.) records the oral law, which is sometimes seen as a commentary upon the written law (the Torah or the first five books of the Bible). The Hebrew word means repeat from the belief that this merely repeats the original law given to Moses by God. The second part of the Talmud is the Gemara, meaning completion. It is sometimes seen as a commentary upon the Mishna, but it also contains additional material. The Babylonian Gemara was completed about 400 A.D. while the Palestinian was finished about 500 A.D. The Talmud remains an important source of moral law for many Jews today. Some of these rules have found their way into general western thinking including legal thought.

Teleology: Greek "telos" means end. See "Consequentialism."

Triage: An emergency procedure in which those who cannot survive are left untreated, those who can wait for treatment are left untreated (or treated only sufficiently) so that those requiring immediate attention to survive are treated first.

Truth: Something actual or real. The opposite of false. May be seen as absolute rather than relative though "facts" change from time to time or at least our interpretations change.

Truth-Telling: The ethical issue of whether health personnel should tell patients everything about their condition or disease, the nature of the research, the prognosis for recovery, etc.

Universalism: Applicable to all. In Kant's ethical system, one of the norms or standards was whether an act, if done by everyone, would result in good. See "Categorical Imperative."

Utilitarianism: An ethic of consequences. Some describe it in terms of the greatest good for the greatest number. Utilitarianism acts are based on consequences and the good results. Utilitarianism rule is the rule that brings the greatest good. Utilitarianism is sometimes described as the ethic that the end justifies the means. This tends to be a derogatory description. Utilitarianism officially began with Jeremy Bentham (1748–1832) and John Stuart Mill (1806–1873).

Values: Worth, esteem, things desirable. Values may range from the most simple (I like ice cream) to ultimate values such as God or Life or Nature. Values often exist in a hierarchy such as God, country, family. As noted in the text, "Values Clarification Theory" elaborates the concept. Values are personal beliefs about ideas, objects, or behavior. Values are personal guidelines providing a frame of reference for relationships, ideas, and events.

Vitalism: Life is the ultimate good. It must be sustained at all times and at all costs. In this regard, the concept is related to Sanctity of Life. An older, more elaborate meaning of vitalism is the philosophical concept that life is a vital principle quite apart from its physical characteristics. It is self-determining and evolving, in contrast to a mechanistic view of the universe.

Wedge Argument: See "Slippery Slope."

ZPG (Zero Population Growth): The idea that no one should produce more children than required to maintain the population at zero growth. Another way of stating it is that the birth rate should equal the death rate or that no one should have more than two children, i.e., enough children to replace themselves.

Index

A

Abortion, 73–104
  attitudes toward, 78–82
  birth control and, 50
  case studies on, 87–89
  counseling, 85–87, 89
  ethical issues and, 82
  historical perspective of, 74–78
  nurses and, 82–87
  personal values and, 83, 87
  religious perspectives, 74–75
  Supreme Court decisions, 73, 76–78, 80, 226
  viable product of, 106–107, 120
Abuse
  adults and, 134, 165, 170
  children and, 134–36
  ethical issues in, 134, 146–48
  historical perspective on, 135–36
  legal considerations in, 142–43
  nurses and, 141–44
  primary intervention in, 141
  secondary intervention in, 142
Accountability, role of nurse and, 4, 116
Adolescent sexuality, 51, 52n, 136–38, 144–46, 149
  ethical aspects of, 144
  historical perspective, 136
  legal aspects of, 144
  pregnancy and, 136–37, 145–46, 148
Adults and bioethics, 161–82. *See also* Allocation of scarce medical resources
  case studies in, 172–74
  ethical issues and, 166–67
  role of nurse, 167–72
Advocate, nurses as, 59, 116, 140
Aging and ethics, 183–209. *See* also Death and dying
Allocation of scarce medical resources, 29n, 161–64, 166, 187n

Allocation of scarce medical resources (*cont.*)
  aged and, 184–85, 187–88
  case studies involving, 195
  concept of social worth in, 164
  ethical issues in, 161–64, 183
  historical perspective and, 162
  how to allocate, 164
  nurse role in, 167–70
Altruism, 9n
American Nurses' Association Code for
    Nurses, 1, 11, 162n, 163n, 165n. *See also*
    Codes of ethics
  abortion and, 82, 84, 85, 88
  adults and transplants, 170
  birth control and, 60
  child abuse and, 142–43
  and death and dying, 186, 190, 191
  discussion of, 3
  genetics and, 33–34, 36
  historical background of, 11
  neonatology and, 118
  research on children and, 140, 221
Amniocentesis
  abortion and, 80
  case study involving, 35–36
  ethical issues in, 27
  genetics and, 32
Artificial insemination, 28–29, 227
  case study of, 37–38
Assault, definition of, 224–25
Autonomy, concept of, 26, 188, 190

B

Battery, definition of, 224–25
Benemortasia. *See* Euthanasia; Death and
    dying
Bioethics, definition of, 2, 8
Birth control, 49–71. *See also* Contraception
  case studies in, 59–62
  ethical issues in, 58
    abortion, 50
    coitus interruptus, 51
    condom, 51
    intrauterine device (IUD), 50–51
    oral contraceptives, 52n, 54, 59–60
    rhythm, 53–54
    sterilization, 56–57, 226–27
  historical perspective on, 49–54
  legal aspects of, 219
  religious views and, 50, 51–54, 55–56, 57
  role of nurse and, 58–59
Birth defects. *See* Genetics

Brain death, criteria of, 186n, 217
Brompton Cocktail, 187n

C

Carrier, 25. *See also* Genetics
Casti Connubi, 23n, 53, 54, 57
Categorical imperative, 8, 9n
Childhood and ethics, 131–59
  case studies in, 146–49
  ethical issues, summary, 138–39
    child abuse, 134–36, 147–48
    children and research, 132–34, 140–41,
      146
    sexuality, 136–38
  historical perspective, 135–36
  role of nurse, 139–46
    abused child, 141–44
    adolescent pregnancy, 145, 148
    adolescent sexuality, 144–46
    research on children, 139–41
Codes of ethics
  ANA, 1n, 2n, 11, 55n
  ICN, 11–12
  personal values and, 3–4
  purpose of, 1, 10–12
Coercion, concept of, 25, 26, 84–85
  sterilization and, 56
  transplant donors and, 162–63
Confidentiality
  child abuse and, 134
  contraception and, 219–20
  genetics and, 27, 33–34
  patients records and, 222–24
Conscience clause, 55n, 84–85
Contraception. *See* Birth control
Cost benefit, 51n, 112, 139, 187n
  transplants and, 163, 168
Covenant
  concept of, 8–9
  nurse-patient relationship and, 3, 7, 186

D

Death and dying,
  attitudes toward, 187–88, 191–92
  care of, 193
  case studies in, 193–95
  definition, 185n
  ethical issues in, summary, 188
    death with dignity, 184
    refusal of care/treatment, 186
    truthtelling, 192
  historical perspective on, 185–86
  laws concerning, 186n

no treatment in, 108*n*, 109*n*, 111, 186*n*
role of nurse in, 188–93
Decision-making
ethical dilemmas in, 4, 107, 110–11, 113
nurses and, 3–5, 115*n*, 115–16, 167–70,
171–72, 189, 191
patients and, 26, 44, 110
team, 5, 110–11, 114, 115, 167–68, 189, 191
Deontology, 8, 113*n*
definition of, 8
ethical systems of, 8–9
Distributive justice. *See also* Allocation of
scarce resources
case study in, 174
principle of, 162, 164, 166, 167
"Do no harm." *See* Primum non nocere
Double effect, principle of, 8*n*, 9*n*, 26*n*, 79*n*,
109*n*, 111*n*. *See also* Secondary effect,
principle of
Downs Syndrome, 25*n*, 34, 80, 110, 111, 114

E

Ensoulment
Aristotle and, 75, 76
concept of, 29, 73, 76–77, 106
creationist view of, 77
Plato and, 76
Talmudic reference on, 75–76
traducianist view of, 77
Ethical codes. *See* Codes of ethics
Ethical hedonism (egoism), 8*n*, 9, 165*n*
Ethics
definition of, 1, 7, 8*n*
history and, 6–8
nurses and. *See* Nurses
principles of, 1*n*, 50*n*, 166*n*, 184*n*
study of, 12–13
theories of, 2*n*, 8*n*, 8–10, 166*n*
Eugenics, 24*n*, 28–29
Euthanasia
active defined, 190
adults and, 185, 187
definition of, 111
neonates and, 108*n*, 109*n*, 110–12, 218
passive defined, 188, 191
role of nurse in, 190–92
Extraordinary means. *See* Ordinary/
extraordinary means

F

False imprisonment, 225–26
Fetal experimentation. *See* Research, fetal/
neonatal

Fetus
concept of, 74*n*
feticide, 75
personhood of, 76*n*, 162
Formal-equality principle, 107–108, 171
Freedom of Information Act, 222, 223

G

Genetics, 23–47
case studies in, 35–38
cloning in, 30
counseling for, 32–33
disease, 34, 38, 119
engineering in, 27
ethical issues in, 31
gene pool, 27–28
gene therapy, 30
historical perspective of, 23–24
nurses and, 30, 31–35
screening in, 25*n*, 33, 227
Geriatrics. *See* Aging
Golden Rule, 1*n*, 8*n*, 9*n*, 10, 171, 186*n*

H

Harvard criteria of death, 185*n*, 217
Hippocratic oath, 78, 106, 111*n*, 187*n*. *See also*
Primum non nocere
Historical perspective of ethics, 6–8
abortion and, 74–78
birth control and, 49–54
child abuse and, 135–36
death and dying and, 185–86
distributive justice and, 162
increased understanding with, 7–8
neonatology and, 108–109
Hospice, 187, 188, 193
Humanae Vitae, 54, 55, 77*n*
Hyde Ammendment, 74*n*, 164

I

Incest taboos, 24, 36
Incompetent practitioners, 227–28
Infanticide, 23, 24, 49–50, 106, 134*n*
Informed consent
abortion and, 81*n*
adults and, 165–66
age of, 132–33, 140, 220
case study on, 61, 146–47
children and, 111*n*, 132–33, 138–39
definition of, 8*n*, 214
genetic screening and, 25*n*, 33–34

Informed consent (*cont.*)
  mature minor and, 220
  research and, 30–31, 116–17, 140–41
  role of nurse in 216–17
  trends in, 214–16
International Code for Nurses, 11–12
Intrauterine device, 50–51
In vitro fertilization, 29–30
Is-ought, 9n, 28, 76n

J

Judeo-Christian tradition
  abortion and, 73n, 74–75, 76–77
  artificial insemination, 28
  birth control and, 24n, 50, 51–54, 55–56, 57
  child abuse and, 135–36
  dying and, 186, 187
  genetics and, 26
  incest and, 24
  infanticide and, 50, 106, 108–109
  organ transplants and, 162–63
  quality of life and, 109–10
  research on children and, 133
  rule ethic and, 8, 10
  women and, 166
Justice and Fairness. *See* Rawlsian theory

K

Kidney disease
  dialysis, 162n, 169–70, 72
  transplant, 162–63, 168, 172–73

L

Law
  abortion and, 77–78, 226
  allocation of scarce resources, 164n
  artificial insemination and, 28–29, 227
  child abuse and, 134, 142–43
  death and, 186n
  ERA and, 166
  euthanasia and, 218
  genetics and, 26n
  helpless and, 219–20
  hemodialysis and, 162
  incompetent practitioners, 227–28
  informed consent and, 214–17
  nurses and, 172, 216–17
  patients' rights and, 212–14
  viable fetus and, 106–107
  wrongful life and, 26n, 75n, 110n

Lifeboat ethics, 164, 164n
Living Will, 186, 217–18

M

Malpractice, 186n, 212, 218
Masturbation, 51
Mercy killing. *See* Euthanasia
Metaethics, 2
Moral development, stages of, 8n
Morals/morality, 1, 2, 162n

N

National Center for the Prevention and
    Treatment of Child Abuse and Neglect,
    134n, 141
National Commission for the Protection of
    Human Subjects, 132
National Research Act, 221
Natural Death Act, 186n, 218
Natural fallacy. *See* Is-ought
Natural Law, 8n, 25, 26, 51n, 52–53, 55, 76n,
    105, 113n
Nazi experience, 29, 30, 56n, 111n, 186n, 215
Neonatology, 105–30
  case study in, 117–20
  ethical issues in, summary, 113
    NNICU's, 105, 110, 114
    no treatment decisions, 111–12, 117–18
    ordinary vs. extraordinary means, 107
    quality of life, 110
    research, fetal 112
    research, neonatal 112–13
    treatment, 111
    viable product of abortion, 106, 120
  historical perspective in, 108–109
  role of nurse in, 113–17
Normative ethics, 2n, 8n
No treatment decisions. *See* Death and dying;
    Neonatology
Nuremberg Code/Laws, 30, 135, 215
Nurses
  abortion and, 82–87
  adults and, 167–72
  birth control and, 58–59
  childhood and adolescence, 139–46
  conscience clauses and, 84–85
  death and, 188–93
  ethical codes for. *See* Ethical codes; ANA
    Code for Nurses
  ethics, reasons for study 2–6
  genetics and, 30–35
  legal responsibilities of, 217–18, 228–29
  loss of license, 227–28

making health care decisions. *See* decision-making
neonatology and, 113–17
professional competence of, 6, 8*n*
rights and responsibilities, 4*n*, 10–11, 228–29
roles and relationships, 3, 5, 83, 143, 166, 169–70, 171

O

Ordinary/extraordinary means, 8*n*, 80*n*
aged/dying and, 185, 186*n*, 188–89, 190
neonatology and, 107, 111
transplants and, 163

P

Patients' Bill of Rights, 32*n*, 212–13
Patients' rights, 212–14
access to records, 222–24
Personhood, concept of 106*n*, 110*n*, 135–36, 167
fetus and, 162
Population control, 56, 81–82
Power
fighting for, 5
patients and, 165–66
Prenatal diagnosis. *See* Amniocentesis
Primum non nocere ("Do no harm"), 1*n*, 31, 78, 106, 111, 132*n*. *See also* Hippocratic oath
Privacy, right to, 33, 224. *See also* Confidentiality
Privacy Act of 1974, 186*n*, 222, 223
Pro-choice, 74*n*, 80, 81. *See also* Abortion
Prolife movement, 74, 79, 80, 81
Proxy consent, 132–33

Q

Quality of life ethic, 110
abortion and, 81, 82
adults and, 163
aged and, 184*n*, 186*n*, 187, 190
birth control and, 50–51
children and, 131, 136
genetics and, 25–26, 31, 34
neonates and, 105, 108*n*, 109, 111*n*

R

Rawlsian theory of justice, 9
Recombinant DNA, 30

Research
children and, 132–33, 146–47, 221
ethics of, 132–34
fetal/neonatal, 112–13, 146
guidelines for, 140–41
rights of patients in, 221–22, 132*n*
role of nurse in, 30–31, 34, 116–17, 140–41
Rights and Responsibilities
children and, 26, 131–32
clients and, 133, 165, 212–14
to die, 112, 194, 217–19
employer's, 228–29
fetal, 73, 75*n*
genetics and, 25, 31
to health care, 162
helpless and, 219–21
human, 25, 73
legal aspects of, 211–43
privacy, 186*n*
to refuse treatment, 216
reproduction, 28*n*, 74*n*
societal, 56, 74

S

St. Christopher's Hospice, 187*n*
Saline abortion, 107
Sanctity of life ethic
abortion and, 81, 82
aged and, 184–85, 186*n*
children and, 131, 136
genetics and, 25, 34
neonatology and, 109
Self-determination, 189–90, 193
case study in, 194–95
no code orders, 218
Sexual discrimination, 29*n*, 165*n*
case study in, 173, 174
nurse and, 228
and women as patients, 165–66, 170–71
Sexuality, adolescent, 136–38, 2*n*
Sickle cell disease, 25
Situation ethics, 9–10, 74
Slippery Slope argument, 79
Sterilization, 56–58
compulsory, 23, 25, 61, 219
genetics and, 24, 226–27
volunatry, 51, 61, 227
Suicide, 186, 188
Supreme Court, U.S.
abortion and, 73, 76, 78–79, 80, 106, 226
committing children to mental hospital, 133*n*, 219
contraception and, 53, 57*n*, 220

T

Tay-Sach's disease, 25,80
Teleological ethics, 9
Test-tube babies, 29. *See also* In vitro fertilization
Triage, 28, 29*n*, 112*n*, 164*n*
Truthtelling, concept of, 188, 190, 192–93, 194

U

Utilitarian ethics, 1*n*, 2*n*, 9, 10, 113*n*, 164, 184, 185, 186*n*

V

Values
    abortion, 83
    concept of, 2*n*
    conflict of, 33, 59, 142, 185
    human life, 183*n*
    nurses and values clarification, 2–3, 113, 144, 145–46, 169–70
    personal, 191
Viability, definition of, 107
Vitalism, doctrine of, 109–10

W

Women
    abortion and, 78–79, 81, 85
    allocation of resources, 184
    attitudes towards, 29, 2*n*, 78–79
    birth control and, 57
    ethics and, 74*n*, 164–66
        as health care providers, 166, 171–72
        as patients, 164–66, 170–72, 173
    sexuality and, 137–38
Wrongful life concept. *See* Law